Stories from ICU Doctors

Diane Dennis • Aaron Calhoun
Rahul Khanna • Cameron Knott
Peter Vernon van Heerden
Editors

Stories from ICU Doctors

Navigating and conquering adversity

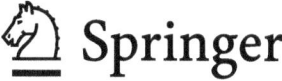 Springer

Editors

Diane Dennis (iD)
Department of Intensive Care and
Physiotherapy
Sir Charles Gairdner Hospital
Perth, WA, Australia

Rahul Khanna
Department of Psychiatry, Phoenix
Australia
University of Melbourne
Melbourne, VIC, Australia

Peter Vernon van Heerden
Department of Anesthesiology, Critical Care
and Pain Medicine
Hadassah Medical Center
Jerusalem, Israel

Aaron Calhoun
Department of Pediatrics, Division of
Critical Care, University of Louisville, and
Norton Children's Medical Group
Louisville, KY, USA

Cameron Knott (iD)
Department of Intensive Care
Bendigo Health
Bendigo, Australia

Monash Rural Health Bendigo
Monash University
VIC, Australia

Rural Clinical School
University of Melbourne
Australia

Department of Intensive Care
Austin Health
Heidelberg, Australia

ISBN 978-3-031-32400-0   ISBN 978-3-031-32401-7   (eBook)
https://doi.org/10.1007/978-3-031-32401-7

This Springer imprint is published by the registered company Springer Nature Switzerland AG
The registered company address is: Gewerbestrasse 11, 6330 Cham, Switzerland

Preface

Upon receiving a small grant in 2018 from the Raine Medical Research Foundation in Perth, Western Australia, Diane Dennis and a subset of the editorial team set about collecting qualitative data pertaining to the mental health and well-being of doctors working in intensive care. At first, the context provided to participants was the occurrence of adverse events, errors, and other difficult care experiences. As data collection evolved, this context expanded to include any stressors pertaining to the intensivist's work in the intensive care medicine setting. Initial interviews were undertaken in Australia and Israel. The dataset was then extended by including researchers and a cohort of participants from the United States of America.

In 2021 and 2022, two other grants were awarded in Perth, Western Australia: a North Metropolitan Health Service Building Allied Health Research Capacity Grant and a Sir Charles Gairdner Osborne Park Health care Group Research Advisory Committee "Charlies Research Foundation" Grant. These grants built the capacity to complete the work and allowed the team to sample a population of allied health professionals. Collating and analyzing this data took time, and by July 2022, the group had published 7 scholarly papers around the topic [1–7]. This book came about following a conversation lamenting the limitations of succinctly reporting our results from an abundant qualitative data set in just a few peer-reviewed scholarly articles. We collectively agreed that these papers represented only snapshots of the full dataset. How could we portray the holistic experience of intensive care doctors more richly and deeply? "What about a book?" we said… and here we are.

All editors gratefully acknowledge the generous contribution of research study participants who gave up their time freely and with vigor, to share their reflections about their work in the intensive care specialty. We have used their unidentified verbatim quotations throughout the text to support the statements made and the conclusions reached. Although the original context of medical error and adverse events feature prominently within the book, other stressors were also explored and are described in some detail.

Our participants are the heroes of this book, and we hope we have represented their views and their stories with integrity and respect. We recognize there are still many voices unheard and unrepresented, as well as biases and heuristics unexplored. Most participants voiced an appreciation of the opportunity to contribute and offer a way to hear others' truths, with one saying:

I feel added value by having been asked to share these observations. If it helps a programme or perspective. To me, it's neither been threatening nor cathartic. I share these kinds of experiences freely with my trainees because I want my experiences to be as widely shared as possible, just as I want their experiences to be widely shared back to me as possible. I'm richer if I hear their story. If you can't tell your own story then you are not going to be good at hearing other people's, so I'm usually first in line to tell my story. Make yourself feel vulnerable so that others will feel vulnerable in your presence.

We hope that the messages contained within this book reach the wide range of people embroiled in intensive care medicine. It is for the consumers of care—whether patients or their families—so they can appreciate the human side of the doctors working with them. It is for the non-medicos (nurses and others) who work alongside ICU doctors, so that they might walk for a moment in the shoes of their colleagues, with renewed patience and understanding. It is for the families of these doctors themselves—that they might better comprehend how their loved one navigates their workplace, and perhaps forgive the inevitable absences that may occur with more frequency than in other specialties. It is for doctors working outside of intensive care medicine—that they might understand the stressors peculiar to a different and relatively new specialty. It is for junior doctors considering a career in the specialty themselves—that they might reflect on their own suitability for the choice and be as prepared as possible for the challenges and the rewards. Finally, and not least importantly, the book is for doctors already working within the specialty. We hope that you might be reminded that both your experiences and your thoughts and feelings about your experiences are valid and not unique. Most of all, we hope you realize that are not alone in navigating and conquering the adversity that is often found within intensive care medicine.

References

1. Dennis D, et al. Behavioural responses of Intensivists to stressors in Intensive Care. Occup Med (Lond). 2021;71(8):343–5.
2. Dennis D, et al. The nature and sources of the emotional distress felt by Intensivists and the burdens that are carried: a qualitative study. Aust Crit Care. 2021.
3. Dennis D, et al. Mitigating emotional responses to stressors: coping strategies, modifiers and support. Australas Psychiatry. 2022;30(2):247–53.
4. Dennis D, et al. Characteristics of the Contemporary Intensivist: a qualitative study. J Emerg Med Critical Care. 2022;8(1) (in press).
5. Dennis D, et al. Advice for doctors working or planning to work in intensive care: summation from a qualitative study. Anaesthesiol Intensive Ther. 2022;54(1):85–90.

6. Dennis D, et al. The different challenges in being an adult versus a Pediatric Intensivist. Crit Care Explor. 2022;4(3):e0654.
7. Varker T, et al. Intensivist's responses to potentially traumatic events: a qualitative study. Traumatology. 2022. https://doi.org/10.1037/trm0000402.

Perth, WA, Australia   Diane Dennis
Louisville, KY, USA   Aaron Calhoun
Melbourne, VIC, Australia   Rahul Khanna
Bendigo, VIC, Australia   Cameron Knott
Jerusalem, Israel   Peter Vernon van Heerden
February 2023

Contents

Part I:
A Travel Guide to the Intensive Care

Foreword: A Tale of Seven Cities

Diane Dennis (iD)

It was the best of times, it was the worst of times.
  —*Charles Dickens, A Tale of Two Cities*

How do you describe and explain the characteristics of the intensive care unit (ICU) to someone who has never experienced it before? Perhaps likening the description to a travel guide, with the tales of seven cities serving as a metaphor for the sights, sounds and energy of the ICU, and the people who reside there...

New York, United States of America

In the quiet corridors of most hospital wards at night, the lights are dimmed and most of the patients sleep. Nurses creep silently through the hallways making their rounds to review and care for their charges, who are often oblivious to their care. Not so in the ICU. It's like New York, the city that never sleeps. In the ICU, the lights are on, the alarms continue to sound, and the intensity and pace of care is unremitting 24/7. Patients continue their journey amidst the noisy bells and whistles that herald their acuity. Just as the New York subway never closes, the pathways and doors to the ICU are constantly open to receive any acutely deteriorating or critically ill patients. New admissions appear both from within and beyond the hospital itself. They arrive with an array of equipment and a fanfare of personnel who support the transfer.

> *... when there is nobody else to take care of the 'sickest of the sick', this is where they come. We are the problem solvers; we are ones who get jobs done; we take care of everything.*

D. Dennis
Department of Intensive Care and Physiotherapy, Sir Charles Gairdner Hospital,
Perth, WA, Australia
e-mail: Diane.Dennis@health.wa.gov.au

Monte Carlo, Monaco

The flashing lights, and the noise and excitement of the Casino de Monte Carlo is perhaps an appropriate analogy to the glare and buzz of the ICU. In the window-less casino, day becomes night, and night becomes day, on an endless continuum. So too, the ICU is a place where time is curiously indeterminable. It is fast-paced, exciting, ever-evolving. There is a carefully calculated degree of risk and benefit associated with every intervention. The environment itself is not the only element of ICU reminiscent of Monte Carlo. The people who end up in the ICU might also be viewed as similar to the punters who frequent the Casino de Monte Carlo. A portion of patients seen in the ICU are arguably people who have been gambling on life and death over their lifetime with the choices they made and the paths they have travelled. Of course, the jackpot is when they are able to cash in their chips and leave, but not every patient has that opportunity. Some patients win and are discharged to return to their normal life again; others lose and are left bereft of anything.

> ... the person who has been smoking and drinking, and a bunch of other less-than-ideal lifestyle choices comes in sick and says, 'Fix me'. I can't undo 30, 40 or 50 years of poor choices.

Perth, Australia

More than 2000 km from the nearest city, a little metropolis known as "Perth" on the western side of Australia is the most isolated city in the world. Intensivists might perceive ICU to be the Perth of the hospital in that practice is often quite remote in relation to other wards and departments, particularly in the middle of the night and on weekends, when there is skeleton staffing throughout the remainder of the hospital. Being an intensivist can therefore be a lonely existence, and this seclusion can be emotionally draining.

> I think, from a personal... like being on at a weekend at night-time as an intensivist, you feel quite isolated in that situation. You know it's you who's dealing with it. You are also trying to deal with the ramifications for the patient, her husband, and the staff who obviously all feel upset. And then you also worry that you could have done something different, at the same time that you are having to deal with the other 23 or 30 patients in the unit, who are also sick! And so, from a personal point of view, I think that it puts quite a lot of emotional strain on you in those situations...

Jerusalem, Israel

The ICU is consistently a place of high emotion. Many times the environment is filled with grief and wailing, just as at the Western Wall in Jerusalem. Sometimes there is a quiet reverence; sometimes there is an outpouring of sorrow. It is a place of pilgrimage where people come from all over the world to see and make peace with a family member or friend for one last time. It is sometimes a place where people reach for solace from their religious beliefs.

> *…the family had an acute grief response at the time; and the Dad was screaming 'Murderers! Assassins! You killed my baby…' I mean just openly screaming… But again, to me I recognised that… I mean you always warn your team that the acute grief response can look like a lot of different things. You can think that the family is in lockstep with you, and then they have an absolutely different response when the death happens… I certainly tell you it had an impact on my staff, and it felt intense at the time. You know, when you have someone screaming at you…*

Tokyo, Japan

The extent of the technology and equipment utilised within the ICU make it the "Tokyo" of the hospital. The automation involved in mechanical ventilation; extracorporeal membrane oxygenation (ECMO); continuous veno-venous haemodiafiltration; telemetry; cardiac pacing; cooling; heating; oxygenation…. the list goes on. Perhaps the home of automation and sociotechnical integration, Tokyo represents the ICU.

> *The ICU is one of the most technologically advanced places in the hospital, with any number of ways to support the body as it heals—ventilators, renal replacement, ECMO, multiple medications. It takes an extraordinary degree of attention to detail to make sure it all works in harmony.*

Geneva, Switzerland

In the context of the tiny Alpine nation of Switzerland adhering to a policy of armed neutrality in global affairs, the intensivist often acts as the negotiator between the patient and family and other healthcare professionals. They advocate for the patient and navigate mutually agreeable patient-centred healthcare plans among competing interests, especially around the proportionate escalation of a person's care involving multiple organ support systems.

> *Like when a patient is bleeding to death, they should just go back to theatre. Or you know if a patient needs a particular treatment, and just the to-ing and fro-ing about the negotiation about something like that, that should just happen quickly.*

Paris, France

And finally, and perhaps most importantly, the ICU is also a haven of great love—it is perhaps the "Paris" of the hospital. Individuals don't come to work in the ICU environment without a passion for people and a human kindness that allows them to interact with those who are experiencing one of the worst times in their lives, offering dignified care with grace. In fact, they often perceive their role to be one of privilege. A basic love of humankind underpins the intensivist and a resilience around the fragility of life. People drawn to work in ICU have an appreciation of human vulnerability, and often an acceptance of the foibles of human nature. This love extends beyond the bedside. The ICU interprofessional team is a close-knit family, with trusted relationships built over time and through shared perilous high-stakes experiences. Intensivists perceive overarching responsibility for the well-being of the ICU team members, providing multi-dimensional cross-professional support.

> *It's the job I love and the job I have chosen to do, and although dealing with people in end-of-life situations is tough, it's also a rewarding part of the job because you have the opportunity to meet people at this awful time for them and make a positive difference, I guess. And I think also that it is kind of life affirming in a way.*

This love of humankind was deeply evident in the generous reflections and observations provided during the interviews that underpin this book, and in the eagerness of co-authors to contribute with insight to the chapters you are about to read.

Diane Dennis Dr Diane Dennis has been employed as a researcher in the ICU setting since 2008, with an interest in simulation and human factors in the safe delivery of healthcare services. She has been exploring the well-being of medical staff in the specialty since 2018. With a background in clinical training as a physiotherapist, she has taught as Co-Lead of Simulation and Senior Lecturer at Curtin University and is currently acting as Deputy Head of the Physiotherapy Department at Sir Charles Gairdner Hospital in Perth, Western Australia.

Chapter 1
The Sights; the Sounds

Caleb Fisher, Natalie Henderson, and Chrystal Rutledge ⓘ

> *This is the reality of intensive care: at any point, we are as apt to harm as we are to heal.*
>
> —Atul Gawande

The ICU is a unique work environment, as anyone who has ever walked through one is aware. Many things seemingly occur simultaneously, with an abundance of alarms, buzzers, equipment, and lights constantly "on." Additionally, there are many people crossing paths, including doctors from multiple teams, nursing staff, personal care attendants, cleaners, physiotherapists, and speech therapists, together with family members crowding the unit. As confronting as these experiences are for patients and their families, these environmental factors present a never-ending barrage of stimulation for those working within the ICU. Patient needs are complex, as in our ICUs they have likely never been sicker. For an individual to successfully work in this environment, several challenges need to be surmounted. The following chapter explores the environment within the ICU that impacts and drives emotional responses in ICU staff, focusing specifically on the nature of the acuity of care

C. Fisher (✉)
Department of Intensive Care, Austin Health, Heidelberg, VIC, Australia

Department of Critical Care, The University of Melbourne, Melbourne, Australia
e-mail: Caleb.FISHER@austin.org.au

N. Henderson
Division of Critical Care, Department of Pediatrics, University of Louisville, and Norton Children's Medical Group, Louisville, KY, USA

C. Rutledge
Division of Paediatric Critical Care, Department of Paediatrics, University of Alabama at Birmingham Heersink School of Medicine, Birmingham, AL, USA

Simulation Center at Children's of Alabama, Birmingham, AL, USA

© The Author(s), under exclusive license to Springer Nature Switzerland AG 2023
D. Dennis et al. (eds.), *Stories from ICU Doctors*,
https://doi.org/10.1007/978-3-031-32401-7_1

required, the factors surrounding decision-making, and the impact of on-call requirements on the individual clinician.

Unwell Patients

Patients in ICU are by their very nature, the sickest patients in the hospital. They represent a diverse group, with care requirements that vary significantly.

> … We admit very, very, very complicated medical patients… [they] usually, have a lot of background illnesses and a lot of medications and poor reserves to start with. When something critical happens, they end up at the end of their capabilities.

Balancing these individual needs around patient care, coupled with the internal of the dynamics of the ICU, raises many challenges. For example, patients recovering from routine, elective cardiac surgery are alongside patients with undifferentiated, acute, critical illness. Therefore, ICU clinicians must have a huge breadth of knowledge and skill set to manage patients optimally. With the patient mix in the ICU being varied, multiple things are often occurring simultaneously. In addition, the situation is dynamic and can also change quickly, with the potential for emergent situations to arise at any time. This leads to significant difficulty with planning workflow within the unit. Planning for the ward round, associated tasks, and other meetings will change many times during the day. The impact of the constantly changing priorities of the unit can make for the treating clinician, a seemingly piecemeal approach to the day, with often, no patient fully "sorted out" at any time.

On an individual level, patients in the ICU are very unwell with multi-organ system illnesses that require complex therapies. Due to the multi-organ involvement, treatment decisions are not always straightforward. The importance and impact of their comorbidities upon functional levels of reserve and subsequent impact upon outcomes becomes more apparent. This impact is evident in the quote above by the manner that the pre-existing health of the patient ("poor reserves") and the outcome of critical illness ("end of their capabilities") are qualified throughout the statement.

The condition of a patient can also change dramatically and unexpectedly. For example, sudden deterioration may occur, and the clinician needs to act in a decisive and timely manner. ICU clinicians need to be always flexible, and this unpredictability presents a constant challenge.

This acuity brings a range of emotions and cognitive responses in those who care for this type of patient group. The gravity and importance of the care provided for many patients is apparent and felt by all members of the ICU team. The fragility of many patients, and consequential decision-making, frequently elicits the realization that admission to the ICU is the last line of restorative care for many patients, further increasing the weight of clinician responsibility.

> It's established and I would say that the scariest kid is the one that doesn't have enough 'plastic'. By that I mean, plastic in the IV lines,… intubation… Once they're 'plasticised',

yes, they can be sick or not, but you have pseudo control. But if they are limping along…not quite intubated yet…, are they going to tip over (into respiratory failure)?

By having patients, described as "plasticized" above, the ICU clinician now has access to almost endless stream of information in the form of arterial blood pressure monitoring, oxygen monitoring, metabolic control, renal function, and conscious state. The control over these aspects of a patient's physiology and care allows for the accurate and timely application of therapeutic interventions and also allows for the early recognition of deterioration or deviation from expected recovery trajectory. This self-described "pseudo-control," and it is possibly a fallacy that we have any control, is evident in the quote above.

Furthermore, the quote gives a sense of the inner tension and pressure felt by the clinician when providing care to those within the ICU. Regardless of the clinical severity, the intensivist may now feel more competent and calmer once "pseudo-control" has been obtained. The importance of pseudo-control on managing these cognitive and emotional struggles is further highlighted by the final sentence, whereby in the absence of control (if they are limping along, not yet intubated), greater clinical concern and their potential consequences (are they going to tip over into respiratory failure) manifest as greater intensivist uncertainty and anxiety.

Interdisciplinary Interactions

Dealing with the acuity of critically ill patients is one of numerous challenges particular to the ICU environment. Another potentially even more complex challenge among the ICU staff is the interdisciplinary nature that working together with the treating "home" teams brings. Patients of the ICU are usually under the care of a "home" unit. This is the medical specialty team who admits the patient to hospital, provides ward-based diagnosis and therapies, and then discharges the patient from hospital.

When a patient comes to ICU for higher intensity of therapy exceeding that provided on the wards, or organ failure support systems, they continue to be cared for by their home team. The ICU team integrates negotiating and sharing the care goals and expectations of the patient, family, and home team while they are inside the ICU.

Thereby, ICU clinicians need to work together, with potentially all the general and subspecialty teams in the hospital. Some of these teams are well-known to the ICU staff; however, other teams will be less known. Of course, for the treating "home" teams, the patients in the ICU will be among their most unwell and complex patients. Patients admitted to the ICU remain nominally under the control and decision-making of the treating "home" unit. There is considerable worldwide variation in the degree that an ICU is "open" (treating "home" doctor-led decision-making) versus "closed" (intensivist-led decision-making). This shared-responsibility dynamic frequently leads at times to tension and conflict:

I use the words 'joint custody'. So, by 'joint' I mean we sort of, we both claim ownership of (our) areas, now if there is a misunderstanding, then there is conflict.

Conflict within the ICU has a wide range of causes, with the most common reported being communication issues, inappropriate mode of information delivery, and inappropriate approaches to patient management. These issues are discussed more deeply in chapter "Calling the Play," but suffice to say, some situations are fraught with emotional complexities as they are based on the grief, disappointment, and frustration felt by individuals from numerous care teams when a patient charts an unexpected deteriorating clinical course.

The role of the intensivist in negotiating these situations is also explored in the chapter "The Looking Glass" and requires the ICU clinician to be self-aware of their own emotional responses to a situation and capable of understanding and responding to other clinicians' emotional responses. This is imperative in developing an appropriate course of action while simultaneously advocating for the patient in their care. A common theme from the participants regarding the strategies used to negotiate is below:

We do the same dance every time, but that's okay I know where he is coming from, he means well.

Understanding and developing an individual relationship also appears to be a very important additional element to manage conflict and tension:

If we don't know each other you have to do the dance, you have to get to know each other.

The numerous peer-peer interactions that are negotiated by ICU clinicians daily highlight the unique, frequently heightened, emotional, and cognitive challenges the ICU environment brings to clinicians.

These quotes highlight the need for ICU clinicians to have highly developed empathy and emotional intelligence skills, to negotiate complex decision-making with peers, not only in relation to a singular event but in a sustained and repeated pattern.

The cost of these tensions and conflict within the ICU environment can be considerable for ICU clinicians and their patients:

I've experienced it. I don't feel like it's usually been directed at me, I didn't bear the brunt, but you could see other staff finding it tough, stuff like not being listened to, people not hearing your voice.

Clinicians who experience regular and sustained conflict in their workplace are more likely to develop stress-related mental health disorders and experience burnout, which is a topic discussed in detail in the chapter "Baggage and Burnout." At a patient level, these conflicts have the capacity to negatively impact patient-doctor and doctor-family interactions and patient-centered care. At an organizational level, increased staff turnover, patient safety problems, and increased healthcare costs are possible outcomes. Subsequently, it is highly important that exploration of the ICU environment takes into consideration the potential high costs of interdepartmental conflict.

Decision-Making

The need to make numerous, often important, and life-impacting decisions is a characteristic of the ICU environment. These decisions can occur in the setting of routine ward rounds; interactions with other medical and surgical specialties, administrative and institutional authorities; and emergent resuscitation on the wards, emergency room, or within the ICU.

Key features of these decisions are the time limitations and perceived pressure in which they conducted, as evident by the quote below:

Then suddenly he had rapidly rising oxygen requirements, and I said to him once intubated, he is going to look very average.

This quote highlights the nature of the decision-making within the ICU and the need for a rapid decision in response to a deteriorating patient. The consequences of that decision, often associated with urgently performing a high-risk or high-stakes procedure, and with full understanding that the consequences of that decision, even if successful, may see the patient experience further deterioration. In many cases, an intensivist making the decision may not have the opportunity to review all information available to make the best choice in the moment:

I think we have the onerous job of having to make decisions, sometimes, with available information – which may be limited sometimes, even the extent of the information. Sometimes it is incomplete, but you don't have the luxury of time to wait to confirm everything.

Rapid decision-making in the absence of full available information, in a time-critical manner significantly, contributes to the cognitive and emotional load that each decision extolls on the decision-maker. While cognitive load has been shown to improve clinical judgements (i.e., thinking before one acts), cognitive overload has been shown to significantly impair clinical judgements.

But I have caught myself in moments, where I am like, I can feel my dander getting up, and I'm like "I am getting triggered now; just take a deep breath."

As the participant above demonstrates, the physical and emotional responses to time-pressured decision-making can be exhibited by potentially all ICU clinicians. The ability to exhibit self-thought, self-control, and situational awareness can all address these responses.

The reality is in the unit, there's only two things that you have to think about, right now. Everything else you can have at (least) three seconds to think about.

Decision-making within the ICU environment is not solely impacted by time pressure; it is also heavily influenced by the volume of decision-making. Decision fatigue is a well-recognized phenomenon and is influenced by the number of decisions and the complexity of the decisions an individual makes.

The complexity of ICU decisions is evident by the responses discussed previously, but the number of decisions is not discussed as frequently. Recent evidence suggests that intensivists make over 100 decisions daily, over a median time of approximately 4-hours, over a standard 10-patient ward round.

This can be compounded by after-hours on-call whereby:

And then on Sunday, the second Consultant goes home, and you are responsible for the rest of the 30 patients ... patients you don't really know.

Impact of Shift Work and the Isolation Experienced by ICU Doctors

While intensivists gain immensely personal and professional satisfaction in caring for patients within the ICU, the requirement for 24-hour coverage "on-call" for an ICU can create an enormous sense of social isolation among many ICU clinicians. The lack of sleep and insidious assault on the personal reserves of resilience seem to be an important factor in the impact of after-hours on-call:

I think certainly taking the on-call, taking calls at night, that's stressful because it decreases your reserve to cope with everything else when you are tired, and you're woken up

I think from a personal.... like being on at a weekend as a night-time intensivist, you feel quite isolated in that situation. You know it's you who is dealing with it (that issue) and while you are having to deal with 23 or 30 other patients who are also sick.

The above quote demonstrates the cognitive pressure and frustration at looking after numerous critically ill patients' after-hours. Even routine events, such as family meetings, offer challenges when conducted after-hours on-call:

I had a family meeting with this family for like an hour and a half with an interpreter. That's a lot of time out of the weekend, and you've done everything you could but still haven't given them what they want...like how you do that out-of-hours?.

In addition to the sense of professional frustration that the increased on-call workload can provide, after-hours on-call is strongly associated with increased stress, job dissatisfaction, burnout, and potential long-term health effects.

Further compounding the isolating and health effects of after-hour on-call, certain groups within the ICU community potentially experience further isolation due to attitudes and perceptions towards their specialization.

Somebody will ask you "What do you do for a living? and I say to them don't tell them you're a paediatric intensivist, just say you are a paediatrician and let it go."
I try not tell my kid's friends Moms'. Like I try to stay out of it, what I do

These quotes suggest many pediatric intensivists may be reticent to discuss the nature of their professions that may further compound the emotional intensities of their workplace. However, this must be balanced by the strong sense of purpose and belief in their vocations, as evident by:

I feel like I have been given a gift to be able to do this

Conclusion

The ICU environment has many unique characteristics that separate it from other areas of medicine. ICU clinicians gain great satisfaction in utilizing their skills to care for those critically ill. However, the high acuity of patient illness, numerous pressures on decision-making, the complex and frequently confronting interactions with other medical specialties, and isolating effects of after-hours and on-call patterns of work all combine to create an exceedingly challenging vocational environment. Of critical importance is the immense emotional and cognitive toll that his environment has upon ICU clinicians. This summary highlights that in many aspects of unique ICU environment, the negative and demanding factors may not only significantly impact ICU clinicians' ability to provide optimal care at the bedside within the ICU but also potentially have impacts outside the ICU.

Caleb Fisher is an intensive care physician at Austin Health, Melbourne, Australia. He has completed dual overseas fellowships in liver disease and extra-corporeal support systems. Outside of work, he is the father of two highly active children, who indulge in his passion for the outdoors.

Natalie Henderson is an attending critical care physician at Norton Children's Hospital. She spends her time in the Just for Kids Pediatric Critical Care Unit as well as well as the Jennifer Lawrence Foundation Cardiac Intensive Care Unit. Clinically, she participates in multiple committees related to cardiac critical care. She serves as the Associate Fellowship Program Director for the pediatric critical care fellowship program. She has an interest in education and, along with two colleagues, has developed an end-of-life curricular to improve the education around end-of-life for trainees. She serves as the Medical Director for the palliative care service line at Norton Children's Hospital. She also spends time teaching at the medical school where she also serves as an advisory dean for more than 30 students each year.

Chrystal Rutledge is an associate professor of pediatrics in the Division of Pediatric Critical Care. She is Vice Chair of Diversity, Equity and Inclusion (DEI) for Pediatrics and Co-Director of the Simulation Center at Children's of Alabama. She is also Assistant Program Director for the Pediatrics Residency program. She is a graduate of the University of Alabama at Birmingham (UAB) Heersink School of Medicine. She completed her pediatric residency at the University of North Carolina—Chapel Hill and her pediatric critical care medicine fellowship at UAB. Her non-clinical interests focus on improving equitable healthcare through simulation, DEI initiatives, and community outreach.

Chapter 2
The Thoughts; the Feelings

Z. Leah Harris (iD)**, Aaron Calhoun** (iD)**, and Tracey Varker** (iD)

> *Responsibility does not only lie with the leaders of our*
> *countries or with those who have been appointed or elected to*
> *do a particular job. It lies with each one of us individually.*
>
> —*Dalai Lama*

As I sit in the surgical ICU room, keeping guard and keeping company with a young training specialist doctor who has been in a bicycle accident 24 hours earlier, I reflect on my responsibility to this member of my larger healthcare service delivery team. I sit here because I have a responsibility and an unspoken obligation: I am the Chair for the training program that recruited this trainee. I promised and pledged to make sure the environment that the trainees and the teaching faculty work within is safe and is meeting their professional needs. This sense of responsibility has not waivered over the years.

Decades earlier, I sat in the preoperative area, the hospital's Critical Care Fellowship Director, with a trainee who had suffered from a herniated spinal disc, causing numbness in his legs. The need to operate was semi-emergent. I remember calling his mother, as she was preparing to board a plane many miles away, and she asked me to stay with him and to put a $20 bill under his pillow to ward off evil spirits. She believed this would protect him and so I obliged. This sense of

Z. L. Harris (✉)
Dell Medical School at The University of Texas at Austin, Austin, TX, USA

Dell Children's Medical Center, Austin, TX, USA
e-mail: zena.harris@austin.utexas.edu

A. Calhoun
Division of Critical Care, Department of Pediatrics, University of Louisville, and Norton Children's Medical Group, Louisville, KY, USA

T. Varker
Department of Psychiatry, University of Melbourne, Melbourne, Australia

Phoenix Australia-Centre for Posttraumatic Mental Health, Melbourne, Australia

© The Author(s), under exclusive license to Springer Nature
Switzerland AG 2023
D. Dennis et al. (eds.), *Stories from ICU Doctors*,
https://doi.org/10.1007/978-3-031-32401-7_2

responsibility defined me as a resident, Chief Resident and as a teaching faculty member. I used to think that this was a uniquely pediatric approach to taking care of each other, but it is not.

I have witnessed incredible acts of selflessness and generosity over the years. There is a recognition of the bond that is formed through training together and working in a clinical space together that makes this a natural extension of who we are. If we are dedicated to taking care of our patients—people we often don't know until the moment they are admitted—how could we not have the same desire and commitment to take care of each other if ever called upon? Perhaps being a specialist doctor pre-selects for a personality that already feels the need to serve others. This baseline attitude forms the frame of reference we will use to consider the responsibility of healthcare service delivery in this chapter.

Sense of Responsibility for Staff

> We have such a close relationship with the nursing staff and with allied health. We work very closely together on the same patient at the same time sometimes, and that bond is unique. It's one of the things that attracted me to the ICU, but also a responsibility from my point of view, is more than from the medical point of view, it could be the person cleaning for floor, it could be the registrar, the nurse, the physio, you know.

A recent article in *The New York Times* raised the ethical conundrum of how we take care of bigoted patients who use profanity and address healthcare team members using gender slurs, vulgar racial slurs, and obscene gestures [1]. How much stress should be allowed to enter the workplace? Who has the responsibility to "protect" the staff? How do we navigate these challenges? Besides the fact that hate speech is never to be tolerated, it makes the workplace environment threatening and staff that feel unsafe are more likely to commit medical errors.

While clinicians have a duty to care for all patients, we also must do our utmost to create a respectful and responsible care environment. If you are the physician leader of a care team, it is your responsibility to provide a safe, respectful, supportive, and data- and science-driven clinical environment that strives for excellence, rewards intellectual curiosity, and provides ongoing education and supports people speaking up:

> I think we have full responsibility for all those people's mental well-being in stressful events or difficult clinical events. As I said before, I don't think we do it enough to call everybody together and have a full debriefing. Either people think that they don't need it, or people think they are on the other side of the spectrum and don't feel comfortable to discuss what they feel. And it definitely is our responsibility to bring everybody together, and discuss the event, let people vent their emotions, their issues, and come to a positive way of moving forward. I think the problem in ICU is that we are so busy and we move from one fire to the next that we sometimes don't have that time to stop.

The ICU adds a level of difficulty to these responsibilities due to the complex nature of the medical issues encountered and the emotionally charged nature of the environment. The ICU team is made up of many different skill sets and levels of training and has a personality make up that reflects the culture of the unit.

There is a hierarchy in medicine that places the most senior positions as the presumed leaders: the charge nurse and the intensivist. In truth, however, there are many units where a more aged and experienced staff member—usually a nurse—is the eldest member of the team. This individual may be many years older than the intensivist. Usually that level of experience is acknowledged and tapped for advice, but at the end of the day, it is the intensivist that bears the weight of the unit's function on their shoulders. This is a daunting task.

Ideally, the rounding (ward round) process serves to unify the care team for each patient and outline the goals of the day. In essence the intensivist—with or without trainees—develops a plan. This is the first level of responsibility. When there is an escalation of emotions with a family, the intensivist and colleagues trained in managing difficult social situations such as social workers, chaplains, and nurses will share the responsibility of de-escalating the situation. When a medical error occurs, it is the intensivist and the charge nurse that once again oversee the conversation. When there is an acute clinical deterioration, it is the intensivist that takes responsibility for the management of the crisis. The ability to manage these events is cultivated by watching, participating and apprenticing during training. It can also be augmented by structured teaching and leadership sessions that involve clinical simulation education and professional development.

The leader is also responsible for taking critical events and turning them into teaching moments for the entire team. As a profession we have fortunately come to recognize the importance of a standardized approach to this learning process, and many ICUs have scripted forms that assist staff members in debriefing these situations. Clinical incident debriefing is a tool used in most ICUs to educate staff and thereby address the responsibility to educate and develop the team. There are two types of debriefings: "hot" debriefings, where the debriefing occurs in the immediate time frame and focuses on the overall timeline of clinical events, and "cold" debriefing, which consists of a detailed review of all contributing events, often aligned with hospital patient safety and system improvement processes. The latter is hopefully less emotionally charged and is often framed as an opportunity to learn from the event and to assess the outcomes through the lens of implementation science [2, 3]. These are discussed in more detail in chapter "Actions After the Moment."

Intensive care leaders can also check on their team members individually following critical incidents, offer emotional support, and provide information to the team member on where they can get further support if they feel that they need it (e.g., from an organizational psychologist). Leaders are in an important and unique position to offer support and non-stigmatizing responses to any adverse psychological reactions that their team members may experience [4].

In some instances, the leader may also share their experiences of similar situations and let their team member know that they too have been impacted by a critical incident at some point in their career. We now know that while support from the ICU leader/team is valuable, it cannot replace professional mental health support and that psychological therapy needs to be done with a professional and not by the ICU team leaders. The notion of support is a topic discussed in more detail in Part V:

I think it's important. As the lead doctor should check in and maybe debrief, although obviously the evidence surrounding debriefing in critical incidents is not great. In terms of that it actually helps to reduce post-traumatic stress and problems. I think there is generally awareness surrounding that as well so I think that is why some healthcare professionals just want to avoid debriefs altogether. Nevertheless, I think the culture is one where we are trying to have at least a mini-debrief without it being all too structured. So, as I alluded to before, I see my role as checking in with nurses and doctors that were part of a critical incident or a "bad day at the office", and to see how they go, but is probably at a superficial level, and maybe my role should be more than that, as opposed to just mentioning it fleetingly.

.... most of us feel like we need to take that role on. Of checking in to make sure everyone is okay with maybe, with the event, maybe what came out of the debriefing, in checking in about things afterwards. I know I personally feel that responsibility and I think many of my colleagues feel the same way. That we are... I think a lot of times in the same way that I might doubt my decision-making, the nurses who is pushing meds at the bedside might think about, did I push that too fast, or did I flush enough in for that to go... So I think everyone is reliving it and second-guessing, and I see, in the same way that everyone kinda looks to me when we are running a resuscitation to give the next decision or instruction, that after the event is over, I kinda feel it's my responsibility to check in and make sure that people are processing in an okay way.

Sense of Responsibility for Patients

Becoming a first-year Fellow was easy compared to becoming a second year Fellow; because becoming a first year Fellow, you could just be a baby, you didn't have to know stuff and there were senior Fellows to clean up your messes. But when I was a second year Fellow, I had to make sure that the first years didn't screw anything up. You see what I'm saying? And then when I began as an intensivist, I had to make sure everyone didn't screw anything up.

One of the most challenging adjustments associated with the transition from critical care fellow to intensivist is the sense of responsibility for the entire intensive care unit: the trainees, the families, and the patients. The weight of the patients' outcomes rest on your shoulders! The buck stops with you!

Many training programs implement "Pre-Attending" or "Pretending" rounds where the senior fellow is given the responsibility for running the unit with the actual intensivist being present but not running the events of the day. These experiences are invaluable especially when the attending intensivist and senior fellow are able to meet ahead of rounds to develop a plan and again at the end of the day to review the events of the day. These meetings provide the framework for constructively sharing skills and techniques for prioritizing issues, addressing questions from other members of the team and learning how to maintain a safe culture among all the individuals in the ICU. It is often the first time a trainee rides with their "training wheels" off and is an important part of the transition to intensivist.

Learning how to shoulder the responsibility for managing many patients at once is an important part of the transition to independence. Time and experience help the intensivist learn that while they oversee, and hold ultimate responsibility for, the activity in the ICU that occurs on their watch, events will still happen outside of their control. Our responsibility to our patients takes priority first and defines who we are. It is our job to provide the best care we can for the patients in our charge.

A recent conversation I had with an internationally respected pediatric cardiovascular surgeon helped me put this responsibility in perspective. He was one of the first pediatric CT surgeons to offer corrective surgery to children with Trisomy 21. From his perspective, it wasn't for him to decide who should live or who should die. Rather, if the cardiac repair would give the child a better quality of life—less heart failure, less pulmonary hypertension, less pulmonary edema—and he had the tools to perform the surgery with minimal risk and the recovery period would be tolerable, then his duty was to perform the corrective surgery. If a family didn't want the care, he never pushed. But if offered a chance to weigh in personally, he would let them know he felt it was his responsibility to alleviate any suffering the child may have. Fast forward three decades and we have a new approach to children and young adults with Trisomy 21 in which the majority undergo corrective cardiac repair.

Most clinicians remember the first patient they examined, the first patient they drew blood on, and the first patient that died on their watch. We also remember conversations with families and patients we wish we could "do over." Ultimately, we entered medicine to take care of the patient. This is both the burden and the blessing of caring for another human being when making their quality of life our focus. We must accordingly develop management plans to get the patient, the medical team, and the family to that point:

> ...irrationally you feel responsible, you know because we are doctors and we are supposed to fix everything, or we think we can fix everything, which is not true.

Our new lexicon in healthcare includes the term "burnout." Burnout is defined as a syndrome resulting from chronic workplace stress that has not been successfully managed. It is characterized by three dimensions: feelings of energy depletion or exhaustion, increased mental distance from one's job, or feelings of negativism or cynicism related to one's job [5]. The perceived responsibility for staff and patients can result in stress that can cause this form of workplace stress. It is important for the ICU leaders to have a watchful eye and be ready to support staff as needed. This is discussed in more detail in chapter "Baggage and Burnout":

> I think ultimately if you are the intensivist in charge, everything comes back to you, and you are the one who is responsible, ultimately. I don't think there's... No one comes to work thinking I'm going to do something nasty to a patient today. Everyone is there trying to do their best and often when mistakes like that happen it's a system's problem more than anything.

Conclusion

The intensivist responsibility is manageable because we learn how to share and compartmentalize the gravity of the moments, and we surround ourselves by incredibly dedicated and well-trained teams. We develop evidence-based approaches for presenting data, identifying severity of illness, initiating therapies and treatments, and proportionally escalating or de-escalating the intensity of these treatments. We also learn from each other via clinical simulations and ongoing interpersonal interactions.

Our teams are made up of experts across many fields, and telemedicine now offers consultation across many time zones. While we may feel we are alone, we never really are. The stress of ICU work is very real. Every professional wants to perform not only within the scope of their practice but at the top of their game, and it is vital that we fully embrace the responsibilities inherent in caring for another human being. This is what makes the practice of medicine both an art and a science. It is a noble calling. The ability to make a real impact, to be a part of a patient's recovery, or to support a family during the darkest moments is our reward.

References

1. Appiah KA. Can I withhold medical care from a Bigot? NY Times; 7 June 2022.
2. Sweberg T, Sen AI, Mullan PC, Cheng A, Knight L, Del Castillo J, Ikeyama T, Seshadri R, Hazinski MF, Raymond T, Niles DE, Nadkarni V, Wolfe H, Pediatric Resuscitation Quality (pediRES-Q) Collaborative Investigators. Description of hot debriefings after in-hospital cardiac arrests in an International Pediatric Quality Improvement Collaborative. Resuscitation. 2018;128:181–7.PMID: 29768181.
3. Wolfe HA, Wenger J, Sutton R, Seshadri R, Niles DE, Nadkarni V, Duval-Arnould J, Sen AI, Cheng A. Cold debriefings after in-hospital cardiac arrest in an International Pediatric Resuscitation Quality Improvement Collaborative. Pediatr Qual Safety. 2020;5(4):e319. PMID: 32766493.
4. Kolbe M, Schmutz S, Seelandt JC, Eppich WJ, Schmutz JB. Team debriefings in healthcare: aligning intention and impact. BMJ. 2021;374:n2042. PMID: 34518169.
5. World Health Organization. International classification of diseases 11th Revision; 2022.

Z. Leah Harris currently serves as Professor and Chair of the Department of Pediatrics for the Dell Medical School at The University of Texas at Austin, Director of the Dell Pediatric Research Institute, and Physician-in-Chief at Dell Children's Medical Center. She is a proud practicing pediatric critical care medicine physician, lifelong learner, and multidisciplinary supporter.

Aaron Calhoun is a tenured professor in the Department of Pediatrics, Division of Pediatric Critical Care at the University of Louisville, and is an attending physician in the Just for Kids Critical Care Center at Norton Children's Hospital. He received his MD from Johns Hopkins University School of Medicine in 2001, completed general pediatrics residency at Children's Memorial Hospital/Northwestern University Feinberg School of Medicine in 2004, and completed pediatric critical care fellowship at Children's Hospital of Boston/Harvard School of Medicine in 2007. Dr Calhoun is the Associate Division Chief of Pediatric Critical Care and has numerous publications in the field of simulation and medical education.

Tracey Varker is a senior research fellow in the Department of Psychiatry, University of Melbourne, and Phoenix Australia—Centre for Post-traumatic Mental Health. Dr Varker leads a team of researchers who focus on improving the lives of those affected by occupational trauma and stress. This includes emergency services and military personnel, healthcare professionals, and those working in heavy industry (e.g., mining and construction). Her research interests center on improving the lives of those impacted by occupational trauma and stress; using evidence synthesis to promote the recovery of those affected by trauma; and improving our understanding of, and the treatment of, problematic anger.

Chapter 3
Patients on the Edge

Bradley Wibrow ⓘ **and Denise Goodman** ⓘ

> *Wherever the art of Medicine is loved, there is also a love of Humanity.*
>
> *—Hippocrates*

The intensivist has many roles and must be adept at transitioning between them. They include but are not limited to the diagnostician, the healer, the last line of defence, the negotiator, and, just as importantly, the companion and comforter for the dying process. Death is so often unavoidable but still unexpected by patients and families. How to navigate and fulfil these different roles is one of the unique stressors of ICU. The words of Hippocrates are as true today as they were then—'cure sometimes, treat often, comfort always'.

The intensivist must maintain and foster hope and balance this with realism. Getting patients and families through long, complex admissions marked by multiple organ failures, debilitating critical illness weakness, and psychological stress would not be possible without providing realistic hope.

While the role of the intensivist in resuscitation is obvious and, to those not familiar with intensive care, may be seen as the most stressful, it is often less so because it involves dealing with known disease processes and is often structured and formulaic. It is also the role of the intensivist to realise when ongoing intensive and invasive care is unlikely to get a patient well and home. The intensivist must embrace assisting families, as most patients cannot communicate adequately themselves. These decisions are often the most complex and can involve stress over prolonged periods, navigating both the patient's illness and family dynamics.

B. Wibrow (✉)
Department of Intensive Care, Sir Charles Gairdner Hospital, Perth, Australia
e-mail: Bradley.Wibrow@health.wa.gov.au

D. Goodman
Lurie Children's Hospital, Chicago, IL, USA

© The Author(s), under exclusive license to Springer Nature
Switzerland AG 2023
D. Dennis et al. (eds.), *Stories from ICU Doctors*,
https://doi.org/10.1007/978-3-031-32401-7_3

Often, the intensivist will recognise this point long before the family does and, while maintaining the patient's comfort, shift the focus to caring for the family, assisting acceptance of the situation, and providing appropriate and targeted support:

I'm going to transition my focus to the family and try to really focus on being direct and clear with them, but also not being cruel, and being honest; and if I can do that in a way that, by the end, they say 'thank you so much for your care, it really meant a lot'. To me, that is a success.

Consistently, intensivists felt assisting the dying process was very much a part of good intensive care:

…I think that it is probably our role as well [palliative care], because we probably see from the start to the end a bit better than some of the other specialties.

… the goal is not to save them, the goal is to make this awful experience as reasonably positive as it can be. If we can get them to organ donation, then I can help that family and other families… So, it's a different pathway. It's probably like a priest who gives Last Rites. Everybody's gonna die, but if you approach it like that, that would be sad. But if you approach it as what a great opportunity to help them in their death process, then it can be positive…

And most intensivists reported finding fulfilment in this part of the job:

Those kinds of experiences feel good. When you can take a scared and terrified family [who are] about to suffer bereavement and allow them to come to a space where there's communication, that seems to be therapeutic. My job is to create that environment for them. It felt great. Nobody thanked me. That wasn't really the issue. I wasn't seeking thanks, but it felt really good.

Difficult Conversations

Introducing the concept of death and that the patient cannot get better is difficult. When death is a regular occurrence, one does become accustomed to it. However, there are still patients where accepting death is particularly hard, such as those in which it is unexpected, those who are young, and those who remind us of our own families:

I probably seemed to her very nervous because she noticed that and said, 'You seem nervous, what has happened?' And I almost started crying. It was really… I was blushing… I was showing emotional distress. And I told her, and her first response was, 'So, [are] you saying that I am going to die?', so this was her first response.

There are many different techniques of dealing with stressful conversations and many different personalities that choose care for the critically ill as a specialty. There is certainly an art in being able to take a family from the devastation of realising their loved one will die toward reaching some level of peace with that knowledge, having time to spend together and to tell stories. It is not unlike a wake or funeral, yet it is happening before the patient has died:

Then I took the family to the [operating room], and we spent 90 minutes together, and they weren't talking. And so I created conversation. I brought out stories. I said 'Show me those pictures you brought' and they were passed around… By the time we were done, they were chatting and telling stories and laughing; like we had almost lived together.

The Teacher

The intensivist must also lead and prepare the staff for patient deaths. It is standard and expected practice to debrief after stressful and prolonged or difficult resuscitation attempts. However, the subtle and slower change to a realisation that a patient will not recover is something that only experience can teach. Educating the junior staff is another burden, and while it is often a positive one, it is another factor that the intensivist must incorporate into their daily practice:

I've realised, and this is part of their burnout, is they [the junior staff] really, I think, think that we can save them. And to me it was so obvious that I didn't think I should tell them. And I realised, probably sharing it with the staff and the Residents [junior staff]… Now there are nurses who have been there for 5 to 10 years, they know… But the new nurses probably don't.

Is Every Patient in Intensive Care 'Intense'?

Some experienced intensivists reported that it helped classifying patients into three categories—those who were always going to get better with well-established standard intensive care, those who were always going to die, and those where the intensive care team has a chance at saving them using the evidence-informed creativity of the intensivist and the intensive care team.

For those who are going to get better with standard care, some of that responsibility may be delegated by intensivists to the junior doctors—to learn, to foster confidence—while maintaining some supervisory oversight and stepping in to adjust or steady the ship where required:

… but you know in those patients, I really try to let the Residents [junior staff] run the show. Let them make the decisions; make them feel the ownership…somebody once said there's nine ways to skin a cat, eight of which are fine, one of which you shouldn't do… as long as they're not doing that one, they can have full reign; give them some ownership, responsibility, added autonomy and, every once in a while, we'll make little adjustments.

The third group, where good intensive care medicine can really save the patient, is always memorable:

Those don't come along very often honestly. between the PICU, general surgery, interventional radiology, she came back to us really unstable, and we spent three or four hours tweaking stuff. We were able to stabilise her, and she extubated on Saturday and left the unit yesterday, completely normal. That is unique but pretty powerful.

…that I can go home to my kids and say, 'I helped save a life today.'

However, where things don't go well in these patients, where an intensivist feels they could have done something differently to save the patient or improve their outcome—these are the stories that never leave the individual and are not forgotten. These are ruminated upon, where one hopes to learn from the experience and, at the same time, are considered as potentially career destroying through stress and self-criticism:

Those are the ones that happen once or twice a year, that you think, 'God, if I had done everything right, maybe this kid wouldn't have died.' Those are the ones that still... You'd have to be not human not to have that effect you. But those generally are rare...

Intensive care staff at times do end up attending the funerals of patients, particularly for those who have been in ICU for a prolonged period. While this memorial celebrates life, there is no similar mechanism to celebrate successes:

They had a yearly memorial event, it was a beautiful thing. They brought all the families of the children who had died over the past year plus others you know, they had the rabbi and the priest, and they came up and had a whole ceremony. And it was very good. But we don't make a party for the kids who did well. And now this is important. It is truly important.

Even the practice of follow-up clinics in intensive care is a relatively new one. Saving a patient from a severe infection or a surgical issue is often evident over days. However, longer-term positive outcomes are often only evident to ICU staff in research and registry data as once patients depart from ICU they are often not seen again. Seeing long-term recovery can be incredibly rewarding:

She is 22-year-old now and he showed pictures of her at university, and of her getting married... So, you get patients like that, but we don't get enough of that. We don't have true follow-up, the bad cases we all remember but our mortality is only 3 to 5%.

The Big-Picture View

Medicine today is so advanced and sub-specialised that no one can be an expert in every field. It is therefore easy to see how different specialty doctors can suffer somewhat from 'tunnel vision' on their organ-specific problems rather than the 'patient as a whole'. 'Generalism' is often hard to attain and maintain.

Often the role of the intensivist is to maintain an appreciation of the holistic 'big picture', the multisystem interplay, to put the likelihood of cure in context for that particular patient while garnering an appreciation of what the patient would want in their treatment goals.

When finite 'care resources' (time, financial, emotional, and physical) are being spent without a holistic view of the patient and the family, the intensivist finds this difficult. One intensivist recounted seeing a patient with advanced cancer who was being prepared for a subsequent cancer surgery:

I read through the notes and counted seven different specialty teams that had seen her, all who had ordered their own tests, all at a cost to the patient in terms of time and invasiveness and to the health system in terms of cost... and then I sat down with her and her family and was asking them what they wanted, and she said she didn't want an operation, and she wanted to be going to hospice. And the daughter said to me 'you're the first person that has actually sat down with us in the bedspace, explained what was going on, and asked us what we wanted'. So then rather than an ICU bed, I facilitated a palliative care referral and pathway to hospice care.

Standing in the Middle

As a medical leader in the ICU, the intensivist often takes on a lot of the stress burden from the junior doctors and nurses. Death and bad patient outcomes are hard on all staff, but particularly on the nurses who spend hours constantly with the patient and their families along with the junior doctors who follow the patient care progress over several days. The intensivist will often have to point out the disease process and the limited opportunity for recovery when it occurs. Trying to relieve stress from others itself can in itself be stressful:

A few months ago, we had a couple of, like a series of, patients that died in the unit. Not because of errors. But there was a very long process of dying. And the nurses were very stressed.

As mentioned previously, the structure of an intensive care unit does vary around the world. In some places a more 'open unit' culture exists where the autonomy of the home specialty team remains. In other places, a more 'closed unit' culture exists to encourage a collaborative approach between the home team and ICU team, where the intensivists ultimately co-ordinate and direct care.

Dealing with specialty medical teams who are clearly and appropriately heavily invested in the patient's care can be difficult when unexpected complications occur or when the patient deteriorates from their underlying disease or the treatment they have been receiving:

Although they have a poor outcome, we are forced to admit them because the medical environment or the medical specialties that treated them before, invested too much care in them, whether it was a bone marrow transplant or a very complicated course of chemotherapy or the newest biological treatment.

Intensive care can often involve dealing in 'shades of grey' rather than 'absolutes'. Intensivists, too, can be invested to the point that their 'big picture view' is obscured. This is mitigated by working with colleagues, engaging in case discussion at regular multi-disciplinary meetings and collaborative multi-specialty care. However, at times, opinions between intensivists can differ. Strong personalities can make this stressful. Humility is a valuable personal commodity, as it allows valuing other opinions and different viewpoints. One intensivist described a difficult stressful situation having to intervene with a more senior intensivist:

Everybody here, three other intensivists, we agree it should be stopped. You are making this big decision on your own, and you have gotten too involved in it, too emotionally involved in it.

Challenging colleague's views can have long-lasting impacts on those important collegial relationships within the intensivist team.

Morality and Value Judgements

The intensivist must understand clinical ethics, particularly in times of disagreement or conflict, and respect the pillars of autonomy, beneficence, non-maleficence, and justice. Other staff look to the intensivist for guidance. The intensivist must be careful to value and proactively incorporate the views of the patient and their family, along with those of the nursing, medical, and allied staff.

> *They have a really keen moral compass, the nurses. Critical care professionals in general do; that's one of the things I like about being a critical care professional.*

'Futile care' is a difficult construct to navigate. There is some controversy over whether it is helpful or a hindrance to define [1]:

> *To me, something else that adds to my stress, is when I see myself providing what I think is futile care. And unfortunately, we do a lot of that here. So, you're like, 'Why am I putting this child through dialysis and ventilation so that he can just lie in the bed and stare at the ceiling when this is all done? Because that's all he can do. Why?'*

Doctors primarily have a duty of care to their patients, and this duty of care has a stewardship or distributive justice component, whereby we spend public resources responsibly:

> *For me it's stressful sometimes. I'm just like, 'Why am I doing this? What are we really doing here? What's the point of this?' There are times in that unit upstairs where 50% of the patients will be like that. We just have a very... and part of it is... this might sound terrible, but I'm going to say it anyway.... part of me also thinks that this is a waste of resources.*

Stress of Litigation

The stress of litigation in intensive care is very variable depending on geography and local culture. Fortunately critical care is one of the least-sued specialties [2]. However, there is also evidence that in some settings, if intensivists practice long enough, there is a significant chance of being subjected to a malpractice claim. Malpractice claims appear unrelated to skill or knowledge and more related to chance [3]. In another study of malpractice claims involving critical care doctors, only a very small proportion actually related to care provided while in the intensive care unit [4].

Intensive care medicine involves high amounts of stress, unsociable hours, and limited opportunity for private practice. The common reason to choose such a medical specialty is a desire to treat severe illness and save or recover the sickest patients. Patients will die and patients will survive with complications. Thus, in settings where there is a high risk of litigation, intensivists must find a way not to take potential litigation as personal criticism:

And how do you risk assess your own practice when there's been an adverse outcome, and what are the steps that you should take that point? Do you run for the hills screaming, or do you say, "actually, I think I did everything I should have" and we'll just go through the normal processes on Monday.

… we have had families who have wanted to sue us and there was nothing more that we could do, but make sure that we had documented things correctly and had done what we could to help the patient.

Mistakes will happen. However, for doctors who work hard and strive for excellence, it is difficult not to take any mistakes personally:

During the first day after the event and around the lawsuit, and around expert opinion, I take it personally. I think that, okay, I'm sure that I am, like, my children say, "You are saving lives", but you are also sometimes making errors that damage or cause death. At some point when it happens you take it personally.

Being Open and Honest

First and foremost, an intensivist must be aware of their primary responsibility to be carers of the sick. To achieve this end, their guiding principle must be openness and honesty. However, intensivists are often also employees of the hospital and need to have some training in judicial or medicolegal practices so they can understand their legal requirements:

How you manage disclosure is pretty important. State the facts, not their subjectiveness. That's harder to do in practice than in theory. Even for someone with experience, it's really hard to do.

You're careful about what you say… but you also realise the error and you have to disclose the error. And the consequences… If we made the error and there is a lawsuit, then that's the way it is. So that doesn't factor into whether you tell them or not. If there is a lawsuit, there's a lawsuit. You do what's right in informing the family.

Careers and Lives Destroyed

Operating under a very real threat of being sued is difficult and highly stressful. Most intensivists were aware of cases where the doctors were persecuted through litigation. Doctors rarely go into work not wanting to do the best for their patients. However, mistakes will happen and how we manage that as a broader society needs open discussion:

… we didn't really have enough resources to put into education. We have this MET [medical response team] system here, it's supposed to be a skilled team who would respond, but we

didn't have any training or education for them. So again, I think it was just so awful that people who are trying to do their best can then get a conviction for manslaughter.

The stress of litigation can certainly be long-lasting with significant negative impacts:

…that was really, I think, a life-changing, career-changing experience for them and they have not been the same since, from an engagement with the job. They went from someone who I think really loved critical care, to hating it, and being sort of miserable, finishing out their career… It really changed them and affected them very negatively.

In addition, the process of litigation itself may be drawn out, and having to function at a high level in the meantime can be challenging:

Interviewer: And then they sued you. Did they win the case? Presumably not?
    Participant: No, because they couldn't find anyone as an expert to say I did anything wrong… but it took five years…

Does the threat of litigation stop you choosing a specialty? Some thought potentially:

I mean look at our malpractice costs - coverage is so high, and there's lots of states where there's not caps on malpractice suits, and that sort of thing…

While others didn't think it was a factor:

I feel like all through your training you know that it's something that's a potential… I think anything that you go to in medicine…No one that I know of in medicine has not chosen a specialty because they think the chances of being sued is too high.

Conclusion

There are certainly unique stressors in the ICU for all staff. However, dealing with the sickest of the sickest is incredibly rewarding and for this ICU will continue to attract new staff. It is essential to recognise these stressors, support our staff, and proactively find ways to mitigate these stressors so ICU staff can continue to do the work they love—saving lives and helping families.

References

1. Richards S. Exposing futility by searching beneath the concept. Clin Ethics. 2021;16(4):321–9. https://doi.org/10.1177/1477750920983577.
2. Jena AB, Seabury S, Lakdawalla D, Chandra A. Malpractice risk according to physician specialty. N Engl J Med. 2011;365(7):629–36. https://doi.org/10.1056/NEJMsa1012370.
3. Meadow W, Bell A, Lantos J. Physicians' experience with allegations of medical malpractice in the neonatal intensive care unit. Pediatrics. 1997;99(5):E10. https://doi.org/10.1542/peds.99.5.e10.

4. Myers LC, Skillings J, Heard L, Metlay JP, Mort E. Medical malpractice involving pulmonary/critical care physicians. Chest. 2019;156(5):907–14. https://doi.org/10.1016/j.chest.2019.04.102.

Bradley Wibrow is an intensivist and emergency physician in Perth, Western Australia, and works in a neuro, cardiac, and liver specialist intensive care unit as well as a small peripheral Emergency Department. He is passionate about ensuring equal access to critical care for all Australians, ultrasound, research and finding ways to maintain morale in a high stress workplace. His research interests include management of delirium, post-ICU care, and finding ways to aid recovery for our patients and families as they deal with one of the worst times of their lives. In his other life he is a father to four children, attempts to run regularly, and gets down to the ocean whenever possible.

Denise Goodman trained in paediatrics at Cincinnati Children's Hospital Medical Center and paediatric critical care at Children's Hospital of Pittsburgh. Prior to this she had undertaken a BS(Physics) at Niagara University, her MD at the State University of NY at Buffalo (now Jacobs School of Medicine at University at Buffalo), and her MS Epidemiology at Harvard T.H. Chan School of Public Health. She spent 2012–2013 academic year as the Morris Fishbein Fellow in Medical Editing at JAMA. Her interests include delivery of care, outcomes, care of children with medical complexity, and medical editing. She considers it a privilege to accompany children and their families through some of the most difficult experiences in their lives, and to share both their joys and challenges.

Chapter 4
Families in Grief

Deanna Todd Tzanetos ⓘD and Sacha Schweikert

> *Being healthy is the crown that only the sick can see. A lot of*
> *times, we take it for granted.*
>
> —Hasan Minhaj

Patients are admitted to the ICU because they are experiencing an acute threat to their lives, and often, the care provided there is the only thing standing between the patient and death. Due to critical illness, patients are often unable to communicate with the care team themselves and the patient's family assists in this situation.

As intensivists, we meet people on what is often their very worst day. Imagine walking acutely into a world of unfamiliar noises, some of which sound very alarming, full of unfamiliar faces who are serious, worried, and intense. Families may witness other patients' crises such as a cardiac arrest or a family saying goodbye to their loved one for the last time. The family is then told the medical facts of their loved one's condition.

For any lay person, no matter how good the explanation, this can be overwhelming and confusing. "Your son's kidneys are not working. He needs emergency dialysis." "Your mother's lungs have failed, and we are helping her breathe with a machine called a ventilator." Then, we often ask them to make urgent decisions based on this information. "Do you know what your loved one would want in this situation?"; "What were her views on resuscitation?" or consent to emergency procedures, "we need to do a heart catheterization right now," "We need to decompress the pressure on your daughter's brain by doing a craniectomy or removing a part of her skull."

D. Todd Tzanetos (✉)
Division of Critical Care, Department of Pediatrics, University of Louisville and Norton Children's Medical Group, Louisville, KY, USA
e-mail: deanna.tzanetos@louisville.edu

S. Schweikert
Department of Intensive Care, Sir Charles Gairdner Hospital, Perth, Australia

D. Dennis et al. (eds.), *Stories from ICU Doctors*,
https://doi.org/10.1007/978-3-031-32401-7_4

Families are thrust into a world of uncertainty [1]. In times of stress and crisis, people react in different manners. The family's reaction has a direct effect on the doctors, nurses, and staff caring for that patient. Intensivists have numerous patients at any given time and thus numerous relationships and interactions with patient families occurring simultaneously. This chapter discusses the experiences intensivists have shared with us from patient-family interactions.

Positive Family Interactions

In the best of cases, intensivist-family interactions can be positive and contribute greatly to an intensivist's morale and job satisfaction:

So, I like to keep the cards pinned up on my wall in my office. There aren't a lot of them, but I do get a few. One of them that's there is actually an obituary statement from the newspaper because I got mentioned. They thanked me in the obituary which had never happened before. So, there are lots of positive experiences after critical events and deaths.

I think that my experience is that families feel that the intensivists are usually reasonable. We are used to talking to them and explaining things in a way that they can understand. So, I think that that is a rewarding thing, where you can helpfully explain what has gone on, even if it's not what everyone wanted.

I love the interactions with families. I had one a couple of weeks ago with this old lady with a head injury and dealing with her relatives and stuff like that and trying to negotiate a path. Having a conversation and trying to find, to me, a reasonable and human way to deal with this, and it worked out well, and I got a lovely card from her. That's fantastic, you know? That's fantastic.

It is important to note that the complex nature of our humanity can lead to negative feelings, even from positive interactions with patient families:

There are families where things clearly haven't gone well. Patients were going well before and now they're dead. And they've still just thanked the team for what they've done, and that can almost be as hard, because we want, as humans, to convey how sorry we are, or we don't feel like we did our best, and the family is being almost too nice about it.

So, actually the two patients that I carry with me, both of their parents were very forgiving and loving towards me. It makes it harder.

Negative Family Interactions

Due to the highly stressful situations families find themselves in, studies have demonstrated families of critically ill patients to be at risk for acute stress disorder, complicated grief, insomnia, and post-traumatic stress disorder [1, 2]. As intensivists, in addition to providing medical care for the patient, there is an inherent responsibility to develop relationships with families:

And we have to use up a lot of our internal power and resources to work on relationships with our families and patients because it is ICU and because it makes up our worth and our whole as a human being, not as a technocrat who makes mistakes.

Nevertheless, individuals have different stress responses and internal coping mechanisms. Some families can have difficulty expressing their emotions or finding an outlet for their fears. This can turn interactions between families and intensivists into stressful, sometimes scary situations. Families can react with violence or verbally abusive language which takes its toll on the intensivist [3]:

The family had an acute grief response at the time and the Dad was screaming 'Murderers! Assassins! You killed my baby.' I mean just openly screaming. But again, to me I recognized that. I mean you always warn your team that an acute grief response can look like a lot of different things. You can think that the family is in lockstep with you and then they have an absolutely different response when the death happens. I don't think that was a negative outcome, but I certainly tell you it had an impact on my staff, and if felt intense at the time. You know when you have...when you have someone screaming at you.

To complicate the matter, the care in an ICU is continuous with several handovers per day between different mixes of care team members. This occurs on any given day with "changing faces" of medical, nursing, and allied health members. This contributes to the family's stress of constantly meeting new people with slight variation in the care provided. This is especially true for "long-stay patients," where family relatives are increasingly aware of medical details and daily care plans. It is possible in such a scenario for families to increasingly criticize or question variables in the delivery of daily care routines and may sometimes become increasingly hostile towards staff. Complex, repetitive family meetings are usually the consequence:

We tried to convey to the family that we would do everything we can but that the chances were not very high, and they wouldn't hear of it. 'She made it through the last admission. She is strong.' The children were very physically big and attached to her, very adamant that we do everything for her. And we did what we usually do, we ventilated, we put in lines, we gave her inotropes, we did dialysis. Eventually she needed a tracheostomy, so we did the tracheostomy. But, she died, and the family...from the family's point of view we killed her. Before she died, we were faced with an extremely aggressive family. But the aggression was not physical – they did not come and punch us in the face. They were verbally aggressive, and they humiliated us. We sat in family meetings, and they said, 'you are useless, your unit is useless, everything is useless, you killed our mother.' ...and it was very, very aggressive, very violent, very passive-aggressive. They would sit with their notes and take pictures, they would record and take notes, and ask, 'what are you doing now? What do you think you are doing? How the hell do you think this happened? What the hell do you know about managing other patients if you can't manage this one?' A very, very offensive level of discussion.

Once I had a grandmother tell me that she hoped that this would happen to my child. I was a first-time Mom, I was just back from maternity leave, and covering a patient I didn't know. And that was pretty awful.

Family reactions can sometimes turn from the emotionally difficult to threatened or actual occupational violence for the intensivist, the intensivist's family, or associated staff [3]:

One of the nurses said, "hey that family is threatening to hurt you.' I was pregnant at the time…'to hurt your baby.'…and it was one where I sort of looked over my shoulder a little bit; and I would go running all over the place and I'd sort of watch.

I did have a Dad too…and I was actually pregnant… he told the nurse, 'What do you think if I…If that baby she is pregnant with dies; how would she feel?

I did have a gentleman punch a hole in the wall next to my head. That was my first year as a consultant [intensivist]. I was just sitting down to tell him his wife was brain dead. And she was my age.

Probably the one patient who was absolutely definitely not harmed in any way by the surgeon who had a bad outcome had dreadful heart disease before undergoing surgery; the daughters were absolutely vicious, going for the surgeon. Almost had to be held across the table to stop them jumping across the table.

We had a family say that they would bring a gun in and shoot us if their child died. That was not a good environment to work in. I've had families get very physically threatening and up in my face. Yelling, 'You need to fix this.' I did have a Mom call, after her child died, and say, 'If I knew what was good for me, I should leave town and not live in…' You know…she didn't want me practicing medicine here anymore. That was actually, probably, one of the worst experiences, because I mean it's very easy to find out where somebody lives. I was scared that I would be out with my family and see this person. What would she do if she saw my kids? She threatened…there were three of us. [She] called our academic office and asked for us. Finally, they got wise to not transfer her to us, but she threatened us all that, 'If we knew what was good for us, we should leave.' I mean, I didn't know what that threat meant. I did take anything on social media that had any reference to my family off; and I still don't put that stuff up.

Family Presence in Resuscitation

Literature has demonstrated that family member presence at resuscitation can be positive. Family presence allows them to see that everything truly was done in an effort to save their loved one's life. In addition, the family can know that their loved one did not die alone and was in the presence of those they loved [4].

Many intensivists are steadfast supporters of family presence in ward rounds, appropriate procedures, and at resuscitations:

[Family presence at resuscitations] allows them to see how hard I am trying to save their child and how present I am. They just… they see the efforts of the team. And I think that's the benefit of often having parents around for a Code. For them to see how many people are caring for their child and how all of these efforts are not working. So those are positive.

I mean she never jumped on the bed or tried to stop us from doing what we were doing; but her grief. She had to be pulled to the back of the room. Because we try to let families be there; and I believe that's a good policy because, to a degree, if the family sees you doing everything possible to save their child's life, they're going to understand the death more than if they are kept in some room and don't see it.

However, watching the physical act of a resuscitation by the medical team can also be shocking and incredibly difficult for families. The act of resuscitation appears physically very violent—chest compressions and cardioversion can espe-cially be hard to see your loved one undergo. Watching a resuscitation can trigger family members to lash out at the medical team:

I was intubating the child, the child has a cardiac arrest; the mother is standing there screaming, 'You killed my child.' The whole time we are resuscitating the child. She ended up like screaming for an hour straight; and so it's just… The child unfortunately was going to die; regardless of the intervention; but as a Mom, I might have done the same thing, right? You just don't know in that situation. When you are facing so much grief; and while I realized it wasn't a personal attack, for her, I was the face of the death of her child. It didn't make it less… even though I can rationalize it, and understand that side of it, as a parent; it still did not make the experience feel good.

Managing Family Expectations and Reactions

As intensivists, learning to manage families and their expectations is a part of the job that cannot easily be learned in the classroom. It requires experience, persever-ance, and a perspective that can only come from situational experience. In addition to understanding and managing the critical illness, intensivists must cultivate skills for these complex interpersonal relationships and learn resilience to maintain their own mental health and desire to continue to practice:

I think a lot of the stress for me is actually involved in the interactions with the families because I also think that families expect their children to survive the Paediatric ICU stay. Whereas a 90-year-old man, the family may not have that same expectation. And so, man-aging family expectation is one of the hardest things actually for me as an [intensivist]. The love bond that the parent has for their child is probably one of the strongest really, the strongest relationship that exists. So, it's quite stressful to actually manage parents and families. I think it's one of the most challenging and emotionally taxing things for me as an intensivist.

Intensivists have mechanisms for managing family stress reactions. Confronting the behavior and setting boundaries and expectations for respectful communication between the family and the care team is one such mechanism:

I was leading a care conference. But this was a big family. Like two sets of grandparents and Mom and Dad. And so, we are talking about their son needing a trach or something like that. So, it wasn't even end of life, it is just these are the next steps. And the grandma is just being so rude, "you all just want to hurt him.' And saying it directly to me, 'you just want to do this…' And I finally looked at her and I said, 'You won't speak to me this way; if you choose to speak to me this way, then you can leave.' And everyone was like, 'this is awk-ward.' And then she left it alone; she wanted to stay. But it was really uncomfortable. She was always fine with me after that. If you confront the behavior, then they actually respect you a little bit; because if they walk all over you, then they are just going to keep walking all over you.

Other intensivists utilize an approach of allowing the family to be where they are in their grieving process, allowing them space to work through the realities of their situation:

You have to give families the space to go through whatever it is they need to go through and not overreact and not get defensive and not strike back.

So my job is to help manage the family's coping and allow them a chance to vent, to grieve, to heal. You simply have to give the family place to grieve. And the space to be angry. And then you have to give them the tools they need. If it's outside of my control, I just allow the family space to express their concerns and I try to give them the tools they need to follow through. Even if that means following through legally. That's their right. I'm not here to say, 'don't do that.' But I think you have to meet the family where they are. If you're going to manage this job well, you have to give families what they need.

Conclusion

Intensive care units bring together patients, families, diverse care teams, and critical illness in a complex, high stress, sociotechnical environment. Coping mechanisms of family members' and intensivists' reactions to them vary. Family interactions can bring a great deal of satisfaction and joy to the practice of critical care medicine. Conversely, negative, stressful interactions with family can have a negative effect on intensivists and add largely to the burnout often experienced by critical care specialist doctors.

References

1. Minton C, Batten L, Huntington A. A multicase study of prolonged critical illness in the intensive care unit: families' experiences. Intensive Crit Care Nurs. 2019;50:21–7.
2. Nygaard A, Haugdahl H, Laholt H, Brinchmann B, Lind R. Professionals' narratives of interactions with patients' families in intensive care. Nurs Ethics. 2022;0:1–14.
3. Chakraborty S, Mashreky S, Koustuv, D. Violence against physicians and nurses: a systematic review. Z Gesundh Wiss. 2022;30(8):1837–55.
4. Bradley C. Family presence and support during resuscitation. Crit Care Nurs Clin North Am. 2021;30:333–42.

Deanna Todd Tzanetos is a pediatric cardiac intensivist at Norton Children's Hospital, affiliated with the University of Louisville in Louisville, Kentucky, USA. She is a professor of pediatrics and the Medical Director of the Jennifer Lawrence Cardiac Intensive Care Unit. Her research interests include quality improvement in the cardiac ICU and anticoagulation management in patients requiring extracorporeal membranous oxygenation.

Sacha Schweikert studied medicine in Switzerland before moving to Australia to pursue intensive care medicine training. He complemented training with a diploma in clinical ultrasound and undertook a fellowship in neurocritical care at the University of Toronto before returning to Australia. He currently works as an intensive care specialist at Sir Charles Gairdner Hospital in Perth and has a special interest in all things neurocritical care.

Chapter 5
A Whole Lot Going on

Matthew Anstey ⓘ **and Deanna Todd Tzanetos** ⓘ

> *What I dream of is an art of balance, of purity and serenity*
> *devoid of troubling or depressing subject matter—a soothing,*
> *calming influence on the mind, rather like a good armchair*
> *which provides relaxation from physical fatigue.*
>
> —Henri Matisse

To some degree, all professions have significant stresses associated with them. The military, firefighters, and police officers all deal with being exposed to significant threats and responding to changeable situations. The COVID-19 pandemic also illustrated that many people working in service industries (such as logistics, retail, hospitality) can have difficult working environments, with potentially volatile customers and much less financial recompense than other professions.

Nonetheless, working in intensive care exposes clinicians to a multitude of both generic work stressors, but also ICU-specific stressors. Laurent and colleagues [1] surveyed nurses and doctors in France, Italy, Canada, and Spain and, after identifying 99 different stressors, grouped them into seven main categories: (1) significant workload pressure, (2) management of complex/at-risk situations, (3) challenges related to one's personal life, (4) dealing with ethical and moral-related situations, (5) problematic situations with patients and relatives, (6) conflicts with members of the healthcare team, and (7) lack of resources.

M. Anstey (✉)
Sir Charles Gairdner Hospital, Perth, Australia

Curtin University, School of Public Health, Perth, Australia

University of Western Australia, School of Medicine, Perth, Australia
e-mail: Matthew.Anstey@health.wa.gov.au

D. Todd Tzanetos
Division of Critical Care, Department of Pediatrics, University of Louisville, and Norton Children's Medical Group, Louisville, KY, USA

© The Author(s), under exclusive license to Springer Nature Switzerland AG 2023
D. Dennis et al. (eds.), *Stories from ICU Doctors*,
https://doi.org/10.1007/978-3-031-32401-7_5

The generic stressors were felt to be common with other healthcare professions (e.g., high job demands, problematic relationships with other professionals, lack of resources), whereas there were also *specific* stressors to the ICU (e.g., management of complex/at-risk situations, dealing with ethical and moral issues, problematic situations with patients and relatives).

A recurring theme expressed by intensivists was their desire to focus on their clinical roles, without the intrusion of the need to deal with bed management, administrative burdens, or non-clinical roles:

> *My wife made a comment this morning. I said, "I'm looking forward to going to work today", and she goes, "You are so more relaxed when you are on clinical... than when you are ...non-clinical."*
>
> *I mean the real reason why many of us do this is just because of the clinical stuff. Isn't it? In the end, that gives meaning to what we do. Being an administrator to me, in and of itself, is meaningless. Unless it is adding to, or part of what you do. Whether it's trying to make what you do better, or as you get older, trying to make what others do better. So, I see that as a very important role. Do I still enjoy looking after sick people? Yes I do. I love the challenge.*

These opinions may reflect several possibilities. The first is that intensivists are highly trained clinicians and thus feel underprepared for the other roles that they need to take on. Much of the training that occurs for managerial tasks is a by-product of their role, rather than taken a proactive and clear decision to develop this skill set. Second, the medical system is increasingly complicated and challenging to reform or improve, even from within:

> *Yes, the administrative side is a difficult foe, and it's almost a Sisyphean task. It never finishes. Particularly in the recent, here at the [hospital], the sort of chain of managers and executives who change faces so often in the last year, it's almost dizzying. So it is like playing on a team, with a constant number of people, the unlimited number of people on the bench. You know, you've only got so many reserves, but suddenly there's a new person that you don't know, and you don't know what their game is, so I think it's harder.*

This leads to intersections and roadblocks to intensivists carrying out the clinical work that they enjoy:

> *So the fact that I sometimes can't accept the patient [into ICU] because I don't have a [staffed] bed, I can't transfer [a] non-critically ill patient out of my unit because I don't have a bed; I am trying to figure out what four elements of something need to go into the note for billing when I got the patient bleeding, there are 15 different steps you have to go through to put in certain orders... You know like a lot of things relate to the electronic medical record....*
>
> *...I think that a lot of the administrative burden becomes very stressful because it detracts from what you want to be doing as a clinician. Or a lot of times, if I need to be... like if there is a bleeding patient and I need to be at the bedside, then it stressful because ... can't not finish all work. So, you're taking it all with you after you've left the hospital, and then you're feeling guilt or trying to like... you've gotta get that work done, but you've missed bedtime five days in a row with your kid. So, I think those things create stress as well.*

Even for those looking to successfully navigate the other components of their career, the academic or managerial advancement, this can be difficult as well:

A lot of my daily stressors, in the majority, are more related to academic stuff, and as I've gotten further along in my career, thinking about how to keep advancing my career can be stressful … I have some leadership positions that I hold, and how to do those and do those well can be stressful. There is not always formal training in how to do that, and I've done a couple of leadership programs… and those things are helpful, but they're still sort of 'boots on the ground'.

As these insights illustrate, intensivists are juggling multiple roles, without discrete barriers between them. The intrusion of one role across into another creates the sensation of constantly being bombarded with requests. One strategy employed by many clinicians is to try and complete one task before moving on to the next.

Fatigue

The backdrop to the stresses faced by ICU clinicians is the fatigue that comes from shiftwork and long work hours:

We all know your coping skills get smacked by fatigue.

While clinical hours are averaging out to be more reasonable than our predecessors worked, within that the average still exists long periods of work (such as runs of sequential days or nights of work, and then days off):

But the days of intensivists doing what we do, which is seven on, seven off, and seven on, is just ridiculous. Your decision-making with the fatigue on Saturday, Sunday and Monday morning is just appalling. It's like putting the barriers up and saying, "Just stop hitting me around the head anymore!" So that's got to change. And that's a work-rostering issue.

Rostering practices do differ across centers, and it appears that shorter blocks of shifts are also associated with better patient outcomes [2]. Nonetheless, we know that these long hours lead to fatigue, sleepiness, reduced vigilance, and increased errors [3, 4]:

…at midnight I finished, and I slept okay that night. And then I woke up yesterday morning and had things to do, had to come into the hospital for some meetings. And I'm behind in a million and a half things. I could tell that I was emotionally and physically very fatigued. I just didn't have a lot left in the arsenal, you know?

The irregularity of shiftwork can also make it hard to have regular activities outside of work:

I also had an awareness of the effects of cumulative sleep deprivation, loss of circadian rhythms, on focus; on interpersonal commitments; on clinical acumen; on relationships outside of work; on physical well-being….

As one participant put it:

I think I have trouble finding the hours to sleep! Once I find the hours to sleep, no, I don't have trouble sleeping! (laughs).

There are strategies that have been identified that intensivists use to mitigate and cope with fatigue [5]. Lifestyle strategies include protecting sleep before on-call shifts, limiting alcohol, and getting adequate exercise. Some useful workplace strategies suggested were prioritizing tasks that need to be done immediately and postponing tasks that could wait and having a structured approach to dealing with problems.

Interpersonal Issues

Interpersonal conflict in intensive care can be between the workers (within the ICU department or with other specialist departments) and with intensivist's families. Many intensivists see their role as taking care of "the whole patient" and thus need to coordinate the different specialty teams that may be involved in patient care. At times, that might require careful diplomacy or work-arounds to achieve what you think is best for the patient:

> *"I used to have times where the surgeon just never listened to me, so I eventually I built this model." I waited until he went home. I waited until 5:15 PM when he had gone home and I went to the head of surgery and I said, "I'd like you to come see this case". Inevitably the patient who was supposed to be operated on during the day got operated on at night. I have lists of cases like that, where I had to bypass this particular surgeon, and it wasn't fun, it wasn't good and every case like that is still in my memory and is traumatic.*

It is important to recognize that conflict between doctors can be a common issue [6]. Shrepel and colleagues found that "preconceived perceptions of their colleagues' specialty and misalignments in expectations around clinical care primed the learning environment for conflict" in North American general medicine and emergency medicine settings. Their solutions were to "focus on honesty, empathy, teaching, and active team formation to resolve or avoid conflict."

A review by Rogers and Lingard [7], from surgeons' perspectives, points out that many solutions to reduce conflict, such as taking time to calm down, might not be possible in the time-pressured environment of a medical emergency. Behaviors that they found to be helpful were maintaining calm, focused problem-solving and being flexible in the solutions offered. Providing more communication and rationale around decision-making when there was conflict, such as taking time to explain your analysis of the situation to the team, and their plan, was also helpful:

> *When the conflicts are between doctors in the unit, I feel it is very important to sit down and discuss it. Instead of just being hot-headed and walking around with this frustration all of the time. The importance of sitting down with the departmental head or myself and a colleague if it was us, or myself and nursing staff... the importance of sitting down and discussing the issue if things have been said in the heat of battle, so to speak, and people have been offended, is to sit down afterwards and apologise, and discuss how we can go forward. Again, sitting down, communicating how to go forward. This is what I have found to be vital.*

Interestingly, while conflict with family members does occur, concordance between the perceptions of family members and medical staff is less common. For example, medical staff might perceive conflict with family members, although the family does not perceive this [8, 9]. Inviting patients or their surrogate decision-makers to provide their opinions and assessment of the situation can help allay this disconnect.

Gender Inequity

Only about one-quarter of practicing intensivists in the United States and Canada are women. In addition, women experience slower career advancement than their male counterparts [10]. This lack of gender parity can be highlighted by the real-world example of an important published guideline in the field. In 2016, the Society for Critical Care Medicine and the European Society of Intensive Care jointly created the Third International Consensus Definitions for Sepsis and Septic Shock without a female intensivist on the 19-person panel [11]. In addition to the academic discrepancy, the lack of gender parity in critical care can be acutely observed at the bedside in several different ways.

Implicit bias can be defined as a prejudice that unknowingly influences thinking and reactions. Both male and female participants shared that consulting services may have implicit biases toward female intensivists:

So, I think there are significant challenges over, on top of, those basic ones and that's unfortunate. I think a lot of it comes down to dealing with interactions with other treating teams particularly some other treating teams that have a more heavy male bias to them. [They] are, or can be, dismissive and not take the female intensivist with the same gravitas as they would, particularly a young female intensivist, as they would an older grey-haired male intensivist.

I do think there are certain families and other providers who are more responsive to the authority of a male intensivist than a female intensivist. When I first became a fellow, I remember one of my intensivists making a big deal about how I was too quiet, too introspective. You know, I wasn't extroverted enough.

I think there are significant challenges for female intensivists. That's over and above the normal challenges that most female doctors have which is, 'I'm not the nurse.'

Again, being a man, I cannot fully identify, but there are any number of times that people assume that female [doctors] are not [doctors], they are nurses. I have some colleagues that wear their white coat all the time because of that.

In addition to biases female intensivists may experience at the bedside, intensivists shared those perceptions of responsibilities outside the hospital may be different for men and women as well. This may play a role in women not choosing critical care or being in the slower advancement of career compared to male colleagues:

One thing I do notice about the men, is that I think that women in their life support their personal life a bit more. How can I say this? I find that women tend to be more organized and more on top of mulit-tasking different things. I find the men are the ones who sometimes forget that they are on-call or that they have a meeting.

I think the biggest challenge probably relates to the responsibilities that we have outside of being an intensivist. I think as a Mom or as a wife...I mean it depends on what the social situation is…but I think in a lot of ways we do a lot of other things. There are a lot of other things we are responsible for.

In our interviews, intensivists relayed clear differences in both in hospital and out of hospital experiences between male and female intensivists. These discrepancies represent unique non-clinical factors related to gender which influence the experience of intensivists.

Conclusion

As much as some intensivists may wish that these non-clinical stressors would not intrude as much as they do, they are unavoidable. Conscious reflection on their reactions to these stressors and designing strategies that work for them is an important protection against any distress that they may cause.

References

1. Laurent A, Fournier A, Lheureux F, Martin Delgado MC, Bocci MG, Prestifilippo A, et al. An international tool to measure perceived stressors in intensive care units: the PS-ICU scale. Ann Intensive Care. 2021;11(1):57.
2. Gershengorn HB, Pilcher DV, Litton E, Anstey M, Garland A, Wunsch H. Association between consecutive days worked by intensivists and outcomes for critically ill patients. Crit Care Med. 2020;48(4):594–8.
3. Bihari S, Venkatapathy A, Prakash S, Everest E, McEvoy RD, Bersten A. ICU shift related effects on sleep, fatigue and alertness levels. Occup Med. 2020;70(2):107–12.
4. McClelland L, Plunkett E, McCrossan R, Ferguson K, Fraser J, Gildersleve C, et al. A national survey of out-of-hours working and fatigue in consultants in anaesthesia and paediatric intensive care in the UK and Ireland. Anaesthesia. 2019;74(12):1509–23.
5. Henrich N, Ayas NT, Stelfox HT, Peets AD. Cognitive and other strategies to mitigate the effects of fatigue. Lessons from staff physicians working in intensive care units. Ann Am Thorac Soc. 2016;13(9):1600–6.
6. Schrepel C, Amick AE, Bann M, Watsjold B, Jauregui J, Ilgen JS, et al. Interspeciality othering: a qualitative analysis of physician interpersonal conflict at the time of admission from the emergency department. Acad Med. 2021;96(11S):S215.
7. Rogers DA, Lingard L. Surgeons managing conflict: a framework for understanding the challenge. J Am Coll Surg. 2006;203:568–74. https://doi.org/10.1016/j.jamcollsurg.2006.06.012.
8. Anstey MH, Litton E, Jha N, Trevenen ML, Webb S, Mitchell IA. A comparison of the opinions of intensive care unit staff and family members of the treatment intensity received by patients admitted to an intensive care unit: a multicentre survey. Aust Crit Care. 2019;32(5):378–82.
9. Ashana DC, Parish A, Jan A, Olsen M, Cox CE. Factors associated with physicians perceptions of interpersonal conflict with families in the intensive care unit. In: B102 professional training and stakeholder perspectives in chronic and serious illness. American Thoracic Society; 2022 [cited 2022 May 15]. p. A3503–A3503. (American Thoracic Society International Conference Abstracts). http://www.atsjournals.org/doi/abs/10.1164/ajrccm-conference.2022.205.1_MeetingAbstracts.A3503.

10. Mehta S, Burns KEA, Machado FR, Fox-Robichaud AE, Cook DJ, Calfee CS, et al. Gender parity in critical care medicine. Am J Respir Crit Care Med. 2017;196(4):425–9.
11. Singer M, Deutschman CS, Seymour CW, Shankar-Hari M, Annane D, Bauer M, et al. The third international consensus definitions for sepsis and septic shock (Sepsis-3). JAMA. 2016;315(8):801–10.

Matthew Anstey is an intensivist and researcher at Sir Charles Gairdner Hospital, Curtin University, and University of Western Australia in Perth. He has a Master of Public Health from Harvard University, and was the 2010–2011 Harkness Fellow in Health Policy, based at Kaiser Permanente in California. He was the past chair of Choosing Wisely Australia advisory group. His research interests focus on improving outcomes for ICU survivors (and built the survivors website mylifeaftericu.com) and improving the quality of care received by patients.

Deanna Todd Tzanetos is a pediatric cardiac intensivist at Norton Children's Hospital, affiliated with the University of Louisville in Louisville, Kentucky, USA. She is a professor of pediatrics and the Medical Director of the Jennifer Lawrence Cardiac Intensive Care Unit. Her research interests include quality improvement in the cardiac ICU and anticoagulation management in patients requiring extracorporeal membranous oxygenation.

Chapter 6
Sick Kiddies

Aaron Calhoun ⓘ **and Efrat Orenbuch-Harroch**

> *Our most basic common link is that we all inhabit this planet.*
> *We all breathe the same air. We all cherish our children's future.*
> *And we are all mortal.*
>
> —*John F. Kennedy*

As we have seen, the ICU environment is replete with stressors. Clinical stressors range from the momentary increases in intensivist's cognitive load imposed by changes in patient physiology to the more existential concerns that arise as ICU clinicians deal with the long-term trauma caused by poor patient outcomes. Some non-clinical stressors include the systems within which team members function—rostering, shiftwork, and fatigue management—as well as the interpersonal relationships and the impact of societal beliefs around gender roles. There are also the stressors imposed by families. This chapter explores each of these stressors through the two lenses of adult versus paediatric intensive care practice.

The paediatric intensive care unit (PICU) represents a distinct area of practice with a different patient population and disease physiology. These distinctions result in different patterns of intensivist stressors. During the qualitative study described in this book, both adult and paediatric intensivists were interviewed, allowing us to gain deeper perspective on the most significant of these differences.

Different perceptions were noted in overall patient care experience, including both the reason for the admission and mortality, the unique clinical overlay of child abuse, the relationship established between intensivists and their families, and the personal attitudes and orientation of the intensivists.

A. Calhoun (✉)
Division of Critical Care, Department of Pediatrics, University of Louisville,
and Norton Children's Medical Group, Louisville, KY, USA
e-mail: aaron.calhoun@louisville.edu

E. Orenbuch-Harroch
Medical Intensive Care Unit, Hadassah University Medical Center, Jerusalem, Israel

D. Dennis et al. (eds.), *Stories from ICU Doctors*,
https://doi.org/10.1007/978-3-031-32401-7_6

Patient Care Experience: The Reason for Admission

Despite the often-quoted adage "children are not small adults", the underlying physiologic states treated in the PICU and adult ICU were not perceived as notably different in many cases [1]. As one participant, who has practiced in both arenas, stated:

In terms of a physiological perspective, no, it's pretty much the same.

Differences were perceived, however, in the causal factors that lead to admission. Prominent here is a sense that adult ICU patients may have had some role to play in the disease processes that brought them to the ICU. Critically ill children were perceived as innocent in this regard. Participants described this in a number of ways:

It's harder in my mind to do paeds critical care because most of the time, it's not because of an accumulation of self-inflicted disease. Whereas the person who has been smoking and drinking, and a bunch of other less than ideal lifestyle choices comes in sick and says, 'Fix me'… I can't undo 30, 40 or 50 years of poor choices.

I think you can get tied into your patients a little more in paeds than what you do in the adult side. I think it's a little bit easier to be a little bit more objective and say, you know, 'They didn't make their clinic visit today, it's not my fault.' Or if they have not been taking care of their diabetes for the last five years, and they come in post infarct secondary to bad vascular disease, there's only so much I can do for that.

Another quote directly illustrates this dichotomy as perceived across the paediatric and adult intensivist communities, providing further insight into how each group perceives the work and stressors experienced by the other craft group:

When I worked in (another Hospital) the PICU was attached to the adult unit. There were six adult beds, so I had to walk through the adult unit all the time to go to my patients and the adult intensivist would come and say, "How can you do this?" … And then I would walk through their unit every day and see all of the old people and would cry every day. I couldn't look at them because all I saw were all of these people's wonderful lives, this is how they are ending up…

I see this guy who was a university professor, I see this guy you know, with all his grandchildren coming to visit him and to me that was tremendous sadness. I didn't know how they could do it…

This perceived difference is often a double-edged sword, however, with the "innocence" of PICU patients at once attracting intensivists of a certain temperament to the field while simultaneously challenging them with a greater sense of moral weight that can enhance the pressure intensivists place on themselves to achieve the best outcomes. As one stated:

That's also a challenging part of paediatric critical care. Kids did nothing to get themselves here.

A final complicating factor affecting these perceptions is whether or not the intensivists themselves have their own children. One adult intensivist movingly described the internal change they experienced after having children themselves:

My first specialty was anaesthetics, and I avoid paediatric anaesthetics now as well. I don't like it. I just feel like… I feel like I'd come to work and upset kids and torture them, and see the look on their faces.

And then Paediatric ICU, I could never do it. That's why I have deliberately chosen an adult hospital.

A Unique Stressor: The Role of Child Abuse

One cause of admission that was addressed multiple times by participants was caring for victims of child abuse. Given the perception of innocence noted above, it is perhaps unsurprising that caring for critically ill children suffering the sequelae of abuse is seen as particularly stressful. As one participant stated:

We have one of the higher rates of child abuse or abusive injuries relative to a lot of other [places] in the country. I have two responses. One is, the sadness of 'How you could do this to a kid?'; the other is anger. Just being angry at the perpetrator, whoever that may be.

This anger places intensivists in a state of ongoing moral distress or cumulative moral injury. Caring for critically ill children involves acting with a great deal of compassion toward potentially culpable family members while they cope with the devastating circumstances they face. As the legal investigation of potential child abuse moves forward, this culpability is often replaced by certain knowledge as to the identity of the perpetrator. Despite this, the intensivist must maintain the same compassionate attitude toward the situation as they would offer to other families. Intensivists often will deliberately attempt to avoid reflection on this difficult tension:

At the same time, it's not my job to figure out 'who did it?' My job is to just identify it and pass it on to the police and let them do their investigation.

Emotional distress from these situations often does not resolve after the case ends and is frequently internalized and subsequently triggered by future child abuse cases. One participant used the analogy of placing that emotion safely within an interior "cabinet," which is then forcibly opened when another abuse case is encountered. This re-emergence of the emotions surrounding these difficult cases is seen as a significant ongoing stressor that is particular to the paediatric intensivist population.

Prognostic Differences in Children: Comfort and Responsibility

Perhaps the most significant perceived difference in the patient population is the drastically lower mortality rates for paediatric ICU patients when compared with adult ICU patients. Recent studies estimate a 19% mortality among adult ICU patients and a 2.4–5% mortality rate in the paediatric ICU context [2, 3]. For paediatric intensivists, this was often seen as a source of comfort which reduced the stress of practice, as most parents can be assured that their child will survive their illness:

> *I think that in paediatrics because our mortality rates are so low, just 3 to 5%, whereas in the adult ICUs, a third of patients are dying, I can imagine there would be a difference in how death and morbidity is approached. Because for us, it is a relatively infrequent event, and so we expect our children to survive most of the things that they come in with.*

Paradoxically, however, this expectation of survival can also become a source of significant distress if the death of a patient is felt to be preventable, imminent, or unavoidable. The same participant described this as a sense of "weightiness" inherent in the death of a child, and another gave a sense that children were "special," full of potential in a way that adults are not:

> *I look at my patient who is nine months old, and wonder, 'Could this kid be the president some day?*

Intensivists also perceive this survival statistic as a hard-won fact of PICU practice, not simply a matter of course, and described the significant ongoing expenditure of physical and intellectual effort required to maintain these outcomes:

> *One of the stressors that I perceive is that while that mortality rate should be 3%, that mortality rate doesn't maintain itself. It is 3% because we work really hard, and we think really hard, and I think sometimes paediatric intensivists can be lulled into complacency about that.*

Additionally, this lower mortality rate contributes to a perception among paediatric intensivists that their adult colleagues, to some extent, "expect" the death of their patients, and therefore the event has a lesser psychological impact:

> *A lot of the deaths in an adult ICU are somewhat expected, in elderly people who have hopefully lived a great life… So it feels less heart wrenching even though their loved ones are probably still mourning and grieving in the same way.*

> *There is more sadness when a child has a bad outcome as opposed to an adult. Particularly if it's an elderly adult, for whom the outcome is relatively expected. You know, the 70-year-old who has congestive heart failure and COPD, and who develops a pneumonia and dies. Well they've had 70 years, and you know, hopefully a good life; whereas the baby with congenital heart disease; infection; or any number of diagnoses that give them reason to come in; they never had any chance.*

> *People expect their parents to die; they don't expect their children to die… People who are seven months old, most people aren't ready for that.*

This differential in mortality rate also affects clinical decision-making, as paediatric intensivists describe a greater perceived willingness to offer "heroic" advanced therapies, such as extracorporeal membrane oxygenation (ECMO), in more dire clinical situations than their adult colleagues. One paediatric intensivist that trained alongside adult intensivists, and hence had frequent encounters with the adult environment of care, described this as follows:

> *I trained in an environment where we trained alongside of adult intensivists, and yes, they think that some of what we do is insane, because they just wouldn't offer that to some of*

their patients on their way in through the door… So there is a fundamentally different start-ing point. Whereas, we, every patient that comes in, I think, many Intensivists, oftentimes ask the question, 'what are we doing?', 'What's the endpoint for this child?' But 97% of our patients leave the unit… alive. So the expectation for us, is that every person is going to get everything to help them survive that.

In contrast, adult intensivists caution that the experience of these paediatric intensivists is no more than a perception and may not necessarily be reflective of the reality experienced within the adult ICU. One adult intensivist, when asked whether they felt that the stressors involved with death in the paediatric context differed from their experience, answered as follows:

I think the same things are probably there because a life is a life. How can you say more valuable for a mother of three versus someone who has not had children versus a child versus someone who has raised three generations and been married for 60 years or some-thing that? I think again some of it is how you relate personally. I think sometimes I find it really quite emotional talking to the surviving partner of an old couple who have been together forever because I think how it was for my mother when my father died and she was kind of left. But then someone who's got a teenage child might relates to a situation when you're dealing with a teenager or someone who is just have a baby looking after that.

In this view, the sense of loss and value attributed to lost life is unrelated to patient age. Rather it seems related to the personal relationships present between family members and between the intensivist and family. It is important to under-stand that the perceptions of one group do not necessary equate with the lived expe-rience of the other.

Family Relationships: Decision-Making and Dysfunction

While family relationships are vital across the spectrum of ages, the particular dynamics present in the parent/child relationship represents a somewhat unique cir-cumstance. Parents frequently need to function as surrogate decision-makers for their children. While in most cases this is not a barrier to care, moral distress can arise when families must address life-changing diagnoses or make decisions regard-ing end-of-life situations for which they may not be prepared. One participant com-mented specifically on this issue, comparing it to an adult situation in which an advance directive may be present:

The way the families respond will be different; their expectations are different because it's a kid; you're always dealing with surrogate decision-makers as opposed to somebody who left, you know, a piece of paper behind that said, 'pull the plug'.

The essential observation here is that many children have not yet reached a level of cognitive development or legal status at which they could speak for themselves regarding goals of care. In this context the surrogate decision-making process, which ideally revolves around determining what the patient would wish for them-selves were they able to make that decision on their own, takes on a more specula-tive light. When coupled with parental lack of experience regarding the types of long-term post-ICU care that children in these situations require, decisions can be made that lead to significant moral distress in intensivists.

This situation is amplified further in situations in which the parents are not themselves of adult age or are of adult age but are cognitively limited and/or have limited adult coping skills. Often in these situations a grandparent or friend of the family is present to offer support and counsel, but cannot themselves formally make the needed clinical decisions on behalf of the child. One participant described a situation in which they were caring for an infant with severe congenital heart disease whose mother was 14:

> I was like, 'I have a 13 year old. How would I explain this?' Because you are always taught to explain things to the parent, not the grandparent; but this girl is like my son's age, and she is having to care for a baby who has, like, very severe…[illness].

This quote illustrates the struggle this intensivist experienced as they tried to explain difficult medical concepts to an individual who has not yet achieved cognitive maturity in an effort to assist them in reaching a decision that only they were legally allowed to make. These familial scenarios represent a unique stressor for paediatric intensivists.

Personal Orientation: The Inner Compass of the Paediatric Intensivist

When asked to describe the makeup of the typical paediatric intensivist as compared to adult colleagues, a number of key perceived differences were raised. As the vast majority of paediatric intensivists are drawn from general paediatrics training programs (a specialty with a current female majority), one participant observed that more intensivists are women than in the adult field [4, 5]. They also noted a generally similar personality type to others in that field; one centred on team orientation and caring attitude:

> Paediatric critical care is different than adult critical care on so many levels. Many more women; and I think that there is a greater sense among the people who go into this field that recognizes teamwork and caring and sharing in a very unique way.

> … like the medicine world… people would be considered to be more blunt… In the paediatric world it's more touchy-feely soft…

In contrast, however, paediatric intensivists also discussed a sense of perceived difference from their paediatric generalist colleagues, mostly attributable to the difficult clinical situations they are often called to address. One participant noted that much of general paediatrics is focused on well child-care and advocacy, whereas the intensivist is focused on only the most ill of cases:

> I think in general, paediatrics isn't… it's a field of advocacy, and 'well-care'. We're trying to get children from birth to adulthood, with a maximal level of wellness. Which is one of the things I love about paediatrics. But that doesn't lend itself … on a one-to-one transla-

tion… into the [paediatric] ICU, where you're not dealing with wellness, we're dealing with the opposite of wellness, and it requires a different way of thinking about things.

When coupled with a personality type that may be more oriented toward the general paediatric thought process, this dichotomy appears to result in a sense of emotional separation, a feeling that the paediatric intensivist lives in a grey space between the world of the wellness-oriented paediatrician and the disease-defeating world of general critical care.

Conclusion

While all intensivists experience an array of stressors, paediatric intensive care intensivists seem to experience a unique subset of these differently. By highlighting and understanding these potential stressors, paediatric intensivists can engage in more informed self-reflection, in turn enabling them to better manage personal burnout and enhance resilience. In addition, knowledge of the differing stressors present in the adult and paediatric domains could be used to assist young intensivists as they explore potential careers [6].

References

1. Gillis J, Loughlan P. Not just small adults: the metaphors of paediatrics. Arch Dis Child. 2007;92(11):946–7.
2. Burns JP, Sellers DE, Meyer EC, Lewis-Newby M, Truog RD. Epidemiology of death in the PICU at five U.S. teaching hospitals*. Crit Care Med. 2014;42(9):2101–8.
3. Capuzzo M, Volta C, Tassinati T, et al. Hospital mortality of adults admitted to Intensive Care Units in hospitals with and without Intermediate Care Units: a multicentre European cohort study. Crit Care. 2014;18(5):551.
4. American Academy of Pediatrics. Percent of AAP members who are women increases from 28%-63% over 30 years. 2017. https://publications.aap.org/aapnews/news/12848. Accessed 25 Feb 2022.
5. American Medical Association. How medical specialties vary by gender. 2015. https://www.ama-assn.org/residents-students/specialty-profiles/how-medical-specialties-vary-gender#:~:text=Based%20on%20key%20findings%2C%20women,Pediatrics%20(about%2075%20percent). Accessed 25 Feb 2022.
6. Dennis D, van Heerden P, Khanna R, Knott C, Zhang S, Calhoun AW. The different challenges in being an adult versus a pediatric intensivist. Crit Care Explor. 2022;4(3):e0654.

Aaron Calhoun is a tenured professor in the Department of Pediatrics, Division of Pediatric Critical Care at the University of Louisville, and is an attending physician in the Just for Kids Critical Care Center at Norton Children's Hospital. He received his MD from Johns Hopkins University School of Medicine in 2001, completed general paediatrics residency at Children's Memorial Hospital/Northwestern University Feinberg School of Medicine in 2004, and completed paediatric critical care fellowship at Children's Hospital of Boston/Harvard School of Medicine in

2007. Dr Calhoun is the Associate Division Chief of Pediatric Critical Care and has numerous publications in the field of simulation and medical education.

Efrat Orenbuch-Harroch completed her training in internal medicine, intensive care, and infectious diseases and works as an intensivist at the medical intensive care unit and as infectious diseases consultant at Hadassah Hebrew University Medical Center, Jerusalem, Israel. She is currently doing a clinical fellowship in transplant infectious diseases at the University of Alberta hospital in Edmonton, Canada, and plans to combine the knowledge she acquired in order to provide accurate care to transplant patients in the intensive care unit.

Chapter 7
And Then, a Pandemic

Christopher Danbury ⓘ **and Peter Vernon van Heerden** ⓘ

Be safe, be smart, be kind

—*Tedros Adhanom Ghebreyesus, WHO Director General*

Introduction

In medicine we declare a disaster when the number of casualties or cases exceeds the available resources to deal with them [1]. This may be a sudden emergency, such as a bomb blast, or a more gradual, but nonetheless devastating, emergency such as we have all recently experienced with surges of viral COVID-19 pneumonitis caused by the SARS-Cov-2 virus. Health administrators routinely plan for acute surges in critically ill cases as may occur after a sudden natural event or terrorist attack. Such an occurrence may temporarily overwhelm the healthcare system, but it is soon over—usually in a few days.

We have much less practice in planning for and dealing with a situation where medical resources are inundated and indeed overwhelmed for a long time (weeks, months and years). This chapter will address some aspects of dealing with limited

C. Danbury (✉)
University Hospital Southampton, Southampton, UK

University of Southampton, Southampton, UK

Kings College London, London, UK

University of Reading, Reading, UK
e-mail: chris.danbury@nhs.net

P. V. van Heerden
Department of Anesthesiology, Critical Care and Pain, Hadassah University Medical Center, Jerusalem, Israel

resources during a prolonged assault on intensive care services, with special reference to how these services coped in the UK and in Israel.

Intensive care units have expertise in adaptive capacity and iterative system improvement practice in everyday work. The challenge for sustaining adaptive capacity in sociotechnical healthcare systems and continuous system redesign is an over-arching thread of the COVID-19 pandemic response. It can be seen from other chapters in this text how this might overlay "everyday intensive care work" and how teams of intensivists would handle this combined public health and critical care disaster with a "broader-than-normal" group of collaborators.

Going with the Flow

In any healthcare system, it is true that no amount of planning will foresee all eventualities. We have all learnt that we need to heed warnings and to be flexible in the response to the perceived load of cases expected. The warning period may be short (from minutes to a few hours) in the event of a bomb blast. It may also be longer, as we have seen during the COVID-19 pandemic, when we were able to see what was happening in the rest of the world and plan accordingly.

We all heard about the cases of a new form of viral pneumonitis appearing in Wuhan, China, months before the appearance of the first cases in our own countries. During the subsequent pandemic, the healthcare system needed to accommodate for increasing and decreasing morbidity, as surges came and went and thus be able to expand and reduce resources as required. This lesson was learned 100 years ago with the so-called "Spanish flu" pandemic. Several waves of the virus affected the global population over the course of a few years. The speed at which the waves/surges appeared was affected by the slower modes of transport in that era (boat and train) versus the rapid spread of the SARS-CoV-2 virus by today's widely accessible air travel.

Although in the recent COVID-19 pandemic we all had weeks to prepare for what was to come, what we didn't know was the scale of what we would have to deal with, especially during the first wave of the pandemic in Spring 2020. Thus, the healthcare system had to be adaptive, able to "go with the flow" [2, 3]. We may have planned to receive thousands of ventilated patients in our ICUs and only received tens or hundreds, or vice versa. The uncertainty about the nature of the disease and the expected numbers of patients had profound consequences, such as a "run" on mechanical ventilators around the world.

Suppliers and logistics teams were not able to meet the demand, and factories were re-purposed for the manufacture of these devices in several countries [4]. Within hospitals, there was anxiety both in departments expecting to receive patients with COVID-19 and those who were not expecting to manage such patients. The communication of plans from a strategic (international and national) and local level made a huge difference to the confidence of clinicians waiting to receive patients with COVID-19.

Distributive Justice, Information and Difficult Decision-Making in Continuing Societal Resource Limitation

To provide for all the new cases presenting during the pandemic, we had to rapidly develop a just and fair system for distribution of limited resources, as well as ways to limit damage to the population and the economy at large—triage and public health measures. This was carried out at all levels.

Nationally, there had to be a decision to limit the spread of the disease with a system of lockdowns and curfews balanced against keeping businesses open and the economy active [5]. Strict lockdown measures had severe economic consequences in most countries, but especially in countries where citizens work as day labourers and depend on their daily income to feed their families [6]. In some countries, this process became politicized, with demonstrations against lockdown measures [7].

Politicians also had to deal with issues such as border closures, whom to let into the country and how to deal with new arrivals, such as the location and duration of quarantine. This led to many heartbreaking stories of people not able to attend happy (e.g. weddings) or sad (e.g. funerals) occasions of family members. Countries, such as Australia, New Zealand, Singapore and South Korea, who were successful in reducing patient numbers placed their resources into strict lockdowns, limiting entry to the country and extensive "test and trace" procedures.

All of these measures required resources or had an economic cost, but resulted in less burden on the healthcare system and less lives lost, these all being economic upsides of this approach. Time has shown that the low burden of disease due to these measures resulted in complacency in some of the countries and increased resistance to vaccination. As the borders opened up, there was a predictable surge in cases.

In the health economy, decisions had to be made as to whether to try to continue work other than that which was COVID-19 related. In the UK, most elective operating ceased, and in high-stress areas of the country, operating rooms, recovery rooms and general wards were converted into extensions of the intensive care unit. This has had the predictable impact of extending waiting times for elective surgery, with 6,725,633 people waiting for surgery in June 2022. Over 355,000 have been waiting in excess of a year in the UK.

Other countries took a different approach and favoured keeping the general economy going at the expense of a greater burden on the healthcare system and subsequent greater loss of life. The USA and Brazil are examples of this approach.

Nationalism in the management of resources was an unwelcome by-product of resource limitation. Examples of this were wealthier nation states paying a premium for medical equipment, such as mechanical ventilators, personal protection equipment (PPE) and vaccines, at the expense of poorer countries. There were also instances of altruism such as the transfer of cases between France and Germany and other European countries to spread the burden at the height of the pandemic.

Internationally, resources were mobilized for the rapid development of vaccines and treatments for COVID-19, for the benefit of humanity in general.

Regionally, resources had to be allocated appropriately for the care of COVID-19 patients. Not every hospital could, or needed to, receive patients requiring strict barrier isolation and intensive care services. In some countries, hospitals could be set up as COVID-19 hospitals, with the required equipment and staff to receive high numbers of these cases, whilst other services were moved to nearby hospitals [8]. This approach made the logistics of providing oxygen, medications and PPE and essential supplies to fewer locations easier. This also placed a burden on patient transport systems in order to get patients to regional COVID-19 centres from further away.

Sometimes COVID-19 hospitals were set up de novo (e.g. a 1000 bed hospital was constructed in Wuhan, China, in a matter of weeks to deal with COVID-19 cases). Similarly in the UK, Nightingale hospitals were set up. The theoretical advantage of this approach, besides concentrating resources, is the ability to continue providing regular services at "unaffected" hospitals, this being of benefit to the populace (e.g. not cancelling elective surgery or cancer treatment) and providing ongoing income for the institutions, depending on the funding model. In countries where this approach was successful, it reduced the number of secondary victims of the pandemic, i.e. those patients not able to receive urgent, life-saving, treatment for their condition (e.g. cancer, heart disease) because resources had been diverted to treatment of COVID-19 patients.

However, the approach was not universally beneficial. In the UK, there was insufficient equipment to fully equip the Nightingale hospitals to the standard of the existing infrastructure, especially modern ICU ventilators. More importantly, there were insufficient trained critical care staff to provide anywhere near the manpower needed. This approach is estimated by the King's Fund to have cost the UK £530 billion, and it is questionable as to whether this was money well spent.

At the institutional level, resources had to be prioritized to deal with the COVID-19 pandemic. This required "buy-in" from hospital management, divisional re-organization and departmental (intensive care) re-organization and expansion within each institution dealing with COVID-19 patients.

Hospital management had two main priorities: deciding on which services to retain during the pandemic and then providing the resources to expand the intensive care services in the hospital to deal with COVID-19 patients. In healthcare economies such as the UK, the priorities were nominally set by a national body, but implementation left to the institution.

One positive side effect of the pandemic was that intensive care services received the recognition due to them from hospital management, and the general population at large, as being essential to the care of critically ill COVID-19 patients [9]. There were large public shows of appreciation in several countries for intensive care personnel. As an aside, in several places this gratitude turned to blame against the medical establishment as the cause of discomfort due to mask mandates and lockdowns—as if doctors were responsible for the pandemic!

Surge Capacity Through Pre-existing and New Networks

Providing the infrastructure, space, beds and equipment to provide these services was expensive and paid for out of existing funds, diversion of funds from other services or new budgets provided by funding bodies such as state or national funding bodies. In addition, the extension of the infrastructure was temporary, as the extra critical care beds were created out of existing wards, operating rooms and recovery rooms. As each wave of the pandemic passed, these areas had to be returned to their original use at additional cost. Although other specialties were initially very supportive of the need for critical care expansion, they understandably wanted to return to "normal" as quickly as possible, generating internal tensions within institutions.

There were many instances of misuse and misappropriation of these funds, and indeed blatant corruption, around the world in health systems usually chronically underfunded and then suddenly having access to "excess" funds. The UK "Test and Trace" policy is arguably an example of such waste, with the Public Accounts Committee of Parliament saying, ""Unimaginable" cost of Test & Trace failed to deliver central promise of averting another lockdown." The programme cost the taxpayer £37 billion over 2 years.

Hospital management also had to oversee many aspects of the clinical management of COVID-19 patients. In some countries this involved setting up a committee to specifically review changing information from around the world and advise on current and acceptable therapeutic approaches or setting up committees to manage difficult triage decisions. However, this approach was not universal, and many critical care clinicians felt left to make these decisions on their own. This was particularly stressful due to the relentless nature of the pandemic; deciding who to admit and who to refuse admission at 3 am has left a heavy toll on senior clinicians.

Hospitals had trouble finding suppliers and supply chains able to provide essential equipment such as oxygen and mechanical ventilators due to the increased worldwide demand [10]. Some thought about purchases had to consider not only the immediate needs but also "what about the day after" i.e. how the equipment would be utilized in the future after the pandemic had passed. Equipment had to be purchased responsibly and not in a panic. In many instances ICUs had to be set up de novo, or existing ICUs had to be rapidly expanded. This required equipment and manpower. The utilization of oxygen within hospital was also a problem, as the flow rates were sufficiently high to cause freezing of oxygen pipes. In effect hospitals had to work out their maximum possible flow rate with the result that patient flow was dictated by where it was possible to administer oxygen therapy.

"Staff" or "Stuff": Prioritizing and Providing Means for Safe Intensive Care in a Pandemic

A survey of European intensive care units in 2020 (personal communication) showed that once the equipment needs had been satisfied, the major resource missing was trained intensive care nurses. Nurses from areas used to dealing with acute medical cases (such as recovery room and operating room nurses) were drafted in to help with COVID-19 cases. Indeed, nurses with no experience of acute medicine and untrained workers were also drafted in at times. Clearly, they were not initially able to provide the same level of service to the critically ill patients as their intensive care-trained colleagues. It took time for their integration into the intensive care therapeutic teams and for them to become familiar with equipment and procedures.

Often the number of patients cared for by each nurse at any one time was increased (less time per patient, staff exhaustion), and intensive care nurses may have been taken from their regular units to care for COVID-19 patients. This reduced the level of care to non-COVID-19 patients, resulting in so-called "collateral" damage to these patients.

Many hospitals also instituted urgent training schemes (courses and on-the-job training) for non-intensive care nurses, as well as re-hiring nurses who had left or retired from the profession. There was also an increased use of support staff to reduce the workload on nurses, such as student nurses, aides etc. [10]. It became apparent that developing teamwork between new intensive care team members takes time before there is smooth functioning of the team (i.e. all the elements of the team may be in place, but it takes time until the team works well together). One lesson from this is that nursing staff need to be continuously trained and refreshed in their knowledge of critical care, even in non-pandemic times, so that there is a known reservoir of trained nursing staff that can be called upon in times of emergency/disaster. They may be deployed to their usual places of work between refresher courses. However, since the pandemic, it is clear that there has been an increased exodus of trained critical care nurses, and doctors, from the workforce. It is likely that there are now fewer trained critical care nurses available than before the pandemic started. This is a problem which will need to be addressed.

There was also a shortage of intensive care medical personnel during the pandemic. This resulted in longer shifts, more patients per doctor, use of non-specialist doctors and more use of support staff (e.g. medical students). Resident medical staff from all other specialties (e.g. radiology, dermatology, orthopaedics) were required to work in the intensive care units.

Caring for the Carers: Occupational Mental and Physical Injuries

Counselling services for burnout and post-traumatic stress [11] had to be provided for medical and nursing staff. Staff had to cope with a much higher initial death rate amongst patients (e.g. 50% of ventilated COVID-19 patients died, many more than regular intensive care patients), often whilst being exposed to an increased risk of being infected with the virus as well as also witnessing their family, friends and colleagues getting sick or being in isolation. More recently, the mortality from patients critically ill with COVID-19 has reduced and now appears to be similar to the general population of critically ill patients. The mortality from COVID-19 in the first 6 months of 2022 in UK ICU was 23.8%. Therefore, the high initial mortality is most likely to be related to the fact that it was a new disease and that resources were exhausted.

There was a definite evolution of the use of resources at the institutional level during the pandemic. Young working mothers in the medical teams were heavily impacted by the burden of the work as well as having to care for children at home, either in isolation or because of school closures.

Existing ICUs or newly established ICUs were staffed with medical and nursing staff able to care for COVID-19 patients whilst working with full barrier precautions. Working in full personal protective equipment (PPE) gear is challenging for everyone. Working in PPE does not negate attention to usual infection control measures, especially when dealing with invasive procedures such as central line insertion and maintenance and tracheal intubation or tracheostomy. There are many other challenges working with COVID-19 patients, such as communication between the "inside" and "outside" environments of closed COVID-19 intensive care units. Dedicated radio, intercom or telephone systems were needed. Communication with relatives of patients in critical care was particularly hard and for many clinicians the most difficult aspect of the pandemic. Having to call relatives to tell them their loved one was dying or had died and not being able to be in the same room to pass on such dreadful news proved an enormous stressor to healthcare staff. Even when visiting policies were relaxed somewhat, giving bad news whilst in full PPE is very hard.

Clergy, social workers, psychologists and lay volunteers were asked to help deal with the large numbers of critically ill patients and their distressed relatives [12]. These additional human resources all came at an economic cost and sometimes to the detriment of their regular services. Unexpected human resources that had to be found and enrolled in the service of patients affected by the pandemic were additional support services such as laboratory personnel, clerical staff, medical engineering staff to deal with medical equipment, respiratory technicians and others.

Regular polymerase chain reaction COVID-19 (PCR) testing of the staff identified those who were infected or exposed to the virus [13]. This led to sudden absences of many staff members and an increased burden on those left behind.

In some countries medical and nursing staff were rewarded for the extra work engendered by the pandemic, such as in France, but in most other countries, this was not the case. In any event, the knock-on effects of having to "catch up" with normal elective work means that the stress on the system remains, whilst the massive waves of COVID-19 have gone. Healthcare workers feel forgotten as they continue to struggle with a larger than normal workload.

Day-to-day care of patients COVID-19 patients in the ICU is a challenge, requiring more time and patience. Examples are as follows: obtaining specialist consultations takes more time and performing bedside investigations such as echocardiography is more difficult (needing a separate machine or delaying the investigation until the end of the day when the machine could be cleaned and decontaminated).

Care of COVID-19 Patients Outside of the ICU

None of the following groups of patients were anticipated when planning for the pandemic:

- Some patients became sick at home and either couldn't or wouldn't come to the hospital for treatment. Many such patients were cared for by home carers and/or visited by doctors and nurses at home. They also required resources such as oxygen therapy (supplied via cylinder or oxygen concentrator), medications, radiology and laboratory tests [14]. It was estimated that at the height of the pandemic in Israel, there were more than one thousand such patients being cared for at home. The number of patients who never reached hospital because of lack of transport or lack of hospital or intensive care beds in other countries is not known. The excess death rate is a crude measure of deaths probably due to the pandemic but not recorded as such. This was up to several-fold higher in some countries, notably in some South American countries. Anecdotal stories of bodies being washed up on the banks of rivers also support the probability of large numbers of patients dying outside the hospital system.
- Other patients who have recovered from acute COVID-19 required prolonged mechanical ventilation and rehabilitation, either in hospital or in dedicated chronic ventilation institutions. These patients represent an ongoing burden on resources.
- Many patients were treated with extracorporeal membrane oxygenation (ECMO) when all regular treatments failed [15]. This is an extremely resource-intense activity.
- Critically ill patients also clearly require support before admission to the ICU and after discharge from the ICU. This treatment falls to the regular wards in the hospital, be they medical or surgical wards, placing an additional burden on them also.

Triage When Resources Are Limited

When there is no possibility of increasing resources to meet demand, then in extreme cases, the demand has to be reduced to meet the current resources. This is done by instituting a system of triage, where the patients most likely to benefit from intensive care are selected above those with a more limited prognosis [16]. In order to deal with this, many national institutions or peak bodies in the specialty of intensive care drew up triage guidelines for use during the pandemic [17]. There was much debate in the popular press about these guidelines and not to base them on factors such as age or disability. What was not generally available was a mechanism for patients, relatives or clinicians to challenge any of the triage decisions made.

Patient Survivors

Along with other survivors of critical illness, patients who have recovered from COVID-19 are at increased risk of other disease processes. Some authorities consider "long COVID" a form of post-intensive care syndrome or post-sepsis syndrome. If this is correct, then patients with long COVID will be expected to need increased access to healthcare for years to come.

The Burdens Carried by Pandemic-Affected Frontline ICU Staff

Briefly, the intensivists working in the ICU during the COVID-19 pandemic expressed the following emotions:

- Exhaustion, both physical and emotional, at having to deal with many more patients than usual, often in unfamiliar settings and with limited resources. Triaging patients to the limited resources was also emotionally exhausting.
- Despair, at having to see so many patients die, despite their best efforts, and not being able to comfort their families due to the restrictions placed on visitors.
- Fear, of contracting the illness and/or transmitting it to family members at home.
- Anger and frustration, at seeing patients being admitted to the ICU in critical condition, not having adhered to self-protective measures such as social-distancing, hand-washing and mask-wearing and later on not being vaccinated. It was very hard at times to remain empathetic when a patient who had refused vaccination then turned up in extremis and demanding to be treated—and him/her not grasping that there were no effective cures available. These emotions were also hard to control at times in the general public, dealing with all manner of "Internet experts" wanting to tell the intensivist what treatments to use such as hydroxychloroquine and ivermectin—and if only they would use them they could cure the illness and stop making money from selling vaccines, etc.
- Dehumanization (and other signs of burnout), just not caring anymore and doing one's best to get through the shift.

All of the above have taken a heavy toll on intensivists, with many leaving the specialty after the pandemic and retreating to their base specialties such as anaesthesia and internal medicine or leaving medicine altogether.

Conclusion: Remembering and Using What Have We Learnt

Vaccination and the emergence of new anti-viral treatments, as well as increasing herd immunity means that the pandemic is now abating. Because we are human and have essentially short individual and institutional memories, we may be tempted to put the whole pandemic experience down to bad lack and try to "move on". The next pandemic is inevitable [18], and we should take the lessons in continuous preparation for future pandemic and disaster management whilst incorporating ongoing, systematized collaboration between public health and critical care resource allocation. Further qualitative analysis of intensivists' responses to the pandemic and their learnings would be valuable to inform future actions.

References

1. Farmer JC, Carlton PK Jr. Providing critical care during a disaster: the interface between disaster response agencies and hospitals. Crit Care Med. 2006;34(3 Suppl):S56–9.
2. Harris G, Adalja A. ICU preparedness in pandemics: lessons learned from the coronavirus disease-2019 outbreak. Curr Opin Pulm Med. 2021;27(2):73–8.
3. Machi D, Bhattacharya P, Hoops S, Chen J, Mortveit H, Venkatramanan S, et al. Scalable epidemiological workflows to support COVID-19 planning and response. medRxiv. 2021.
4. Iyengar K, Bahl S, Raju V, Vaish A. Challenges and solutions in meeting up the urgent requirement of ventilators for COVID-19 patients. Diabetes Metab Syndr. 2020;14(4):499–501.
5. Alfano V, Ercolano S. The efficacy of lockdown against COVID-19: a cross-country panel analysis. Appl Health Econ Health Policy. 2020;18(4):509–17.
6. Besley T, Stern N. The economics of lockdown. Fisc Stud. 2020;41(3):493–513.
7. Ferraresi M, Kotsogiannis C, Rizzo L, Secomandi R. The 'Great Lockdown' and its determinants. Econ Lett. 2020;197:109628.
8. Adam EH, Flinspach AN, Jankovic R, De Hert S, Zacharowski K. Treating patients across European Union borders: an international survey in light of the coronavirus disease-19 pandemic. Eur J Anaesthesiol. 2021;38(4):344–7.
9. Emanuel EJ, Persad G, Upshur R, Thome B, Parker M, Glickman A, et al. Fair allocation of scarce medical resources in the time of COVID-19. N Engl J Med. 2020;382(21):2049–55.
10. Casafont C, Fabrellas N, Rivera P, Olivé-Ferrer MC, Querol E, Venturas M, Prats J, Cuzco C, Frías CE, Pérez-Ortega S, Zabalegui A. Experiences of nursing students as healthcare aid during the COVID-19 pandemic in Spain: a phemonenological research study. Nurse Educ Today. 2021;97:104711. https://doi.org/10.1016/j.nedt.2020.104711. Epub 2020 Dec 17. PMID: 33418340; PMCID: PMC7744273.
11. Dewey C, Hingle S, Goelz E, Linzer M. Supporting clinicians during the COVID-19 pandemic. Ann Intern Med. 2020;172(11):752–3.
12. Montauk TR, Kuhl EA. COVID-related family separation and trauma in the intensive care unit. Psychol Trauma. 2020;12(S1):S96–s7.
13. Oster Y, Wolf DG, Olshtain-Pops K, Rotstein Z, Schwartz C, Benenson S. Proactive screening approach for SARS-CoV-2 among healthcare workers. Clin Microbiol Infect. 2021;27(1):155–6.
14. Luks AM, Swenson ER. Pulse oximetry for monitoring patients with COVID-19 at home. Potential pitfalls and practical guidance. Ann Am Thorac Soc. 2020;17(9):1040–6.
15. Dreier E, Malfertheiner MV, Dienemann T, Fisser C, Foltan M, Geismann F, et al. ECMO in COVID-19-prolonged therapy needed? A retrospective analysis of outcome and prognostic factors. Perfusion. 2021;36:582.
16. Booke H, Booke M. Medical triage during the COVID-19 pandemic: a medical and ethical burden. J Clin Ethics. 2021;32(1):73–6.

17. Iacorossi L, Fauci AJ, Napoletano A, D'Angelo D, Salomone K, Latina R, et al. Triage protocol for allocation of critical health resources during COVID-19 pandemic and public health
emergencies. A narrative review. Acta Biomed. 2020;91(4):e2020162.
18. Arabi YM, Azoulay E, Al-Dorzi HM, Phua J, Salluh J, Binnie A, et al. How the COVID-19
pandemic will change the future of critical care. Intensive Care Med. 2021;47(3):282–91.

Christopher Danbury   trained in general internal medicine, microbiology, virology and anaesthesia before switching to intensive care medicine. Appointed as a consultant in 2002, his practice
is in general and neuro intensive care medicine. His current clinical base is at University Hospital
Southampton, UK. He has academic roles at the University of Southampton, Kings College
London and the University of Reading. His research interests are in complex decision making
related to serious medical treatment and the interface between law and medicine. He has held
national leadership roles and sat on a number of national guideline development groups.

Peter Vernon van Heerden   qualified as an anaesthetist and intensive care specialist and has
practiced in South Africa, the UK, Australia and Israel. He is the Director of the General Intensive
Care Unit, Dept. of Anesthesiology, Critical Care and Pain Medicine, Faculty of Medicine,
Hadassah Hospital and Hebrew University of Jerusalem, Israel.

Part II:
Winning the Game

Foreword: Understanding the Game

Kenneth Catchpole (iD)

In school we learn that mistakes are bad, and we are punished for making them. Yet, if you look at the way humans are designed to learn, we learn by making mistakes. We learn to walk by falling down. If we never fell down, we would never walk.
  —Robert T. Kiyosaki

In the late 1990s it became increasingly clear that healthcare delivery had a huge problem.

Studies from all over the world reached similar conclusions: that the number of patients harmed accidentally during their care episodes was unacceptably high, and several factorials higher than broadly comparable accident rates in other industries. The traditional ways of looking at performance and outcomes—as a function of the practitioner and the patient—needed to be updated to reflect the influence of the wider systems of work that shape care delivery.

This became known as the "systems approach" to understanding healthcare delivery. Initially framed by the "Swiss Cheese" conceptual model of accident causation [1] which integrated findings from studies of industrial accidents with those of human performance and cognition, this opened the door for the introduction of human factors engineering (HFE) principles into healthcare research and practice. Cemented by seminal reports from the USA, UK, and similar findings across the world, this has driven a profound change in the way in which those working in healthcare have come to understand the nature of the work we do.

HFE (also known as Ergonomics) is defined as *"the scientific discipline concerned with the understanding of interactions among humans and other elements of a system, and the profession that applies theory, principles, data, and methods to design in order to optimize human well-being and overall system performance."* [2]

K. Catchpole
Medical University of South Carolina, Charleston, SC, USA
e-mail: catchpol@musc.edu

This discipline arose initially from a combination of the scientific management principles of Taylor and Gilbreth and the applied cognitive science during the mid-twentieth century. It was applied most notably to aviation in the 1940s and then to an enormous range of industrial processes, consumer products, software designs, and safety perspectives over the following 80 years. The application within healthcare was initially dominated by a desire to understand how healthcare could achieve similar levels of performance, reliability, and safety to those found in other industries, especially aviation.

One of the first applications of this was in the translation of teamwork and Crew Resource Management (CRM) principles from aviation into acute care contexts. Observation and intervention studies of clinical behavior—rather than technical and patient-oriented approaches—showed the importance of these interactions and skills on clinical processes, performance, and outcomes. Substantial investments in simulation facilities and training followed.

However, it has become increasingly clear that while there are some surface similarities, healthcare has its own unique challenges. A focus on human behavior alone belies the deep and often poorly understood influence of context—the tasks, technologies, working environments and organization—on behavior and performance. Meanwhile, making change in complex systems that may never have been engineered remains difficult and often poorly understood.

Leveraging clinical knowledge, design, engineering, and human behavior to create successful, and avoid unsuccessful, patient outcomes requires many more resources and a broader range of perspectives than perhaps was originally understood by anyone.

Healthcare is vastly more complex, adaptive, opaque, and variable than any other industry in which these principles have been applied. Those of us who have made a commitment to introduce and deepen the knowledge, understanding and practice of HFE in healthcare have often faced an uphill battle to overcome the more traditional views of care that are still often dominant. Recently legal cases in the USA, where individuals are still blamed for organizational and design problems, demonstrate how far we have to go.

These chapters are an important contribution to that growth in knowledge and practical applications of systems thinking in general, and HFE in particular within the intensive care setting. They demonstrate the range of theoretical perspectives, professional backgrounds, and practical expertise that can now be brought to bear on these challenging problems, ultimately for the benefit of everyone involved in receiving or delivering healthcare. I hope that this excellent work will achieve the wide audience that it deserves.

References

1. Reason J. Human error: models and management. BMJ. 2000;320:768–70.
2. International Ergonomics Association. Human Factors/Ergonomics (HF/E) The International Ergonomics Association is a global federation of human factors/ergonomics societies, registered as a nonprofit organization in Geneva, Switzerland. | International Ergonomics Association (iea.cc). Retrieved 21 Nov 2022.

Kenneth Catchpole   Professor Catchpole has spent the last 20 years applying human factors principles to improve safety and performance in acute care in UK and US hospitals. He has authored over 130 peer-reviewed journal articles exploring and implementing systems engineering approaches to healthcare improvement and has pioneered embedded clinical human factors practice as a way to spread and apply these principles, working alongside clinicians at the front line of care to understand everyday challenges and address a broad range of reliability, safety, and performance concerns from a human-centered perspective.

Chapter 8
Who's on First?

Carl Horsley ⓘ **and Diane Dennis** ⓘ

> *If everything seems to be going well, you obviously don't know what's going on.*
>
> —*Edward Murphy*

Intensive care operates at the junction of urgency and complexity, where practitioners navigate life-threatening clinical problems in the face of dynamic conditions and high degrees of uncertainty and ambiguity. Within this setting, ICU clinicians must rapidly perceive the changing conditions, create meaning from them, and use this to inform their future actions. This ability to build and maintain "situational awareness" is therefore fraught with difficulties. Identifying when to move quickly and when there is time to pause and consider is one of the most important skills an experienced intensivist can learn:

> *I think situational awareness is particularly important. You can have people getting too stressed and anxious or it can go the other way where people aren't realising that this is a critical time, and we need to crack on.*

As well as perceiving the situation for the individual patient, intensivists also need to build an appreciation of the wider ICU and beyond, understanding the demands and constraints across the system and how these create new pressures and risks:

> *Keeping a situational awareness, if you like, I think it's very important. Not just about a particular patient, but also about the unit itself. Because when it's busy and there are a lot of admissions, other errors and things can occur.*

C. Horsley (✉)
Critical Care Complex, Middlemore Hospital, Auckland, New Zealand
e-mail: Carl.Horsley@cmdhb.org.nz

D. Dennis
Department of Intensive Care and Physiotherapy, Sir Charles Gairdner Hospital, Perth, WA, Australia

D. Dennis et al. (eds.), *Stories from ICU Doctors*,
https://doi.org/10.1007/978-3-031-32401-7_8

Central to these discussions is the idea that in complex and dynamic settings such as ICU, it is the ability of practitioners to recognize changes and respond flexibly that is central to creating high-quality care. Yet, this approach is often at odds with the highly linear and proceduralized approaches that may be imposed on some of the team:

> *Nurses are very protocol driven and that's regardless of the situation, whereas medical staff should be, and are expected to be, aware of special circumstances of a particular situation which might change the way things should be done.*

This chapter explores what intensivists tell us about navigating these dynamic realities and what this in turn tells us about how they see their role and that of the wider ICU team.

What Is "Situational Awareness"?

Despite the ubiquitous use of "situational awareness" (SA), it remains a contested concept in human factors research, and the understanding of it has evolved over the last 30 years [1]. SA provides a description of problem-solving in complex environments and the way practitioners perceive relevant information, interpret the meaning of this information as it relates to their tasks and goals, and anticipate likely consequences, so as to respond appropriately to the dynamic demands they face [2, 3]. Crucially, it is not only making sense of the situation, but projecting the next steps for patient care. Moving from "where we are now?" to "where will we be in 10 min, or 3 hours, or 12 hours from now?"

> *If you have some critically-ill patient, and you are not really thinking through the next steps, you know, what else you need to do in that situation, like call Blood Bank, get the surgeon to come in, all those other things, then you miss the time-critical steps that are important in critical incidents.*

Early research focused on SA as a cognitive phenomenon, that is, something that resides "in the heads" of individuals. Testing of an individual's SA was built on tacit assumptions that there was some "ground-truth" available to be known and that "good SA" could be determined by reference to expert or normative performance standards [3]. This normative model of SA is at that heart of discussions of "losing" or "lacking" SA whereby a retrospective judgement is made of what staff "ought to have known."

This commonly held view of SA was highlighted in the intensivist interviews, with descriptions of other services or more junior ICU staff as having a mistaken sense of the "true situation," as judged by the intensivist.:

> *I would say the lack of situational awareness is what I probably see often playing a role in patient decompensation, and adverse patient events. So, we had a situation not too long ago… The physician team who was managing the patient were 'General paediatric resident [doctors]', who were rotating on the hospital medicine service; and I think that they maybe did not recognise the risk of this patient having a problem… there was not a recognition of*

the fact that her pain which required escalating doses of narcotic medicine, was an indica-
tor of something very bad.

However, retrospective judgements of inadequate SA can quickly become circular: "Why was there a bad outcome? Because they lost situational awareness. How do we know they lost situational awareness? Because there was a bad outcome" [3]. Additionally, normative approaches to SA may be mismatched to the ambiguous and dynamic realities of ICU work.

An alternative and potentially more relevant approach describes SA as *adaptive, externally directed consciousness* [4], examining not only "what is in the head" but how this relates to the task environment and context; that is, "what the head is in." This approach acknowledges that clinicians *actively seek* information based on their knowledge, experience, tasks, goals, role, and context. Differences in these factors create varying perspectives of a situation:

> *I've had situations where I get a phone call, particularly in an outlying facility - and I understand; I see critically-ill children for a living, and I see them every day that I am on clinical service, and so what I deem to be 'on death's doorstep' and what a community paediatrician or emergency physician in a community hospital that sees a dozen critically-ill kids in a year... is very different. They may say, 'This kid looks terrible' and by the time they get to me, they are happy and laughing and really don't need to be in the ICU; but for them, it's sick...*

This view also sees SA as a *dynamic cycle of perception and action* used to develop deeper understanding about the situation. Perceptions inform the actions taken, and the effects of these actions inform further understanding. This approach will be familiar to intensivists who use it to navigate ambiguous and dynamic clinical problems, remaining open to an evolving understanding of the situation:

> *I do think that people that have high EQ [Emotional Quotient] have a gift that way and can appreciate things in a very different way. I think what's more common in our practice here is... people 'bucket' a diagnosis. So, they build a differential that's very narrow, based on a premature assessment of a condition. And will base their decision on interpretations that other people have had... it's just, being open to questioning what you see.*

What About Team Situational Awareness?

ICU care is always delivered by multidisciplinary teams who work together to meet the complex needs of critically unwell patients. The ability to build a shared understanding of the priorities and relevant issues is at the heart of effective support.

Given the multiple competing demands in ICU, it is not possible for team members to attend to all the information available, and teams instead rely on the organization and division of "cognitive labor" to keep track of evolving situations and inform the actions needed:

> *In ICU, you know, if you are taking care of 15 to 20 patients, you obviously, as one person, I'm not at everyone's bedside all day and you rely on a series of other people to be your eyes and ears about changes in the patient status. That starts with the bedside nurse. And I think*

that we rely a lot on their ability to recognise that things are changing or that something worrisome is happening.

As discussed earlier, team members experience a situation in different ways as defined by their own personal experience, goals, roles, tasks, training, mental schema, and so on [1]. Therefore, rather than having a singular SA, teams use communication to develop *compatible* awareness that allows them to coordinate their activities and understand each other's actions. Without this mutual awareness, the team is unable to coordinate their actions effectively:

I was the senior on-call this past weekend. There was one patient that worried me. I did not understand the story and I asked to see a blood smear. I was worried that she was developing TTP. I asked the one [doctor] that was on call in the unit to see the blood smear as soon as possible. It took a while to receive it from the lab. She didn't understand how urgent it was. And so, I called her several times. I was busy. I called again in the late evening. I explained it was extremely important and that I needed it as soon as possible because it may be crucial for the patient. Eventually she didn't have TTP, but it took about eight hours until she saw the smear and she didn't understand the significance of this smear although I tried to explain. So, I think it was that she didn't understand the situation that well.

It is notable in the interviews that examples of poor team SA were often focused on the inability of other services to see what seemed obvious to the ICU team:

And so by the time the rapid response team was called, her symptoms… she was actually still stable in terms of her vital signs, but our Fellow recognised the situation, made recommendations; and then left the room, because the patient's vital signs were stable, expecting that until she was transferred to the ICU that the recommendations would be pursued, and there wasn't a recognition of the fact that this patient was really high risk by the staff that were left to care for her. So, the recommendations were not pursued in an urgent fashion; and unfortunately, by the time the Fellow returned to the bedside, the patient had decompensated, and was in completely uncompensated haemorrhagic shock, and she was not able to be resuscitated.

This highlights how the differentiated backgrounds of the members of teams can create different needs for "transactions in awareness" [1]. Within the ICU team, similar backgrounds mean less coordination activity may be needed, whereas with more divergent teams, there is a greater need for communication to build compatible SA.

Towards Distributed SA

More recent research has gone further, embracing a view of SA as an *emergent property of collaborative systems*. There is a *distributed SA,* formed in the interactions between different parts of the system including not only people but the tools, technology, and culture within the system. It is only by examining the system as a whole that we can understand how SA emerges.

For intensivists, this ICU system is comprised of the intensive care (attending) team but also elements such as technology (monitors, information and communication technology systems, equipment) and artifacts (ICU charts, care plans, etc.). When these elements change, the distributed SA changes too, creating new challenges:

> So, if you have a deteriorating patient on the ward, you have to be aware of the shortcomings of the ward. You know, equipment, interpersonal... You know, other people's teamwork, all those different things... you have to actually be aware that you are in a different situation and adapt to that situation. So often you have a deteriorating patient and people are asking for things that would be normal in the ICU that are not normal on the ward.

This modern view of SA aligns with the idea of the ICU as a complex adaptive sociotechnical system made up of people and technologies. As ICUs incorporate more and more advanced technology, the ergonomic relationships and interactions between these system "agents," both human and technological, will become increasingly important.

How Intensivists Build Situational Awareness

The interviews highlighted some practical ways in which intensivists try to build SA, both for themselves and for the wider ICU team. Rather than concrete rules, these represent reflections from experienced practitioners, sharing the lessons learnt over time.

Intensivists Actively Seek Information and Learn to Recognize Patterns

The interviews highlighted that experienced intensivists are not passive recipients of information, but instead actively seek information that helps to build a richer understanding of the situation. Their experiences and knowledge create a particular perspective attuned to recognizing familiar patterns of critical illness and "what matters" in any given situation:

> I have seen multiple other examples of that where I think under-appreciation of acuity or 'tunnel vision' related to what was told and failure to think beyond the information or diagnoses. 'Tunnel vision' if you will... For the purposes of this discussion, I am typically recalling situations where, as an intensivist, I have looked at a Fellow, or I've got information from say, another consulting specialist doctor, somebody referring me a patient from this or another Emergency Department outside of here, where their look at the situation was clearly different than what I saw when I laid eyes on the patient.

Intensivists Understand the Uncertain and Dynamic Nature of the Work

Given the inherent ambiguity and urgency of the work, intensivists must often act with an incomplete understanding of the problem. This means they must constantly reassess not only the patient but also the response to interventions. Building SA is therefore not a single event but an ongoing process.

Given this "judgment in uncertainty," intensivists must also remain open to considering alternative ways to navigate situations and be open to both self-reflection and feedback from peers:

> And so that feedback is part of the teaching process and helping trainees better understand when they have underappreciated something or missed something, for lack of a better word...I think some of that happens within the group who are intensivists as well. That we get to sign out, and someone says, 'Hey, had you thought about A, B, or C?' and it's like, 'Huh, that's a good [idea]...', you know?

Intensivists Actively Build Distributed Situational Awareness

Despite being leaders in the ICU, intensivists recognize that they are dependent on the rest of the ICU team to build effective SA of both the individual patient and the wider unit:

> If you are not aware that there is a problem, you are not aware of whatever else is going on, then that leads to difficulties with communication, lack of teamwork, and those sorts of things.

This means that they must invest the time needed to build compatible SA within the team, through events that allow the exchange of perspectives such as team huddles. By doing so, the team is better able to recognize and respond effectively to evolving situations:

> ...Sometimes the very skilled or experienced nurses will just jump up and take it further, but that there is that reliance on that person at the bedside to recognise what's happening and if they are inexperienced and they think, like their gut says somethings wrong so they call someone, but that person doesn't recognise that that is a serious change and then it doesn't go any further and that person at the bedside doesn't know to be dissatisfied with that first response.

It is also clear that SA is dependent on the free flow of information throughout the team. It is part of the intensivists role to maintain a social climate where people feel they can contribute to building SA. This requires inclusive approaches that invite and value contribution from the team, rather than projecting judgment or blame:

> So, although we think we can stand at the end of the bed and have a broad view over how things are going, and direct things appropriately, when you start to get an emotional response like being told that you have just killed someone in front of 20 other people, I think your situational awareness narrows, and that can lead to poor performance.

Training for SA

Once we abandon the idea of "good SA" being an intrinsic capacity of individuals, we can explore potential ways to develop expertise in building SA. From the above, we can see that experience is key to making visible the patterns of ICU illness and deterioration. This may be enhanced by intensivists making explicit the way they perceive situations and what they see as important:

> I think situational awareness is a difficult thing to train. And I think it's dynamic. You don't have people who have good situational awareness all of the time. I think that that probably plays a part. I don't know that it is directly actionable on, in terms of a way to fix lack of situational awareness. I don't know if you can make situational awareness better, other than repeated exposure and training.

Additionally, a collaborative style of leadership and communication is central to enhancing team SA. Experiential training through simulation may offer important opportunities to develop pattern recognition, reflexive learning, and team skills that are at the heart of navigating the conditions of ICU care.

Conclusion

Modern ideas of SA are well matched to the realities of ICU. Rather than just being about "what is in the head" of individuals, we come to see a rich applicable and adaptive concept. This has implications for not only how we think about ICU work but also how we design our systems to function together in providing care for those who need us.

References

1. Stanton NA, Salmon PM, Walker GH, Salas E, Hancock PA. State-of-science: situation awareness in individuals, teams and systems. Ergonomics. 2017;60(4):449–66.
2. Endsley MR. Toward a theory of situation awareness in dynamic systems. Hum Factors. 1995;37(1):32–64. https://doi.org/10.1518/001872095779049543.
3. Flach JM. Situation awareness: proceed with caution. Hum Factors. 1995;37(1):149–57. https://doi.org/10.1518/001872095779049480.
4. Smith K, Hancock PA. Situation awareness is adaptive, externally directed consciousness. Hum Factors. 1995;37(1):137–48. https://doi.org/10.1518/001872095779049444.

Carl Horsley is a dual trained intensivist currently working in the Critical Care Complex of Middlemore Hospital, Auckland, New Zealand. He is the Clinical Lead for System Safety at the Health Quality and Safety Commission and is leading work to introduce modern safety science approaches into healthcare in New Zealand. Dr Horsley also recently completed his MSc in Human Factors and System Safety at Lund University, Sweden, with a thesis focused on the sociology of safety.

Diane Dennis has been employed as a researcher in the ICU setting since 2008, with an interest in simulation and human factors in the safe delivery of healthcare services. She has been exploring the well-being of medical staff in the specialty since 2018. With a background in clinical training as a physiotherapist, she has taught as Co-Lead of Simulation and Senior Lecturer at Curtin University and is currently acting as Deputy Head of the Physiotherapy Department at Sir Charles Gairdner Hospital in Perth, Western Australia.

Chapter 9
Knowing the Play

Diane Dennis (iD), **Carl Horsley** (iD), **and Eduardo Salas**

> *None of us, including me, ever do great things. But we can all do small things, with great love, and together we can do something wonderful.*
>
> *—Mother Teresa*

Healthcare is a team sport, and teamwork matters in healthcare, especially in the ICU. Research investigating the contributing, causative and preventative factors for adverse events has shown that team performance is imperative in providing safe patient care [1]. In the ICU, patient outcomes are critically dependent on effective and timely intervention by a coordinated interprofessional and sometimes interdisciplinary team working together, drawing on individual expertise, to deliver care. The form and function of ICU interprofessional teams is not well studied [2], and some doctors reported entering the field somehow expecting that their decisions would be regarded as omniscient:

> *During my training I think [I was] taught… You made it into med school, you made it to being an MD… You're the decision-maker; because of your intelligence, you're going to save lives. And you don't really get the… It is truly a team.*

This may in part be because as healthcare professionals, despite caring as part of a team, we train largely as individuals. With experience, these same doctors

D. Dennis (✉)
Department of Intensive Care and Physiotherapy, Sir Charles Gairdner Hospital,
Perth, WA, Australia
e-mail: Diane.Dennis@health.wa.gov.au

C. Horsley
Critical Care Complex, Middlemore Hospital, Auckland, New Zealand

E. Salas
Department of Psychological Sciences, Rice University, Houston, TX, USA

D. Dennis et al. (eds.), *Stories from ICU Doctors*,
https://doi.org/10.1007/978-3-031-32401-7_9

75

discovered this not to be true, and appreciated the value of a well-coordinated team who worked well together—especially when lives depended on it:

If you like it in intensive care, you have to like to be part of a team; you can't want to be a person who does it on their own. If you have a plastic surgery technique that can fix a cleft lip better than anyone else, the team has a different function, but you're doing the magical part of that procedure. Anaesthesia does their thing, and all that sort of stuff, but in the intensive care unit, I can have the best ideas in the world, it doesn't matter, because I'm not running the ventilator. I need to be able to communicate with my team and help the team on the ventilator understand what we're doing, and what we need to look for...

Modern ICUs sit at the confluence of three major trends in healthcare: *increasing knowledge, specialisation and interdependence. Knowledge expansion* is accelerating and is beyond the ability the absorption of any one individual. This drives *specialisation*, whereby healthcare practitioners develop deep knowledge and expertise within a specific scope. Expanded specialisation leads to increasing *interdependence,* with teams collaborating to bring together and integrate their fragmented expertise:

Rounds are a team sport, and academic medicine is only fun if we do this altogether. If I wanted to have it done with brevity and efficiency, I would round without any of you because I could get done in 30 minutes. So that we have a responsibility to make each other the best we can be, and that's a really important piece, because if you can get a team to believe that we are only good together and that one person doesn't shine, then that takes care of a lot of the classic human factors that contribute to error. So, for me, teamwork is probably the most important...

Diverse perspectives are therefore necessary to deal with the complex demands of intensive care medicine. However these different perspectives can also create barriers to working collaboratively. Different professional values and traditions, as well as differences in approaches and actions, may lead to misunderstandings or incompatible perspectives.

A further challenge arises from the lack of temporal stability, a common feature of teams within ICU [2]. There is constant organisational fluidity around the staff and, therefore, the level of expertise and clinical acumen among the team that assemble at any one particular time. This fluidity creates challenges to promote robust and precise shared understanding (i.e. shared mental modes) of patient care. Furthermore, it can be difficult to build a sense of "mutual trust" when the team composition and expertise is changing. A pragmatic step to ensure a more consistent level of skillsets or competencies was described:

What I need to do is come up with a team that has the same competency value every day. And that may be having me as the more senior person, and I actually may not be the most competent person, the senior Fellow may be the most competent person on the team, but it doesn't make any sense to have all your senior people on Monday night and all your junior people on Tuesday night because then in fact you don't have the same standard of care. And that's just something that has been really important to me since the day I started in medicine. So it wasn't that there was something I observed, it's just always been my practice to be multidisciplinary and interprofessional.

The size and intra-group communication of the multidisciplinary team reviewing patients on ward rounds can present other challenges. There may be miscommunication when things are not heard, or when there is waning attention or distraction. All of these need careful consideration, including an appreciation of individual coping strategies—efficient, robust handoffs are imperative:

> *The other thing that is challenging and stressful... we have a big team that's interprofessional. We have residents, but we also have pharmacy, respiratory therapists, that's one of the things I love about the PICU... I try to position myself in one spot and have like a semi-circle of the team and the parents here... but then what inevitably happens is that some specialist comes in over here, somebody from the team breaks off, or somebody else gets pulled, and I feel like there are times when all this like background noise going around, I'm sort of like, you know what, 'Be quiet, can we just focus?'*

Teamwork is a set of interrelated competencies [3]. Essentially, teamwork refers to the knowledge, behaviour, skills, and attitudes that team members need to navigate and perform when task interdependency is high, as in the ICU. At its core, teamwork requires mutual performance monitoring (i.e. team awareness of their surroundings), supportive behaviours (i.e. back-up), efficient information exchange protocols (i.e. the clarity and timeliness of the information exchange) and team leadership [4]. There are also some emerging processes—psychological safety (i.e. "license to speak up"), shared mental models, and a need for adaptive or flexible behaviours. These dynamic, moment-to-moment (emergent) processes arise as coordination, and cooperation demands are required to complete team goals.

In terms of measuring the effectiveness of teamwork in healthcare, the most important metrics are things like morbidity and mortality rates. In the ICU setting, the goals of care include, but are not limited to, improving these factors. For example, an important additional objective is to manage end-of-life care, and the coordination of the team to enact this role well is difficult to articulate and measure. Added to this is the complexity of competing goals of interprofessional teams within the environment. Coordinating the delivery of care is important, with alignment of individual and team tasks needed [5, 6]:

> *Poor teamwork. We definitely see it. Especially when you are an intensivist from a medical background and you deal with a lot of surgical patients. There is the classic ongoing surgeon-intensivist conflict that happen lots of times. Sometimes that actually comes out with patient damage. I have definitely seen that happen where surgeons won't listen to the medical people and then we have to pick up pieces afterwards. The ability for the medical people to tell the surgeon sometimes, that this or that has to be done. To be able to stand up and advocate for the patient, on the other hand, this is where the teamwork comes in - the ability or inability to listen to another voice. We have multiple surgical services and with some of them we work very well and with some of them it doesn't work well at all. The intensivist-surgical 'thing' is a big problem for intensivist burnout. Stuff like not being listened to - people not hearing your voice.*

Improving teamwork was seen as a shared aspiration of most ICU personnel, although specific-team based training was uncommon. We know that well designed and delivered team training can yield good clinical outcomes [7], and opportunities to "play as you train" are needed:

More team-based training would be useful. Currently often we do scenario-based things that are medical-focused or nursing-focused, and increasingly team-based training, is interesting, but it's very speciality focused. So, we do the ECMO team-based training, the cardiothoracic arrest team-based training, but we don't do the standard team-based training for everyday work. So, I think that would be useful.

Intensivists acknowledged appreciation of their team members. Team cohesion (a sense of "teamness", wanting to be part of the team, satisfied with the team), and mutual trust, matters in the ICU. That is, the "feeling" that you can rely on or count on the support, the expertise and the back-up of your teammates is key to effective teamwork and, thus, better care and engagement:

I am everyday grateful for what the people in the team do every day. [It] is extraordinary. There are crazy heroes out there, all the time. So I don't think I could see any of the successes as my own... and in the same way it helps a little bit to realise that when something doesn't go well, that again, you don't live in a vacuum.

Many intensivists recognised the need to spend time with their clinical team outside of work doing things that bonded them together to foster unity and dispel feelings of isolation when things were stressful at the bedside:

We need to do social integration, so we are a team. If I want to emotionally die because my patient died then no, I'm not alone. We are a team. Everybody is in this together.

There was also acknowledgement that challenging times in the ICU bought with them a degree of team bonding through shared experiences—particularly shared adversity. This was seen as a powerful tool to bolster the resilience of the whole team:

So, after it was all over, we all were like, 'Wow. I can't believe that happened.' And knowing that we functioned pretty well as a team... we worked through it and got every kid admitted and every kid survived; you know all those things that... you really want to be able to take care of patients effectively; have enough manpower to do so; push ourselves enough; and even though people say, 'Well that was a lot, should we have done things differently?' Where else were they going to go? This is the only ICU that can handle this in the state, and so you make it work. And so yeah, it did, it kind of... I think it's the war stories that you have from those situations that you remember for years and years... 'Remember that night when this all happened?' So, you develop camaraderie with people from that, which hopefully makes people like what they do. So that was a good outcome, you know in the end. A horrible thing that happened to those children, however we worked really well as a team.

Whether interdisciplinary teams work well together or not, there is always the challenge of demonstrating team unity to patients and families:

So, I will often share with them that I have a reason to believe that something must have happened [intraoperatively]. So, let's say they nicked the renal artery. 'Creatinine is going up; and I'm not so sure why; it's possible that they might have had something intraoperatively happen to the kidney; when your surgeon comes in tomorrow, we'll talk about it together.' I think it's very easy to splinter. And I also think it's really important for the teams to be perceived with unity, for many reasons.

Conclusion

A team of experts in the ICU does not necessarily make an expert team. Effective teamwork in healthcare does not happen naturally. It requires team training, the adoption of the evidence-based team-based principles (many noted here) that have emerged over the last 40 years the creation of supportive organizational conditions (i.e. leadership that supports, promotes and develops teamwork) and the use of powerful yet simple interventions like debriefing [8]. The complexities in ICU require an infusion of the science (and practice) of teamwork. And that is the challenge and the opportunity in ICU care. The challenge to seek and apply what we know and the opportunity to transform ICU care one team at a time through "learning by doing together".

References

1. Kohn LT, Corrigan JM, Donaldson MS. To err is human: building a safer health system. Washington, DC: National Academy Press; 1999.
2. Ervin JN, Kahn JM, Cohen TR, Weingart LR. Teamwork in the intensive care unit. Am Psychol. 2018;73(4):468–77. https://doi.org/10.1037/amp0000247. PMID: 29792461.
3. Tannenbaum SI, Salas E. Teams that work: the seven drivers of team effectiveness. New York: Oxford University Press; 2021.
4. Salas E, Sims DE, Burke CS. Is there a "big five" in teamwork? Small Group Res. 2005;36:555–99.
5. Østergaard HT, Østergaard D, Lippert A. Implementation of team training in medical education in Denmark. Qual Saf Health Care. 2004;13(Suppl 1):i91–5.
6. Woolf SH, Kuzel AJ, Dovey SM, et al. A string of mistakes: the importance of cascade analysis in describing, counting, and preventing medical errors. Ann Fam Med. 2004;2:317–26.
7. Hughes AM, Gregory ME, Joseph DL, Sonesh SC, Marlow SL, Lacerenza CN, et al. Saving lives: a meta-analysis of team training in healthcare. J Appl Psychol. 2016;101(9):266–304.
8. Reyes DL, Tannenbaum SI, Salas E. Team development: the power of debriefing. People Strategy. 2018;41(2):46–51.

Diane Dennis has been employed as a researcher in the ICU setting since 2008, with an interest in simulation and human factors in the safe delivery of healthcare services. She has been exploring the well-being of medical staff in the specialty since 2018. With a background in clinical training as a physiotherapist, she has taught as Co-Lead of Simulation and Senior Lecturer at Curtin University and is currently acting as Deputy Head of the Physiotherapy Department at Sir Charles Gairdner Hospital in Perth, Western Australia.

Carl Horsley is a dual trained intensivist currently working in the Critical Care Complex of Middlemore Hospital, Auckland, New Zealand. He is also the Clinical Lead for Patient Safety at the Health Quality and Safety Commission and is leading work to introduce modern safety science approaches into healthcare in Aotearoa New Zealand; Dr Horsley recently completed his MSc in Human Factors and System Safety at Lund University, Sweden, with a focus on the sociology of safety.

Eduardo Salas is the Allyn R. & Gladys M. Cline Professor and Chair of the Department of Psychological Sciences at Rice University. A prolific author and active consultant, he has published over 600 articles and chapters and his work has been cited over 120,000 times. He has consulted in a wide range of areas such as healthcare, manufacturing, oil and gas, aviation and aerospace. He is a Past President of the Society for Industrial/Organizational Psychology and the Human Factors & Ergonomics Society and is a fellow in numerous scientific societies. He was awarded the Lifetime Achievement Award from American Psychological Association.

Chapter 10
Calling the Play

Diane Dennis ⓘ, **Carl Horsley** ⓘ, **and Eric Eisenberg** ⓘ

The single biggest problem in communication is the illusion that it has taken place

—*George Bernard Shaw*

As we have learned in the previous chapter, intensive care is a multi-layered, complex environment with a constant flow of people with different roles and specialties, each with different tasks and perspectives, working together to deliver quality healthcare to critically ill people. The environment may be calm or noisy, with emergency situations or delirious patients adding to the commotion, and there are inevitably a range of alarms sounding—coming from monitors, ventilators, and the myriad other technologies that support modern intensive care. There are many modes of communication occurring constantly and often simultaneously—written observations, notes and messages; face-to-face conversations; individuals talking; groups handing over care; telephone exchanges; intercoms; and pagers. There are also the potential issues created by personal protective equipment as well as the barriers arising from providing care in negative-pressure single rooms. Each communication exchange offers the possibility of misunderstanding that may have serious consequences for patients.

D. Dennis (✉)
Department of Intensive Care and Physiotherapy, Sir Charles Gairdner Hospital, Perth, WA, Australia
e-mail: Diane.Dennis@health.wa.gov.au

C. Horsley
Critical Care Complex, Middlemore Hospital, Auckland, New Zealand

E. Eisenberg
College of Arts and Sciences, University of South Florida, Tampa, FL, USA

D. Dennis et al. (eds.), *Stories from ICU Doctors*, https://doi.org/10.1007/978-3-031-32401-7_10

When clinicians and other members of the care team become frustrated, they often cite ineffective communication as the source of their concern. Similarly, when researchers and administrators seek "root causes" of medical errors and adverse patient outcomes, inadequate communication is often to blame. While these conclusions are in some ways understandable, they reflect an undertheorized and overly vague definition of communication that, more often than not, provides little guidance on how to make things better.

There are two fundamental ways in which one can think about communication in the ICU:

1. *Information transmission*, which focuses on how well and how accurately needed information is passed along from those who have it to those who need it to decide.
2. *Social construction*, which emphasizes how individuals use communication to create shared meaning through interaction. Each definitional framework highlights different issues in the environment and suggests different strategies for improvement.

Information Transmission Challenges in the ICU

Some intensivists described situations where there was an overt lack of verbal or written communication that impacted their ability to deliver high-quality care. Examples were given where this happened both within their own team and with groups outside of the ICU:

> The loop is not closed and somebody is talking about, for example, we are asking this specialist "What is the plan?", and he is saying something to one doctor who is telling another doctor, so that the last one understands something else, and nothing has really been written and documented and to check exactly what was the purpose, and at the end, I would say that the origin is different from the endpoint... communication that is passing few people, and is not well documented. It is definitely a source of miscommunication, disinformation and errors at the end.

When information transmission is inadequate, it may impact other human factor domains, to the extent that they are interrelated. Improvement in communication skills and processes will translate to improvement in other areas within the team and patient care. One intensivist said:

> Poor risk management or poor task management all generally result from poor communication or people being unaware of something or not realising that they need to do things a certain way because it hasn't been communicated.

There is also an enormous amount of information that needs to be interpreted, understood, and delivered in prioritised order so as to be relevant and useful for continuing care on a day-to-day basis. In this way, the issue is not only whether what someone chooses to communicate gets to the receiver in a way that they grasp it but *whether they decide it relevant to communicate that information in the first place.* For example, things that will be pertinent for the patient in the long term may not be immediately significant; however, those same things may become relevant during the course of their stay in ICU and must somehow be remembered. During prolonged care this can oftentimes present challenges:

> *Most of the problems occur because people don't talk to one another in the first place, so you don't quite know what's going on or one person does and doesn't pass the information on to another. Or what they deem unimportant maybe actually quite important if you [are] looking at it from a somewhat different perspective.*

> *A lack of critical information available, that may become available in hindsight or was out there, but the individual didn't hear about it, didn't know about it... and I think that that is the background, sometimes, for some of the other potential contributors. You know, maybe there is poor communicating amongst the team and so that the decision-maker isn't aware of a piece of information that somebody else had, but I think, at the moment a decision is made, lack of relevant information that may have changed that course I think is probably the most common experience that I've seen.*

> *Last weekend, one of the specialists told the Fellow something, and I was told in the morning something else. At the end I called the specialist, to ask what exactly he was meaning, because we have different information. I told him, "If you saw the child and decided something, why didn't you pick up the phone and communicate and tell me exactly what you wanted?"*

All of these quotes highlight the fact that handoff communication is never a simple matter. More specifically, effective information transmission requires the sender to understand and anticipate the information needs of the receiver, so that they may share what they need in a fashion that will make sense to them. Organizational theorists call the ability to do this "heedful interrelating" which requires communicators to have a heightened awareness of what others are thinking and acting which can then inform how to best communicate with them. While this mindset informs decisions about transmission, it also applies to social construction (see below), since communication can be improved when considerations of a receiver's role, information needs, and overall state of mind are taken into account.

One of the most common communication errors cited in our interviews were those involved with what was physically written and read, with *illegibility* a frequently contributing factor. The advent of the electronic health record may address some of these concerns, but attention to detail and careful consideration as to the common sense and the broader context of what is written and prescribed was seen to be an important preventative strategy. One intensivist shared how they caught themselves by pausing to reflect on a prescription:

> *I actually copied 10 times the dose because she was receiving a very low dose that did not make any sense to me, but she was a tiny lady and apparently this was the dose... I should have looked better, I think, because the dose did not make any sense. Not the first dose, and not the second dose, so I should have done it more carefully.*

> *We write the chart - handwriting - so not all of the doctors or the residents in the ICU are familiar with the doses. So, because it's handwriting and they copy from day-to-day, it could be that one day it's written... let's say 0.125 of clonidine and the next day it will be 125 - they miss the decimal point...*

I think almost every day, because we are still using written charts there are "almost" events that happen.

Consistent with prior studies [1, 2], transitions of care were seen to be the most vulnerable time-points for communication breakdowns. There were several reasons put forward to explain this: differences in the perceived relevance and importance of the information needing to be conveyed, level of detail required, and fatigue at end of a shift:

There is a lot of stuff that can be missed in that communication from the NICU to the OR to CICU, because people… The thing that is important to me, as the intensivist, when the anaesthesiologist is giving their handoff in the morning - it's not the same. So they may not tell me something that they were told by the NICU because it wasn't an important factor for them. It wasn't something that was going to be important for them to get through the next 12 hours in the operating room. We have tried to create a process where we can communicate these things better from NICU to the ICU, but it's things like that, transitions of care, where things get lost or missed.

So I think what must have happened was that when there was a handoff, the day team - which I was part of - did not… we probably didn't ask the right questions to elicit this information, and neither did the night team offer it to us in a precise way. Rather we just got, 'She was doing okay'. You know, whatever that meant. I don't know how much information the nursing staff got. We weren't present for the nursing handoff so I can't speak to that.

The dangerous period between handover in the afternoon - when everyone is tired - to the evening staff; and then you may be on call or whatever. And that, to me, may be one of the most dangerous periods, for that poor communication…

In sum, the asynchronous and often noisy nature of the intensive care environment and the pervasiveness of shift work can and usually do create serious barriers *to information transmission.* Worse yet, team members may well perceive that they *have* communicated when they have not grasped what was meant. But since they do not know that they actually do not have the correct information, they do not do anything to correct their understanding. From an information transmission perspective, it is absolutely critical that when important information is shared, the sender must not be satisfied until they have checked to see if the receiver has grasped their meaning [3]. Checking for grasping can feel awkward and even onerous in an urgent environment where people are not accustomed to verifying understanding, but once the habit has been created, the benefits are so great that people often report that they can't imagine how they ever failed to do this.

Social Construction Challenges in the ICU

In Chap. 8 when we explored situational awareness, we highlighted the notion that ICU work requires teamwork and that one of the key functions of communication is to create shared situational awareness or a consensus view of reality. Pursuing such a nuanced and agreed upon understanding of "what is happening here" is both critically important and extremely challenging due to the diversity of perspectives that may exist and the many barriers to sharing those diverse views. But teams that pursue dialogue and promote psychological safety across status and professional lines make better clinical decisions [4].

Breakdowns in information transmission may occur in circumstances where personnel do not feel comfortable to speak up to their colleagues when they have an awareness of potential misadventure. It may be that a power differential exists that prevents them from escalating a situation, and this cascades to a mistake or compromised care. Poor outcome may also result when the person to whom concerns were raised does not respond appropriately:

Being satisfied with the response that they [are] getting from the person they escalated it to. And not recognising that they should escalate it more. In general, I think we are all very approachable and very much encourage people to go up the chain anytime, regardless. I think that our culture is such that there is not much fear that would discourage that. But it still... it happens.

The large number of personnel involved in ICU patient care guarantees that there will also be a diversity of viewpoints or frameworks held by individuals and team that see and interpret the clinical picture. These frames may be incongruous with one another and contribute to miscommunication. In addition, what one person sees clearly another may interpret very differently:

I think communication is the hardest thing that we do. And there are so many things that happen, not all of them are adverse clinical events, but things that weren't as ideal as you would hope that they would be. Because of poor communication or just complete lack of communication or, it's always fascinating to me when people don't intuit that they need to communicate something. And I think that as I have been a faculty member, and started supervising Fellows, that has become more apparent to me... that not... it isn't obvious to everyone what needs to be communicated so something that very clearly seems to be obvious to me, isn't necessarily obvious to everyone.

The fact that what is obvious to one member of the team seems unimportant or invisible to others is precisely why developing a shared situational awareness is critical, and why teams that work to do this get a far more complete understanding of what is happening. Intensivists described several strategies to improve shared understanding within the ICU. A frequent approach was to be explicit and prescriptive around the parameters of expected care. This included establishing limits such that deviation from those would be recognised as important by other team members:

I think a lot of people make assumptions about their ability to communicate well. Some of it is not being specific enough. We have, in our minds, we are saying all the right descriptors, all the right words of things that we want to know about, but when we actually say it out loud, I feel like sometimes we lose parts of our ability to communicate well. Because you've said it in your mind, you thought it, and you say it out loud, and then you think, 'Why don't they understand what I'm saying?' and then you think, I left out like a really big piece of this. Another part of it is being explicit when we talk. So that during a code simulation for instance, there's some people who do a lot of non-verbal cues or non-verbal communication. Nodding their heads shaking their heads "Aha" "Nah ha"; things that are more vernacular, that are not specific words. And unless someone is absolutely looking at you, they're not going to see that happen. And when you're in a team that you think is cohesive, you think everybody knows each other, there are still things that are lost in that.

The length and depth of relationships among healthcare team members have in past studies shown to have a counter-intuitive relationship with effective communication. Generally speaking, if a specialist doctor doesn't know well or doesn't think highly of the individual they are engaging with, they will take their opinion with a grain of salt and re-check the facts for themselves (which can sometimes result in a positive change of diagnosis or treatment). If they trust or have a positive and long-standing relationship with someone, they may just adopt their definition of the situation uncritically, which can sometimes be a mistake:

Like if you work with somebody for 10 years, you know their body language. But if you work with somebody for 10 days, you don't really know them well, so you have to be intentional about communicating… and I think that sometimes is lost.

When things don't happen in ICU, very often it is lack of communication… we tell the juniors … "don't believe anybody" because you need to make sure that if the nurse says she has done it, you need to check that whatever the test we wanted sent, was sent. You need to check that it got to the lab. You need to speak to the lab and make sure that they do it. And we do find that when things don't happen in the ICU, that the common denominator in all of this is poor communication. And I have found again and again and again … if you want something done, you better pick up the phone and speak to somebody.

The need to establish a shared mental model of the likely outcomes in any clinically progressive situation was also recognised by intensivists and similarly managed through explicit communication with the team, the patients, and their family. One intensivist outlined their approach in some detail:

I would try to pre-empt all the different things that would happen. So, I would make sure I had all of those different parts so I would say, 'Okay I'm going to intubate. I know that when I intubate potentially there's going to be a vagal response, potentially there's going to be a drop in blood pressure, potentially we're going to need fluids so I'll be the one intubating at this point, but if X, Y and Z happen I want you to do this…' so you kind of pre-plan going into it as to what potentially could happen…

I think the only way you can try to mitigate some of those barriers and challenges is to say, 'I'm gonna be focused on this task but these other things that I think might happen, because of what I'm about to do… this might occur… so if this happens I want you to do this or I want you to do that', so you kind of think through the scenario before and the different potential pathways that you may go down and let the team know if it's this, do that; if this, do that. And then try to get them as ready as they can be.

Another intensivist described trying to create situational awareness by *over-communicating*, which takes extra effort but may be in everyone's best interest:

I decided that I'm going to 'over' communicate… I'm going to make sure that my communication is clear and consistent in just about everything I need to do. And just keep going down that pathway, and just make everything as transparent and informed as we go along, to make sure that there [are] no further opportunities… or to minimise the opportunities, that somebody could have a go at me. So, I guess it's a self-defence mechanism in many ways, but also I think it's in the patient's best interests. That everyone is having a shared model of what's happening…,

A third specialist doctor concluded by saying that the need for explicit and continuous communication is especially important for intensivists who do not have singular control or responsibility for a patient. This example highlights both the challenges associated with shared responsibility for patients and issues with effective transmission associated with multiple receivers:

So you have these patients, you have the 'joint custody' if you like, of these patients, which is fraught in its own ways, sometimes, between yourself and the cardiothoracic team. And if there are no clear goals or understanding or expectations expressed, then deterioration can occur... It may not be said that, "This is the thing I'm worried about", or whatever and then what happens when these slight changes occur, and people are just wondering... And this is one of the problems with a teaching hospital, particularly after hours, is that you have a whole lot of chatter and interaction between junior medical staff, with lack of intensivist involvement directly. Direct communication and a clear understanding, and even the most difficult patient and perhaps even the most difficult cardiothoracic surgeon - it's far easier to deal with them directly, than deal with the chatter and communication and miscommunication in between.

An additional strategy discussed was the value of multidisciplinary team meetings to facilitate shared communication:

We have instituted a weekly multidisciplinary meeting which is specifically designed to have members of all of the teams, so allied health, physio, dietitians, the speech therapists, social workers, as well as the medical and nursing staff. And especially the bedside nurse of the patient that's being discussed, to listen to what all of issues are and so try and avoid that divergence and bring people together and it's generally been extremely successful.

It is difficult to overestimate the value of multidisciplinary dialogue to effective teamwork and quality patient care. The time it takes to have these intentional conversations yields a tremendous return on investment, both in terms of employee engagement and patient outcomes. Unfortunately, those with power are often oblivious to the challenges that others have in speaking up. Research shows that some of the benefits of pursuing multidisciplinary dialogue in a psychologically safe environment are as follows:

- Employee satisfaction with having a meaningful voice in clinical decision-making:

If I go into it "Let's just work through this" and value their opinion, and hopefully they value mine, and we talk it through. I think it works okay.

- A more nuanced understanding of patient history, context, and the various complexities and trade-offs involved in treating a particular individual:

It's not that I don't trust, but I like to get original source information. So, I go back, I review everything, so that I know what's going on myself and try to communicate as early as possible to the family about what's going on. You know, "This is what I think";"I'm worried"; or whatever. Set expectations early on. And even if things have gone wrong, you know, at least early, [I] say, "Look this isn't going as we expected, there's been this...whatever..." - I flag that early. I might not give all the details early, but I flag expectations early. I try to set expectations; I think that's the key to mitigating things is being honest and appropriate.

- The development of a shared mental model that encourages a consistency of action:

We need to understand where the error was and what the event was, so that we can have a collective unified mental model of what the problem is and how to reverse it. If you know what the problem is, then you can devise a solution that's specific to that problem, which is high yield.

• An openness to continuous learning and refreshing that mental model as new perspectives and new data arise:

It's really hard to get angry at somebody for making a decision. I mean, you bring together a team and you hire people, and you trust them to do what is ethically right. And none of us are in that position at the moment as that same person is in. I support them. Very seldom have I ever had to say, 'Psst... I think you made a mistake'. And there are ways to do that, right? Always behind closed doors, you always gripe 'up', you never gripe 'down'; so you never complain to someone who is junior to you about something operational, it doesn't fix things for them. They are allowed to complain about something operational to you, but you come and try and figure out solutions.

I need to be able to communicate with the team that trusts me to listen, and has the right vocabulary to explain to me what happened, so I can figure out how to make it not happen again...

• The encouragement of enterprise-wide thinking that includes all aspects of the patient and provider experience and promotes heedful interrelating:

I try to go through with my junior guys and teach them to be as thorough as they can to make sure that they don't miss something. And that means having a pro forma in their own head... starting with the patient from the top of the head and going down to the heels just working through every single body system and saying with the nurse and with my team, saying "This is what our issues are here; this is how we're dealing with it", so sharing the communication and the same mental model so that everyone is on the same line, but were also going through things in a systematic way so don't miss something.

• The ability to question deeper aspects of the teamwork environment such as issues of asynchronicity, time management, hospital layout and design, and the use of data bases and other electronic resources.

Conclusion

Communication is acknowledged by intensivists as a contributing factor to many of the problems confronting healthcare teams. This chapter has shown how a more precise definition of communication as either information transmission or social construction can lead to better description of the challenges and more actionable paths to improvement.

References

1. Eisenberg E, Murphy A, Sutcliffe K, Wears R, Schenkel S, Perry S, Vanderhoef M. Communication in emergency medicine: implications for patient safety. Commun Monogr. 2005;72(4):390–413.

2. Eisenberg E. The social construction of healthcare teams. In: Nemeth C, editor. Improving healthcare team communication: building on lessons from aviation and aerospace. Hampshire: Ashgate Publishing Ltd; 2008. p. 9–22.
3. Eisenberg EM, Mahar SE. Stop wasting words: leading through conscious communication. Charleston, SC: Advantage Media; 2019.
4. Edmondson AC, Harvey J-F. Cross-boundary teaming for innovation: integrating research on teams and knowledge in organizations. Hum Resour Manag Rev. 2018;28(4):347–60. https://doi.org/10.1016/j.hrmr.2017.03.002.

Diane Dennis has been employed as a researcher in the ICU setting since 2008, with an interest in simulation and human factors in the safe delivery of healthcare services. She has been exploring the well-being of medical staff in the specialty since 2018. With a background in clinical training as a physiotherapist, she has taught as Co-Lead of Simulation and Senior Lecturer at Curtin University and is currently acting as Deputy Head of the Physiotherapy Department at Sir Charles Gairdner Hospital in Perth, Western Australia.

Carl Horsley is a dual trained intensivist currently working in the Critical Care Complex of Middlemore Hospital, Auckland, New Zealand. He is also the Clinical Lead for Patient Safety at the Health Quality and Safety Commission and is leading work to introduce modern safety science approaches into healthcare in Aotearoa New Zealand; Dr Horsley recently completed his MSc in Human Factors and System Safety at Lund University, Sweden, with a focus on the sociology of safety.

Eric Eisenberg is professor of communication and Interim Provost and Executive Vice President of the University of South Florida. Eisenberg graduated Phi Beta Kappa from Rutgers University and received his doctorate in Organizational Communication from Michigan State University. Dr Eisenberg is the author of over 50 articles, chapters, and books on organizational and health communication with his most recent work focused on handoffs and the role of communication in promoting patient safety. Dr Eisenberg is an internationally recognized consultant specializing in the strategic use of communication to shape organizational culture and promote positive organizational change.

Chapter 11
Making the Play

Carl Horsley (ID)**, Diane Dennis** (ID)**, Ragnhild Holgaard** (ID)**,
and Peter Dieckmann** (ID)

> *A leader is one who knows the way, goes the way, and shows
> the way.*
>
> —*John Maxwell*

In the ICU, the role of an intensivist is often seen as that of the leader. A "leader" is a mysterious term, triggering a variety of associations. Are they the expert, who knows it all? Are they the inspirational figure that unites large groups behind a greater cause? Are they the person who organises everything and keeps track of all the different tasks to be done? Or perhaps are they just the boss whose signature is needed?

In the extremely team-oriented environment of the ICU, understanding the nature of leadership is particularly important. The role of leaders and leadership is therefore crucial in how we build functioning teams and effective ICU services, so different points of view are voiced and integrated into clinical decisions. To get a sense of what leadership looks like to intensivists, we explore how they talk about

C. Horsley (✉)
Critical Care Complex, Middlemore Hospital, Auckland, New Zealand
e-mail: Carl.Horsley@cmdhb.org.nz

D. Dennis
Department of Intensive Care and Physiotherapy, Sir Charles Gairdner Hospital,
Perth, WA, Australia

R. Holgaard
Copenhagen Academy of Medical Education and Simulation, University of Copenhagen,
Copenhagen, Denmark

P. Dieckmann
University of Stavanger, Stavanger, Norway

Copenhagen Academy of Medical Education and Simulation, University of Copenhagen,
Copenhagen, Denmark

D. Dennis et al. (eds.), *Stories from ICU Doctors*,
https://doi.org/10.1007/978-3-031-32401-7_11

leadership and combine it with an approach that considers that different situations might require different leadership aspects. As explored in Chap. 9, there is a recognition that the complex needs of intensive care patients can often only be met by bringing together many team members with diverse perspectives and contributions.

> *I do think that a good intensivist has good leadership skills, because like I said, you're running this team. I once took a picture of like my team, because we had some extra medical students, and it was like the residents, and there is the pharmacist and the social worker; sometimes there's like 20 people, it's crazy.*

Establishing Leadership

Intensivists are routinely involved in the treatment of critically unwell patients, both in the ICU and elsewhere in the hospital. Several interviews highlighted how intensivists see one of their key roles as establishing situational leadership of the teams managing these situations:

> *I think it's important for us to take ownership and responsibility for the situation when you walk into the room. You need to gather information fairly quickly and then announce to the room that you are going to lead.*

Where there is an existing leader on scene, the entrance of a more senior intensivist may be a source of hesitation and/or conflict within the team. For example, they may be *informally* perceived to take the leadership role by virtue of their seniority, and this can create uncertainty for the team: who is in charge? The question of who should lead may also be problematic when there are multiple services or specialties involved. Accustomed to assuming their usual leadership role, senior doctors from different specialties who are called to collaborate in managing a crisis might experience difficulties in effectively clarifying roles, responsibilities, and tasks, potentially leading to conflict or ineffective teamwork [1].

> *I think it almost always should be the intensivist [taking leadership]. The problem is, in an out-of-intensive-care-area, when you have a senior registrar and an emergency department Consultant, I think in that scenario, probably the emergency department Consultant is reasonable to run the resus; and then you've got generally a highly skilled ICU fairly advanced trainee who can assist with access and lines, and I think that's probably reasonable. I think in the case where there is an intensivist there, and you have left the emergency department, then an intensivist should run the resus.*

Allocating situational leadership to someone who has arrived late to the situation means they may not be aware of all the relevant issues. Rather than taking over from the incumbent situational leader immediately, intensivists may instead take time to get an overview of the situation before getting caught up in leadership activities. While the impulse to *get going*, to *do something* might feel overwhelming, taking the time to understand the situation may save more time later.

Because the reality is in the unit, there's only a few things that you have to do something about, right now. Everything else you can have at least three seconds to think about it… you could have 10–20 min to think about most things. The only thing you have to do 'right now' is (when there is) a heart rate of zero, which we know exactly what to do for; and you don't even need to think, you go into an algorithm and a protocol. Everything else can have a second.

In some circumstances, intensivists may actively choose not to take on a situational leadership role at all, such as when coaching trainees to develop their own leadership skills. This handing over of leadership also serves to model *active followership* to trainees, showing how the intensivist can contribute as an effective team member without needing to take on the leadership role.

[Followership] shares a lot of the same important communication factors that a good leader can make a good follower as well. I guess that's being able to take direction but also feed-back information appropriately. And most of the time we will be the leaders… But it's also important to teach followership to the team. That is, the nurses, the registrars, the senior registrars, because you want them to be able to do their job without being distracted and being able to feed back when they have completed their job. And sometimes it might be that I will say, you know, we've got good Fellows, so I will say you're going to run this, and you take the leadership and then hopefully I can display some followership and do my bit…

These quotes show how complex the mere "start" of leading can be in the ICU context. This complexity emphasises the need to train the team in how to handle this start of an acute situation and to support this by establishing procedures and agreements between and within departments in a more structured way.

The Conflicted Role of the Intensivist

Intensivists called into a room often bring a level of expertise that was not there before, and it may seem natural that the leadership baton might fall to them. However, the interviews highlighted how this can create tensions with their concurrent role as technical domain experts with specialised knowledge and skills.

If you are in an experience where a patient is deteriorating or coding and there are multiple tasks that need to be done such as placing an endotracheal tube or getting IV access… If you're the most qualified person to do those tasks but you're also trying to lead the code, it can just lead to a compromise in the leadership for a period of time.

Stepping back, keeping an overview, prioritising, and coordinating can still look (and feel) like *doing nothing* to those trained to act in life-threatening situations. This highlights the concept of leadership as a *role* required for team functioning, rather than a *person* with technical expertise or hierarchical authority. This is an important concept, as if the leader is defined solely by being the most senior clinician, then what happens to the leadership role when they are required to engage in a critical task that needs their technical expertise?

Being able to stand back and lead, delegate a task and know that that task will be happening in the background, and then being able to move on rather than going to the trolley and drawing up the drugs yourself, you know like if someone is intubated, going over to… Sometimes you have to, if you are limited by numbers, but in our environment a lot of the time you don't have to be able to do that. As a senior registrar, you're probably always doing the "things" whatever that may be, and taking the next step and allowing others to do those things, you almost feel - sometimes I still feel - you know, you can't get that line in? Like you sort of just want to crack on and get it done [yourself]. But then, that's not necessarily what you're there for.

Leadership may also be questioned when there are conflicting opinions, whereby intensivists are challenged around their legitimacy to make decisions and their power to voice opinion:

We have multiple surgical services and with some of them we work very well and with some of them it doesn't work well at all. The intensivist-surgical thing is a big problem for intensivist burnout. Stuff like not being listened to - people not hearing your voice.

This tension between roles is a reality that is constantly renegotiated during clinical crisis situations. Seeing leadership as a role rather than a person enables the intensivist to take on the role best suited to the needs at that time, including handing over the leadership role if needed. The described social complexity of the role distribution explains why establishing leadership is not just a procedure but is also an interpersonal relationship that needs to consider the different motivations of the parties involved.

What Is the Role of Leadership?

As alluded to in Chapter 9 on teamwork in the ICU, working collaboratively is a hallmark of intensive care medicine. That being said, team members may perceive a significant hierarchy of social status, and this may prevent them from contributing fully due to the *social risk* of being embarrassed or rejected for voicing their opinions. This may lead to self-censoring, particularly in those who perceive themselves as having lower social or professional status [2].

A key role of leadership is therefore about building a shared belief within the team that it is safe for interpersonal risk-taking. This *"psychological safety"* is now recognised as vital to optimal team performance in conditions of uncertainty and high interdependence, such as seen in the ICU [3]. This is what allows the knowledge, creativity, and skills of the whole team to be used effectively.

With high levels of trust, psychological safety and clear team goals, there may be a degree of *distributed leadership* whereby "conjoined individual actions across the team enable shared and complementary leadership" [1]. For example, in a shared crisis, individuals may have specialised skills that enable them to take responsibility for a particular issue or function. A formal leader would typically still have the task of coordinating care and creating the *social climate* that enables the team to function effectively.

I need the nursing staff to understand what we're doing; I need to raise the awareness of the team so that the team can collectively anticipate problems, and then treat them together... By the time I get there, it's all over. I didn't see it. I need to be able to communicate with the team that trusts me to listen, and has the right vocabulary to explain to me what happened, so I can figure out how to make it not happen again...

How then can leaders in the ICU build psychological safety within teams? One important factor is "leader inclusiveness," the words and acts that indicate an *invitation* and *appreciation* for others' contributions [2]. We can now see that what intensivists say and do, at all times, is an important factor in how effectively teams can come together for collaborative work. This extends to how leaders create opportunities for contribution from the team and how they seek and respond to feedback, as well as how they negotiate conflict within the team.

... Try to learn how to see things from other people's perspective; because we are really in the ICU, the team leader; but that does not mean we are the owner of the team; and so to see how other people - whether it's other specialist doctor teams or nursing or respiratory therapists - really trying to stand in their place and see what they're seeing and be more of a cheerleader and not a dictator of the team. I mean clearly putting our part in is important, but I've learned to not take offence when somebody disagrees or says something that you're wondering why, or where did that come from? And being confident in your own... Who you are, if someone disagrees with you, or doesn't really want to do the same plan, to be confident in what you need to be confident in, and be flexible when things can be done in two different ways.

This quote speaks to the reality that although intensivists may see themselves as the leaders of the team, they are in fact *situationally dependent* on those they lead [4]. That is, depending on the situation at hand, the intensivists may be more or less dependent on their team members as they may possess knowledge or expertise at that moment in time that must be appropriately harnessed and utilised. In other words, in the ICU environment, the complex needs of critically unwell patients are beyond the ability of any one individual, no matter how knowledgeable or skilled they may be.

A pretty healthy appreciation that you don't know everything, and that you're going to be wrong some of the time. Because you are definitely in a specialty, we are constantly seeking advice and expertise from other specialties or trying to pull together the expertise of multiple teams. And if you are too convinced that you already know what the right treatment course is, then you are not actually going to benefit from the different expertise that comes through the unit.

Leadership is therefore in part about the ability to unite people in working towards a common goal, drawing out the different expertise in the team and creating a climate that enables everyone to contribute. This speaks again to the importance of the *relational work* required to build high-performing teams and ICU services. It can be easy to underestimate the need for this relational work, especially when faced with competing clinical and administrative demands, yet leadership is built on the repeated everyday interactions we have with those with whom we work.

So, we come to an understanding of leadership that embraces the idea of a multifaceted *activity* that unfolds in an organisational, social, and psychological context.

Leading Beyond the Bedside

The sense of leadership beyond clinical management and well-functioning team-work emphasises the role of intensivists in taking care of the health and well-being of those who work with them.

I really feel at the deepest level that my job as a leader is to take care of the emotional burden of the people who are younger and not to leave them by themselves in the way that I was left by myself.

This side of leadership requires knowledge, skills, an attitude, and dedication for which leaders might need further specific specialised training. Reflective practice with other leaders on their level may be useful in developing leadership practices.

A good leader will be able to deal with the different members of the team. So, for some people, that would be, just having a chat to, "Are you okay?"; other people, that would maybe have a more have a coffee with; other people who.... someone else you might be a bit more concerned about, you might have a formal debriefing process. For that I think [we play] a significant role - a very difficult role, in many cases.

This aspect of leadership also extended to the mentoring and support of others, helping the team grow and reach their potential. Yet, as so eloquently described below, this requires letting go of the view that the team exists to serve the leader to instead embracing the idea that the leader is there to meet the needs of the patient-centred team.

I often say to people when they'll come to me, and I'll say... 'When you grow up, what you want to be?... And once I get a handle on where they want to go, and what they want to do, then we have more fundamental questions about... and we build 'how to get there'. But one of the lessons is that you can't commit to leading a team until you care about the team more than yourself. That if you are still at a stage of your career where moving your own career forward matters more, then you're not ready. And that's not an easy lesson for everybody to hear. It's, 'Are you ready to have your own academic productivity go down?' But how you then take care of everybody also changes; and how you take care of them in their roles.

Part of taking care of the team also involves finding solutions to problems where the solution lies outside the influence of those immediately involved and is instead found in the wider system. The formal leadership role of intensivists may mean they have connections to other parts of the organisation that can solve these wider system issues. Their ability to convince the relevant stakeholders of the severity of the problem and then find solutions relies not only on their formal authority, but also on their ability to navigate the political and relational issues at play within organisations.

The Impacts of Leadership

It is important to acknowledge that many aspects of the leadership role within the ICU may be challenging. While intensivists are trained to lead clinical resuscitations, it is only with time that the wider facets of leadership become apparent. The cumulative impact can be significant as intensivists manage their own sense of responsibility as senior clinicians, while also acknowledging that it is the relational work of leaders that enables the best care to be delivered.

> *Well, there's a multitude of things that are hard. First of all, part of it has nothing to do with medicine. Part of it is the fact that you're the leader on a team and we are a team, but you are kind of where the buck stops in many cases. And managing that is challenging – all the issues related to managing that. Not hurting people's feelings; and interacting with them appropriately; and helping them feel supported; and making sure they're getting education while they're actually taking care of the unit; and how do you interact with someone who does something that you would do differently; and how do you make sure they get the teaching. And how do you make sure they get all of that? And everyone has a personality too and managing all of those personalities. You know, I would say that is probably at least half the challenge of the job, at least. It has nothing to do with medicine.*

Leadership can also be isolating, even lonely, and may create significant demands on intensivists. One approach to staying healthy in unhealthy conditions may be to reflect on the following three aspects of work [5]:

- What sense does my work make (even if it is difficult), and how do I contribute to the benefit of patients, my team, or any other cause that I find valuable?
- How well do I understand the dynamics of the situation? Where are clarifications needed to get a better grasp of the key issues?
- How manageable is the situation? Which parts do I influence over and which are beyond my reach (now)?

Conclusion

In this chapter we discussed different situations relevant to intensive care and how they might pose different challenges to leaders. In intensive care, it is a tricky challenge to find the right balance between a need to act quickly and to be thorough in diagnostic and treatment decisions. We hope that the chapter can contribute to enlarging the search for an effective interpretation of what it means to be a clinical, situational, longitudinal, and systems leader.

References

1. Paquin H, Bank I, Young M, Nguyen LHP, Fisher R, Nugus P. Leadership in crisis situations: merging the interdisciplinary silos. Leadersh Health Serv (Bradf Engl). 2018;31(1):110–28. https://doi.org/10.1108/LHS-02-2017-0010.
2. Nembhard IM, Edmondson AC. Making it safe: the effects of leader inclusiveness and professional status on psychological safety and improvement efforts in health care teams. J Organ Behav. 2006;27(7):941–66. https://doi.org/10.1002/job.413.
3. Edmondson A. Psychological safety and learning behavior in work teams. Adm Sci Q. 1999;44(2):350–83. https://doi.org/10.2307/2666999.

4. Schein EH. Humble inquiry: the gentle art of asking instead of telling. San Francisco: Berrett-Koehler Publishers; 2013.
5. Antonovsky A. The sense of coherence: an historical and future perspective. In: McCubbin HI, Thompson EA, Thompson AI, Fromer JE, editors. Stress, coping, and health in families: sense of coherence and resiliency. Thousand Oaks, CA: Sage Publications; 1998. p. 3–20.

Carl Horsley is a dual trained intensivist currently working in the Critical Care Complex of Middlemore Hospital, Auckland, New Zealand. He is the Clinical Lead for System Safety at the Health Quality and Safety Commission and is leading work to introduce modern safety science approaches into healthcare in New Zealand; Dr Horsley also recently completed his MSc in Human Factors and System Safety at Lund University, Sweden, with a focus on the sociology of safety.

Diane Dennis has been employed as a researcher in the ICU setting since 2008, with an interest in simulation and human factors in the safe delivery of healthcare services. She has been exploring the well-being of medical staff in the specialty since 2018. With a background in clinical training as a physiotherapist, she has taught as Co-Lead of Simulation and Senior Lecturer at Curtin University and is currently acting as Deputy Head of the Physiotherapy Department at Sir Charles Gairdner Hospital in Perth, Western Australia.

Ragnhild Holgaard is a psychologist working in research within the field of cognitive psychology. She is working with education of healthcare professionals at Copenhagen Academy for Medical Education and Simulation in Denmark. Her main focus has been concept formation and adjustment, and how concepts differ between different healthcare professions.

Peter Dieckmann is a work and organisational psychologist, professor of healthcare education and patient safety with the University of Stavanger, Norway; Senior Scientist with the Copenhagen Academy of Medical Education and Simulation, and Assoc. Professor at the University of Copenhagen. He is doing research and development in patient safety, simulation, cognitive and social skills, and innovative teaching concepts.

Part III:
Je ne sais quoi

Foreword: Historically Speaking

Cameron Knott ⓘD

Efficiency is doing things right; Effectiveness is doing the right thing.
—*General Stanley McChrystal*

The specialty of Intensive Care Medicine was started in response to a 1952 poliomyelitis pandemic. In 1953, Dr Björn Ibsen in Copenhagen, Denmark, coordinated the around-the-clock care of overwhelmingly large numbers of patients for artificial mechanical ventilation and holistic coordinated care from the whole hospital healthcare team [1].

These poliomyelitis-affected people, their failing respiratory muscles paralyzed by illness, required continuous and compassionate support to survive. This care was delivered from a highly coordinated team of healthcare students, nurses, doctors and allied health staff who integrated human ingenuity, personal and professional commitment, clinical science and new technologies and devices to solve some of the individual patient and health system problems of a global pandemic virus with a mass paralysis event.

This was the birthplace of the tradition of the committed, innovative, complex sociotechnical environment that is the ICU [2, 3]. The disruption of a pandemic drove science-based and team-based innovation and rapid healthcare system adaptation, which remains a hallmark of the ICU today [4].

By all accounts, Dr Ibsen was a persuasive leader in creating this new way of working in the hospital system. However, leadership cannot function without proactive followership. To harness and reconfigure the whole of the hospital's systems to

C. Knott
Department of Intensive Care, Bendigo Health, Bendigo, Australia

Monash Rural Health Bendigo, Monash University, VIC, Australia

Rural Clinical School, University of Melbourne, Australia

Department of Intensive Care, Austin Health, Heidelberg, Australia
e-mail: cknott@bendigohealth.org.au

provide the right care to the right patient at the right time requires the work of multiple well-coordinated, diverse teams [5]. As the specialization of intensive care medicine spread from the long-term ventilation polio wards in Copenhagen to post-anaesthesia wards near operating theatres, and then to more modern hospital-based and mobile ICUs, the teamwork required remained a key ingredient. Now a 'team of teams' approach is considered normal [6].

The ICU's 'magic' is in the longitudinal and ad hoc inclusion of diverse talented people with well-trained killsets that have been developed to enable contribution to a patient's care plan, whilst simultaneously working toward improving systems of care. This part describes characterizations detected by the researchers from common reported patterns of behaviour and thinking from the participant intensivists.

References

1. Ibsen B. The anaesthetist's viewpoint on the treatment of respiratory complications in poliomyelitis during the epidemic in Copenhagen, 1952. Proc R Soc Med. 1954;47(1):72–5. https://doi.org/10.1177/003591575404700120.
2. Reisner-Sénélar L. The birth of intensive care medicine: Bjorn Ibsen's records. Intensive Care Med. 2011;37(7):1084–86.
3. Wunsch H. The outbreak that invented intensive care. Nature. 2020, last corrected 29 June 2020. https://doi.org/10.1038/d41586-020-01019-y. https://www.nature.com/articles/d41586-020-01019-y. Accessed 14 Nov 2022.
4. Baker AA. Genesis of the College of Intensive Care Medicine of Australia and New Zealand. Anaesth Intensive Care. 2018;46:35–51.
5. Tannenbaum S, Salas E. Teams that work: the seven drivers of team effectiveness. New York: Oxford University Press; 2020.
6. McChrystal S, Silverman D, Collins T, Fussell C. Team of teams: new rules of engagement for a complex world. London: Penguin; 2016. 304p.

Cameron Knott Dr Cameron Knott is an intensive care specialist interested in clinical simulation-based education and person-centered healthcare system redesign aimed at improved workplace inter-professional team performance and healthcare system performance. He is an intensive care specialist in the tertiary Austin Health, Victoria, and the regional Bendigo Hospital, Victoria, Australia. Cameron holds a Master of Clinical Education and is an Honorary Clinical Fellow at the University of Melbourne's Austin Health Clinical School and Honorary Research Fellow at the Health and Biomedical Informatics Centre (HaBIC). Cameron's responsibilities include the Academic Lead of the Clinical Skills and Simulation Centre, Monash Rural Health Bendigo, Austin Health's ICU Education and Simulation portfolio lead, and the Bendigo Health ICU Clinical Performance and Innovation portfolio lead.

Chapter 12
All Things to All People

Aaron Calhoun ⓘ

> *Perfection is not attainable, but if we chase perfection, we can catch excellence.*
>
> —*Vince Lombardi*

As has been described previously, the ICU is a place where information overload is normal, where patient care needs can (and do) change from moment to moment, and where seeming clinical stability can mask imminent physiologic decompensation. Those charged with leading patient care teams in this environment thus require traits that enable them to function within this difficult environment. In this chapter, we review these key traits broadly, as described by the participants in our study.

The first, critical trait is expansive expertise within the field, as well as a plan for the ongoing maintenance of that knowledge base. As one participant stated:

> *[the need for] medical knowledge, is massive. So, understanding the complex diseases that you are treating; having an extremely broad knowledge base; and sort of constantly reading and learning and understanding the new guidelines; and keeping up-to-date on the most relevant literature in your field, is huge.*

The nature of the diseases treated and situations encountered require the mastery of a complex body of knowledge. While this is true for all medical subspecialties, the acuity of the illnesses treated within the ICU environment means that this information must be recalled accurately in short spans of time. This adds to the stressful nature of the environment.

Participants also identified a number of basic attitudes that, in their experience, were core to the experience of being an intensivist.

A. Calhoun (✉)
Division of Critical Care, Department of Pediatrics, University of Louisville
and Norton Children's Medical Group, Louisville, KY, USA
e-mail: aaron.calhoun@louisville.edu

© The Author(s), under exclusive license to Springer Nature
Switzerland AG 2023
D. Dennis et al. (eds.), *Stories from ICU Doctors*,
https://doi.org/10.1007/978-3-031-32401-7_12

> *Driven; reflective; compassionate to the foibles and weaknesses of the human colleagues*
>   *Calm under any situation*
>   *Toughness. We are supposed to be tough*
>   *Self-confidence, [but] not too much self-confidence*
>   *Able to handle stress*
>   *Able to detach a little*
>   *Curious; even a bit playful at times*
>   *Resourceful … Inquisitive and eager to learn*
>   *Comfortable with the skills … comfortable with the acuity … but you're not comfortable*
> *with what's happening*
>   *We're all high achievers; we are all perfectionists*

This is a diverse list, and, at least in some respects, the individual items on it may even seem to contradict one another. For example, consider the characteristics of toughness and reflectivity. The expectation here is that an intensivist is able to look at their own performance and objectively judge whether it is adequate or requires improvement (a sometimes deeply unsettling task), while simultaneously maintaining a detached attitude of confidence. Or consider the need to be both "a bit playful at times" and a "high achiever" or a "perfectionist." In this case, a dynamic balance must be achieved between a more relaxed attitude in some circumstances and a more intense approach in others. These exemplars speak to the inherent tensions present within the intensivist role and the energy required to sustain this pattern of practice over time.

In addition to these internal tensions, the intensivist must also be able to manage external conflict diplomatically. Intensivists must lead interprofessional teams and must interact with multiple differing specialties and provider types. They therefore must possess the communication skills needed both to maintain immediate and longitudinal relationships among these disparate teams and to shape those interactions in a way that advances patient care. As one participant opined:

> *On any given day… I deal with, if I'm on, somewhere around 150 people. I do the ward round; I catch two, sometimes three shifts of nurses, so we're talking about 50 or 60 people; we're talking to the registrars, another 10 or 15 people; then you talk to the surgeons; the physios; the PSA's; all those sorts of people. We're talking more than 100 people. And those people have to feel that I can lead them; I can respond to anything that might go wrong; they have to trust me; and they have to like me.*

Among intensivists, many of the external provider groups are perceived to have competing approaches and agendas even if all are concerned with the welfare of the patient. To direct care in this context, then, requires the navigation of a complex set of social interactions in which multiple needs are dynamically balanced.

Taken together, these observations describe a role in which practitioners must be both aloof and engaged, humble and confident, directive leaders and diplomats, and all in service to the lives of the patients they care for. Like the parasympathetic and sympathetic nervous systems which keep the human organism ready for action by each exerting a constant "pull" on the overall physiology, the ability of the intensivist to respond to the often-chaotic environment in which they practice seems predicated, in these interviews, by the capacity to hold somewhat mutually exclusive roles in ongoing balance. The maintenance of this difficult dynamism requires ongoing effort, placing a significant cognitive load on intensivists.

Above all, the intensivist is expected to effectively and fairly lead the interprofessional team of which they are a part. Without this role, the care that patients ultimately receive will be suboptimal and outcomes will suffer.

> *And if you, as the leader, who is thought of as the leader of the ICU at the time, breaks down, your whole team breaks down, and they all fall apart. So, you have to be the strength; you have to be the pillar; and so everybody can get through it.*

Conclusion

The knowledge base, dynamic tensions, and diplomacy of the intensivist's role are bent toward the ultimate goal of excellence in patient outcomes and patient care. Practicing intensivists see themselves as needing to be all things to all people as the situation, and the dynamically evolving nature of their patients, requires.

Aaron Calhoun is a tenured professor in the Department of Pediatrics, Division of Pediatric Critical Care at the University of Louisville, and is an attending physician in the Just for Kids Critical Care Center at Norton Children's Hospital. He received his MD from Johns Hopkins University School of Medicine in 2001, completed general pediatrics residency at Children's Memorial Hospital/Northwestern University Feinberg School of Medicine in 2004, and completed pediatric critical care fellowship at Children's Hospital of Boston/Harvard School of Medicine in 2007. Dr Calhoun is the Associate Division Chief of Pediatric Critical Care and has numerous publications in the field of simulation and medical education.

Chapter 13
The Looking Glass

Rahul Khanna ⓘ**, Michael Ruppe, Marc Romain** ⓘ**, Caleb Fisher,
Peter Vernon van Heerden** ⓘ**, Bradley Wibrow** ⓘ**, Katherine Potter,
and Nancy Tofil** ⓘ

> *Circumstances do not make the man, they reveal him.*
>
> —*James Allen*

R. Khanna
Department of Psychiatry, Phoenix Australia, University of Melbourne, Melbourne, VIC,
Australia

M. Ruppe · K. Potter
Division of Critical Care, Department of Pediatrics, University of Louisville, and Norton
Children's Medical Group, Louisville, KY, USA

M. Romain
Department of Medical Intensive Care, Hadassah Medical Center, Faculty of Medicine,
Hebrew University of Jerusalem, Jerusalem, Israel

C. Fisher
Department of Intensive Care, Austin Health, Heidelberg, VIC, Australia

Department of Critical Care, The University of Melbourne, Melbourne, VIC, Australia

P. V. van Heerden (✉)
General Intensive Care Unit, Department of Anesthesiology, Critical Care and Pain Medicine,
Hadassah Medical Center, Jerusalem, Israel
e-mail: vernon@hadassah.org.il

B. Wibrow
Department of Intensive Care, Sir Charles Gairdner Hospital, Perth, WA, Australia

N. Tofil
Division of Paediatric Critical Care and Paediatric Simulation Center, Children's of Alabama,
University of Alabama at Birmingham, Birmingham, AL, USA

D. Dennis et al. (eds.), *Stories from ICU Doctors*,
https://doi.org/10.1007/978-3-031-32401-7_13

Introduction

Rahul Khanna

Intensive care medicine is a highly demanding field that requires doctors to wear many different hats. While Chapter 12 described the traits of ICU doctors broadly, in this chapter of the book, we will explore the different personas or roles that intensive care doctors must take on to navigate the complex and often emotionally charged environment of the ICU. These personas emerged organically from our conversations, tying together common (and generally adaptive) personality traits as well as roles thrust upon an intensivist through the expectations of themselves or others. What emerged was a set of sometimes conflicting aspects of an intensivist–some obvious to onlookers and others known only to themselves. "The duck", for example, presents a veneer of necessary calm while paddling furiously under the surface (perhaps balancing "the neurotic" that also resonated with many interviewees). Similarly, though other departments crave the caped "fixer" to rescue them from clinical conundrums, the sensitivities of the situation require the skills of a "diplomat". From "the fixer" who is responsible for stabilising critically ill patients to "the retriever" who must make difficult decisions about life support and "the negotiator" who must navigate the competing interests of patients, families, and other healthcare professionals, the role of the ICU doctor is multifaceted and constantly evolving.

The corollary to these self-perceptions is explored in Chapter 14. These are the personas intensivists believe others attribute to them. The "superhero", "nay-sayer", and "dictator" speak to the complexity of the intensivists' role in a hospital. Though the tools and abilities of the intensivists sometimes enable heroic acts, resource scarcity and clinical futility often require "nay-saying", with the force and sometimes patience of a dictator. No wonder "the Duck" resonates so strongly.

It was also striking how consistent these themes were across borders, genders, and subspecialties. This suggests that certain personality types are drawn to the pursuit of intensive care or that these traits emerge due to the nature of the work. It is likely that both are true to an extent, and an awareness of these traits and tensions can help those who are, work with, or aspire to be intensivists to survive and thrive.

The Retriever

Michael Ruppe

If you can dream it, you can do it. (Walt Disney)

Deep in the murky depths of the trauma bay sits a problem: a limp, ashen baby being eagerly handed off by a panic-stricken mother to anyone in scrubs that would take her. The charge of the emergency response is to stabilise, consider various diagnoses, and expedite a treatment plan and then make the call: "Doctor, we have a really sick baby that I need to tell you about."

It's at that moment that the retriever springs to life.

The intensivist with the "retriever" persona holds the ICU as the cornerstone of the hospital. Their mission is to be a beacon of light to the farthest corners of their world; be it an outlying emergency room 100 miles away or a patient room down the hall. The retriever has no problem putting on their cape, swooping into a room filled with an anxious clinical team and likely an even more anxious patient and family. And as the intensivist swings into action, a small piece of that anxiety melts away. "Phew. The ICU is here."

> *...Because you've got the most likely person that's going to help. I think throughout the hospital, the feeling is that the intensivist is there... Yeah... A sigh of relief, that they're there...*

The retriever intensivist is set up to fall into a trap. It's the unspoken duty of the retriever to carry themselves nonjudgmentally and inclusively. They need to understand how the story has unfolded up to this point. The classic, unintended mistake that the retriever makes is to authoritatively pour out their ICU magic plan. Even that can be met with disdain:

> *And you'll hear other specialist doctors complain 'Oh my gosh, I hate when the intensivists come; they are so unimpressed; they give me all these orders and it doesn't help me manage the patient.*

The retriever has to be mindful of the clinical limitations from which to advise and be conscientious about the tone and inclusivity of their reactions. All too often are these pieces overlooked to the detriment of morale, relationships, and possibly even patient outcomes.

> *We walk in the room and declare, 'Umm, all this patient needs is some oxygen, 2 mg/kg of Lasix, and to be suctioned, like, what's wrong with you people?'...So you have to know that about yourself. You have to recognize that the (the other team) is at the limit of their capacity, whereas you are at the bottom of your capacity. So, then you have to be non-judgmental and welcome.*

Other than providing a higher level of critical care, the retriever intensivist is tasked with avoiding arrogance, judgement, or condescension. The collegiality, respect, and perspective that they carry into those short encounters set the tone for hospital-wide relationships. The social intelligence of the retriever is perpetually on display, for better or for worse.

The retriever thrives on anchoring a hospital and saving the day. They know what "sick" is and what it isn't. They function with an innate ability to filter out the noise and address the most critical issues. They have the backing of their ventilators and vasopressors when needed. They often bring their "friends": the seasoned ICU nurse and allied health team. And then they either propose a plan to treat the patient where they are, or they magically transport this decompensating, terrifying patient to the "Land of the ICU", where a whole new world of possibilities for healing awaits.

The human inside the retriever needs to take caution. If they feed off the power trip, they have free reign to show their arrogance and superiority. Their body language and words spoken and unspoken are on display. Walking into a room inherently in a position of power will all too often have a negative impact on the morale of the whole.

The Negotiator

Marc Romain

> *History is filled with tragic examples of wars that result from diplomatic impasse. Whether in our local communities or in international relations, the skillful use of our communicative capacities to negotiate and resolve differences is the first evidence of human wisdom. (Daisaku Ikeda)*

In order to assist their patients, the intensivist needs to interact with numerous people on a daily basis, including nurses, doctors, support staff, physiotherapists, families, consultants, and many others. Many of these interactions will involve an element of negotiation.

Let's take an example of a common elective procedure like a bedside tracheostomy. The Negotiator needs to explain the procedure to the next of kin so that they understand and accept that the procedure needs to be performed. Once the family is on board, the intensivist needs to negotiate the best timing for the procedure. They need to discuss with the nurse – should the procedure occur before they wash the patient or afterwards? Should it be after the nurse's tea break or before? If the Negotiator works in an academic centre, they may need to negotiate with the junior staff regarding who will do the procedure together with them. Regarding the equipment itself, the Negotiator may need to discuss with the hospital management and agree upon which specific tracheostomy kit should be used and whether the patients require a special tracheostomy that needs to be ordered specifically for them. If the patient has difficult anatomy and a bedside procedure is not possible, then negotiations need to be entered into with the ear nose and throat (ENT) surgeon, anaesthesiologist, and operating room staff:

> *I never say 'no' to anyone, I actually say "Let's talk about it. Let's talk about it." So, I prefer a negotiated settlement where actually… "Okay I'll tell you what, we'll do that, and we'll see how we go, but if it doesn't work out, in the next two hours, I think will do it this way, is that alright?" Or, I find, I think it is a recurrent finding, that I bring them to the bedside and we just say, "Okay this is the issue… what shall we…. " and I find that if you do this, and you don't try to sell your thinking, but you just say, "Let's talk it through", after a while, they agree that they should change the car tyres, or you agree that you shouldn't, and that's okay.*

> *If you go into it "I want to have it my way", but if you go into it as, "Let's just work through this" and I value their opinion, and hopefully they value mine, and we talk it through. I think it works okay. I think it works out all right.*

Being a successful negotiator is one of the most important traits of an intensivist. To negotiate successfully is an art, and it is a skill that needs to be learned.

In the high-stress environment of an ICU, disagreement and conflict are inevitable, and the well-rounded intensivist will need to navigate these conflicts using their negotiation skills – potentially a time and energy-depleting process:

> *...I think you have to be personable in terms of medically. Most intensivists are very personable and good negotiators, and you can't be rigid. When you're a surgeon you can be... Some of them are very rigid. Whereas, if you try to be rigid in this environment, you just wouldn't survive. You'd just get stressed about people not doing what you wanted them to do, and things not going the way you wanted them to be, and I think you can't... That's one of the personality traits that I think is not suitable to be... to do ICU - if you're very rigid and unable to be flexible.*

The well-trained, calm negotiator needs to be able to handle these situations in order to ensure the best possible outcome for the patient.

> *... sometimes it does feel like we spend a lot of emotional energy... not locking horns with people but trying to get people to do what we think is the right thing to do. But it does require a lot of emotional energy, particularly with some of the more... 'pedantic' is not the right... is not a fair word... the more 'micromanaging' style of surgeons. There can be very unnecessary emotional expenditure. I think, to be honest, I think a hard day at work usually involves personal emotional expenditure where I feel it doesn't necessarily... Like when a patient is bleeding to death, they should just go back to theatre. Or you know if a patient needs a particular treatment, and just the to-ing and fro-ing about the negotiation about something like that, that should just happen quickly. Just due to differences or styles of opinion. Yes.*

Negotiation is not always related to conflict. Difficult decisions and treatment options need to be discussed with families in order to respect the wishes of the patient.

> *I love the interactions with families. I had a great one a couple of weeks ago with this old lady with a head injury, and dealing with her relatives and stuff like that and trying to negotiate a path. Having a conversation and trying to find, to me a reasonable and human way to deal with this, and it worked out well, and I got a lovely card from her. That's fantastic you know? That's fantastic. [1]*

The Neurotic

Caleb Fisher

> *The only true wisdom is in knowing you know nothing. (Socrates)*

The neurotic intensivist has a high degree of internal self-talk, self-monitoring, and self-criticism. Often aligned with perfectionistic traits and attention to detail and structure, these experienced internal dialogues, when unearthed for others to see, can provide some insight into the universe of moment-to-moment everyday experiences of the intensivist.

This is demonstrated in a generic introduction to a family such as this, "Hi, I'm the intensivist caring for your loved one. I'm sorry to meet you under these circumstances." The subsequent parts of the initial generic conversation are shown here, with quoted parallel internal self-talk monologue experienced by the neurotic as:

Did I just say sorry, aggh, now they think it is my fault, it is unfortunate that we meet… uggh I need to remind myself that I may be, should be a little bit obsessive, more obsessive about these details. I think I am becoming more obsessive with time, as every tiny detail is important. And barriers, remember barriers.

Come on it's your job, you are the leader. These people are looking to you. You have to give everybody the feeling, even if you don't believe it, that you are in control, that you've got this, don't worry, we are okay. Let's just deal with this. Do I sound like I am the Consultant? Should I be wearing scrubs or formal clothes? Is my name badge on? upside down? God, I have such bad impostor syndrome.

As the neurotic intensivist continues, "Your loved one will get round the clock care by an expert from a range of staff from ICU Consultants, ICU fellows, ICU residents, expert nursing, allied health and pharmacists to cleaners and clerical staff. Each one plays an incredibly important part in ensuring your loved one has the best opportunity to recover".

I am running this team. I am the boss. I think. I took a picture of like my team this morning, because we had some extra medical students, and it was like the Residents, and there is the pharmacist and the social worker; there's like 20 people, it's crazy. And you have to be able to stand for long periods of time because rounds last a long time. Thank God for these comfortable shoes.

The neurotic gives further information, "Your loved one is critically unwell, there are multiple organs that have been affected and we are providing specialised support to each of these in turn. Additionally, we are consulting with all the other specialities in the hospital to ensure that we are doing the utmost".

I don't think I'm an obsessive-compulsive, but I sort of don't like…I like it all to be neat and sorted out, and I like to know… to be able to answer the questions I'm asked, if that makes sense? You know like, "what's this and what's that?", so I like to know all of that, and I don't like to be surprised at handover by stuff that I didn't know, I find that embarrassing. So, umm, I find that, that's probably the most stressful part of the job, is the, is sort of going there and handing over patient that you don't really know, and you're not responsible for really, and I actually, the registrars laugh, because on Sunday night, I will spend about four or five hours in my office reading up on all of the patients, so yeah, they all laugh at me… I think it reflects on, you know, if you look after the patient and somebody takes over, and they find that you know, that the patient has got staph bacteraemia and you didn't know because you weren't actually looking after them, I think then that's … then I still feel that it reflects on me.

The neurotic intensivist continues to negotiate care plans with families and patients in their care, while managing their own approaches to fitting within their professional development, organisational hierarchy, and inter-professional team: "Yes, that is a really good question. Overnight we have senior experienced staff always looking after your loved one. I am usually at home but on-call, and will be notified, along with you, of any significant changes. If I feel that it is significant, I will return to the hospital to assess and manage the situation myself".

It's like this thing that I've been doing for years. It's like, here we go again, here we go again, here we go again. And you can put structures, and you do, and we do, to make it as unlikely as possible, but somebody will still do something wacky, and you can't stop it. You can't stop it. And that comes with a sense of impotence. You know, like we try, we structure, people do, colleagues do, try to create all of these things, documentation, charts, nurses, warnings, and then, at 3 o'clock in the morning somebody decides to do something that is completely...... "Whaaaaat?!" ." And I think we, most time, intensivists are control freaks, who want to control everything all of the time and sometimes you know that it's slipping.

While aiming for high levels of personal responsibility and commitment to excellence in patient care, the neurotic will make sure there are no unexpected deviations from the patient care plan. "I will check in with the team caring for your loved one and to remind and reassure the team that my phone works and if they ring it, I will answer."

As I say to my suffering partner, if they call me, it's tough; but if they don't call me, it's even tougher, because God knows what is going on that I don't know about.

Continual checking-in with staff and constant negotiation with families is a major consideration for the neurotic: "Do you have any further questions? We will continue to keep you updated as information comes to hand. I think the most important place for yourselves right now, is at your loved one's bedside, hold their hand, tell them that you love them, tell them we are on a journey, and though we are unsure of the eventual destination, we are all on it together."

Do I still have a smile on my face? I am completely strong, nobody can break me, not this patient, not this family, not this case. But there is no way of making peace inside with my soul that is shaking. On the outside I am like a rock. I need to get back to those yoga lessons.

The Fixer

Peter Vernon van Heerden

Employ your time in improving yourself by other men's writings, so that you shall gain easily what others have labored hard for. (Socrates)

The designation of being "the fixer" doesn't attach to the main aspect of any intensivist's persona. In other words, in any ICU there is no one fixer, but rather several intensivists who are known to fix things, to various degrees. Being a fixer is one part of the intensivist's personality that comes to the fore when required. For sure, there are some who are better fixers than others, but being a fixer is part of what the intensivist does every day.

So what does it take to be a fixer? The referring specialist places his patient in the care of the intensive care team, and, in the "closed unit" way of doing business, which is typical of practice in Australia and Israel but less so in other parts of the world, they hope that the patient will be returned to their service "fixed". It's important to note that the patient is indeed delivered to an *intensive care team* for specialised care. This is well-expressed in the quote from one intensivist:

> *Acknowledging that this is a team sport. And it's a team sport between both you and the other… If you have other Consultants on but also with the nursing staff, allied health, everyone; it's a team sport, and you need everyone, and you are an important part of it, but so are they, in their own way.*

The team in the ICU is under the leadership of one or more intensivists, who do their best to care for the patient cohort and see them again in an upright, healthy, and independent state. In order to achieve this outcome and be the fixer of sometimes very complex problems, the intensivist has to rely on a set of skills, which on the whole make up the persona of the fixer.

Firstly, a good fixer needs to be *technically competent*. This means having abroad base of knowledge, as well as good manual skills. The intensivist is required to know at least a little bit about many specialties (from gynaecology, to oncology, to trauma, to neurology), in addition to a lot about organ support and care of the critically ill patient.

> *…as an intensivist you sort of want the skills to manage any crisis situation… You know, I'm not going to take someone to theatre and do a laparotomy, but something in the unit, I feel like we should be able to manage.*

Having the knowledge and technical skills is important, but these skills need to be employed in a sensible and thoughtful" way. There is no place for "cookbook" medicine in the ICU.

> *It is important that you have to use your brain as well, as, you know… anyone can stand there and just run through algorithms, but the important thing is that you need to stand there, taking all the visual cues in, and all the things are happening, and think about other things.*

On the background of adequate knowledge and skill, employed in a thoughtful way, the fixer now needs to proceed in the leadership of the team caring for the patient waiting to be fixed. Multiple decisions may have to be made regarding treatment modality, timing of treatments, intensity of treatment regimen, and suitability of treatment. Fixing the patient may not always involve curing the patient, but rather finding a path for the patient to follow which reduces their suffering and the family's suffering. Firm decisions may be required and are expected of the intensivist fixer.

> *I think that you have maybe an ability to kind of go into 'Okay this is what needs to be done' kind of mode.*

Now being an intensivist, fixer or not, making firm decisions is not an easy task as the stakes are very high and may impact the health and indeed the life of the patient. So, a degree of *confidence* is needed to back up the decisions.

> *…self-confidence, but not too much self-confidence…*

Too much confidence can be self-destructive, because inevitably there will be incorrect decisions at times, some with dire consequences. This will erode confidence and could lead to self-doubt. The fixer then has to learn to live in the space between over-confidence and self-doubt yet be able to function and make good decisions.

> *… a pretty healthy appreciation that you don't know everything, and that you're going to be wrong some of the time.*

Other aspects of decision-making are also important. Decisions are not made in a vacuum. Information about the patient's clinical state continues to stream in, as well as how they are responding to the treatments being employed. There is an element of *multi-tasking* involved:

> *Often what happens is in a busy unit, you've got multiple things going on at the same time, and some people just can't do that.*

This quote identifies why being an intensivist is not for everyone – some people and some specialties are much better suited to the thoughtful pursuit of one topic, without outside disturbance. We need to keep in mind also that multi-tasking in the ICU is often undertaken under enormous pressure and competing priorities, such as more than one admission arriving in the ICU, more than one patient deteriorating at the same time, and high-stakes decisions.

> *I think you do need to be able to function under pressure.*

In addition to having the knowledge and skills, and being able to make decisions under pressure, the fixer must also be effective. This means paying *attention to detail* as missed details could have life-changing or fatal consequences.

> *I think we are 'OCD minus'… the anaesthetists can be a lot more pedantic about some fine details - what syringes, how the syringes are positioned, labelled, and lined up. But I find myself becoming more and more obsessed by little details.*

Given the facets of the fixer intensivist, what is the *motivation* for being such?

> *The successes where you've taken someone slowly through, you've had them for months, and they live…*

One great motivator is the gratification of seeing a critically ill patient recover and start their journey back to health. Unfortunately, we may not see the end of that journey of recovery, but at least the fixer is usually able to present the patient back to the referring team in a better state than they arrived.

> *It's a problem in intensive care, that we never see the real patient, or you don't recognise them when they do come because they look different - they're alive and not tubed and with lines…*

The fixer works with great expectations for their success from within themselves, from within the ICU team, from the referring team, and of course from the patient and their family. This is a large part of who the intensivist is. The reward is *gratification*, sometimes instant and sometimes delayed, and being able to *celebrate success*:

> *I would not be in practice if there wasn't something every day that I did do right. You know, to say to myself, "This was good. I succeeded in weaning a patient, I took a patient from 6 feet under and took him back to life." So there is a lot of success.*

The Duck

Bradley Wibrow

Whoever's calm and sensible is insane! (Jalāl ad-Dīn Muhammad Rūmī)

Well, maybe intensivists are all a little insane. Would you voluntarily choose late nights, chaos, and constant sickness? Intensivists do. They are the ones that thrive in such an environment, the ones that can maintain a sense of calm and lead their team into battle.

You have to "keep your head when everyone around you is losing theirs" to quote Kipling. You've got to stay calm, no matter how you feel. Because if you get angry overtly, then it's a real problem. You have to stay calm.

The art of "staying calm" is one that is not easy to master but is almost a pre-requisite to being an intensivist. It requires practice and is certainly aided by experience. The intensive care unit can be a busy, frenetic environment with multiple patients needing critical attention, requiring an ability to triage tasks in order to be effective. Perhaps even more difficult is the critically ill patient outside the ICU environment (the wards, the cardiac catheter laboratory, recovery – areas with less familiar team members and equipment).

Intensivists have an awareness of managing "emotional contagion" in critical care environments. When the team looks to the leader for direction, the leader's calmness will permeate throughout the rest of the team, allowing the team to function as it should.

I think if you show that you are tempered, if that makes sense, it keeps other people calm. If you start getting frazzled and being short and rude, and dropping things, I think that it's very counter-productive. So even if I'm stressed inwardly, I'd deliberately try and outwardly appear to be docile. (Laughs)

Because I'm the leader, so if I looked distressed and angry and upset, then everyone else is going to respond and mirror my behaviour, so it's not going to allow everyone to focus. And they've got to focus, I don't want to make them feel, like, "the boss is here", the boss is saying this is, how can this happen.

While intensive care may suit a personality that is naturally calm, this can certainly be a learned skill. Often the intensivist will feel the weight of multiple coincident situations and requests on their time and cognitive load. They may appear calm on the outside, but their mind is racing and trying to untangle the scrambled mess of information.

And I spent many years trying to get to the point of stopping, being calm, and obviously with practice and being competent with procedures and running the ICU. I've got to the point of not always, but very often, being able to be that calm, clear-headed person. Because everybody else needs that calmness while things are falling apart around them. It's important for the leader to be the calm one. There were times when it was like I was a duck, looking calm on top but kicking hard underneath! (Laughs)

The persona of the duck is a common one amongst intensivists. Often intensivists are asked how they remain so calm. However, while they may see the duck gliding effortlessly along the water, they don't see the scrambling legs under the water, sometimes only just staying afloat.

It's like in the first instance at a cardiac arrest, take your own pulse. What do I need to do? Okay, I need to lead my team. I need to lead my team in psychological first aid. Then I need to think about my own self-care afterwards.

Yes, it might be generous to say that you have a heightened sense of situational awareness, because you can still overlook and miss things, but I think that you have maybe an ability to kind of go into "okay this is what needs to be done" kind of mode.

While calmness, knowledge, and an ability to structure that knowledge and plan for the next steps are essential within the situation, the intensivist must also be able to facilitate debriefing afterwards so that any adverse events positively inform future management rather than act as a burden and stressor.

All four doctors in the room were very calm, because we had planned before that this was a very difficult procedure and at no point did myself or my senior colleague get stressed. And I think that that was a positive side of the really bad adverse event… The Fellow was quite shocked as to how calm the situation was, and that we had managed to maintain the patient and ourselves during the situation. I think this was because we had worked together, we had discussed the case before, and we were prepared for this adverse event. We all had to sit down, and calmly discuss all of the issues that had arisen, and then the family were okay with that situation.

However, that's not to say that ICU requires only those who are naturally calm. In fact, ICU has long benefited from a range of ICU specialists with differing specialty backgrounds. The intensivist must be adept at adopting different personas appropriate for the scenario at hand. Some have to work on being calm and some work on being assertive when needed.

I've always been a reasonably calm person, that is trying to keep everybody happy. That's a personal trait of mine, I try not to upset anybody (laughs). And sometimes it works in my favour and I'm probably not bad at it, but other times it's a problem in terms of assertiveness.

Practicing Intensive care is full of less "intense" moments such as meeting with families, liaising with other specialties, and planning future care. This in itself can be stressful as families deal with stress differently and anger is often forefront in the list of emotions. It is not unusual that patients in ICU end up there due to complications from other care and, being at the coalface, the doctors, and nurses in ICU often have to deal initially with unhappy family members. The water of conflict and emotional intensity somehow needs to spill off the duck's back:

Regarding families - So one of the things is of course when they are angry. That's not pleasant. You're feeling very uncomfortable of course, and the trick is not to get angry yourself of course, because that's not going to help. You get frustrated but you remain calm and try to keep your voice even…

Some experienced intensivists who knew they needed to adopt the duck persona and remain calm to be effective reported finding this a personal challenge during times of severe stress or in dealing acutely with adverse outcomes:

I can see the registrar moving back, scared and in a corner, looking down; the nurses kind of not knowing what to do, and I can see it all coming, all happening around me. But for a period of time, I can't yet extract myself from this. I'm still agitated. So it takes me 3 to 4 minutes... to say, "Okay, that's where we are, we can talk about it tomorrow, but right now this is what I need to do, I'm going to call the surgeon, call the anaesthetist, get the monitors; this guy's got to go to theatre.

So, it was really the awareness that what I was doing and what was happening within me that wasn't helpful to anyone. But I couldn't control it for at least three or four minutes.

While ICU frequently deals with clinical complications from other specialties, things can go wrong in ICU too. Dealing with conflict amongst the medical teams requires just as much, if not more, tact, as well as the ability to maintain a calm demeanour. Intensivists reported they are frequently called to be the wise or reasoned person in the room.

So you try to be the adult in the room... I had to resort to a lot of internal calm and reflection and 'Yes I understand', but trying to be the voice of reason and, '...we will learn from this, we're going to do this, we're going to do that, it's unfortunate'.... But you obviously you feel like 'For God's sake, you guys cock things up all the time, and what about if we could just reverse the roles for a moment and let me tell you how stupid you guys are.'... But you can't do that, of course, it requires a lot of self-control and a lot of energy at least for me, maybe other people do it naturally: to show calm and reasonable thinking when I don't really feel that way.

There has to be a way to articulate the urgency professionally and maintain some decorum. The team anxiety that follows conflict is not of benefit. Intensivists hope they improve and mature with experience. They draw on past experiences, as they have seen most things before, including almost all adverse outcomes that one can list, and hopefully for those who don't master the "art of calmness" early in their careers, they learn to, throughout them.

That was also an age thing too. You do improve on that as you get a little bit more into things. And you find out, 'Hey, that's really not helping, and if I'm standing there tapping my foot for 25 minutes, trying to get that done, that's probably detrimental.' But you learn that over time.

... So you need to be calm; you always need to be truthful; be open-minded; and be willing to learn continuously; learn from your mistakes; and accept when you are wrong...

While easier said than done, the duck intensivist must maintain that sense of calmness amongst the storm of critical illness, feathers for weathering and shedding conflict and pressure, and strong, open-minded, and determined paddling along the currents of expanding clinical care. Being able to listen and be open-minded to change is essential for growth.

The Diplomat

Katherine Potter

Who shall decide when doctors disagree, And soundest casuists doubt, like you and me? (Alexander Pope)

Most intensivists do not have formal diplomatic training: we have never served as ambassadors to a foreign land, and we have (likely) not even been to finishing schools! However, we may have shared meals as a family in which we learned manners, and we may have siblings with whom we were forced to learn negotiation and diplomatic tactics. Our medical training provided education in physiology, diagnosis, and treatment, but much of our communication style has been learned "on the fly" during difficult encounters, occasionally with our co-workers:

I have had to grow into being assertive and taking leadership. I used to work in the cardiac ICU where there's a lot of interactions with surgeons… it wasn't the best fit for my personality … I'm on the introverted side, but I don't have trouble getting along with most people… But… when you are dealing with a frustrated short tempered surgeon … it just makes me uncomfortable…I didn't thrive in that environment, pushing back or whatever. I'm more of a peacemaker!

Assertiveness and leadership skills can be learned through roleplay and clinical simulation and particularly through the lived experience of fellowship training, during which we must learn to navigate the differing management styles of our mentors while we are developing our own identities as specialist doctors and decision-makers.

Similarly, the role of the intensivist frequently requires both good and careful communication and collaborative management with multiple subspecialties. The diplomat must commonly navigate disagreements between the groups of medical caregivers, and in particularly discomforting situations, disagreements between parents and other subspecialists. It is then that the intensivist may find themselves negotiating a conversational minefield, particularly if they are in agreement with the family instead of a medical colleague.

I do find it hard where I am on the same page as the relatives, and I find they are absolutely right in what they are saying, but I cannot "bag" my colleagues. In this regard, I do find I have tried to defend them [the surgeons] to the family in the past, some of these decisions have been made and they have had a good think about it, whereas deep down I'm not convinced that's this is true. It might have just been that it was 2 o'clock in the morning, and the decision-making was part of a junior service-registrar making a decision with poor communication. Not specifically for the surgeons, there's other teams as well. And yeah, I find that hard to deal with that appropriately, and keep everybody happy. We want to mitigate it to some degree and keep the family happy, but I'm not sure… sometimes I'm not sure how to do that appropriately.

These diplomatic skills of the intensivist are particularly useful when managing the highly emotional situations that commonly arise in the ICUs. Leading care conferences with multiple caregivers and family members require careful navigation with highly invested stakeholders who may not be in agreement regarding the treatment plan.

Not just interpersonal skills it's EQ [Emotional Quotient] skills. It's the ability to be able to read the emotions of a room and be able to respond to them appropriately and try and understand where somebody else is coming from, so I see it as that step above empathy. Empathy is understanding that you are upset. EQ is understanding why you're upset, and where you're gonna be, how you how I can help you with your upset state. And we don't choose that. So, I think they're the crucial skills for intensivists.

At times, diplomacy can involve repressing our initial instincts in order to act as peacemakers. It also leads to self-criticism and the concern that, had we acted differently, the communication would have been more direct and less time-consuming.

If I would have been more assertive… I would have just yelled at the surgeon down the phone to say this was inappropriate, and at the end of the day for that case it probably would have been advantageous. It would have led to the same outcome in the end … Because I'm calm, I just navigate my way in between, keep things level and happy on all the sides, I think I managed to manoeuvre myself reasonably well in this regard, it is not always easy. But yet, to some degree, I find that specific trait also gets me in trouble. Where I'd rather be a person where I take a side, and I take the right side, to know what's the wrong and the right thing, and I just stick with that and again, I don't necessarily have to defend somebody that's done something that wasn't exactly up to scratch. That probably would be easier and would come with more assertiveness, and being more to one side.

In the ideal situation, the diplomat finds themselves in a group where communication is recognised as a cornerstone of quality patient care and each member of the team gives and receives criticism without judgement or denial allowing patient care to move forward without interference from ego.

We argue, but we don't have any significant conflict. We don't agree about everything. Everyone tries to give their own opinion and we try to decide together the best option. We don't fight about things. There's not a lot of ego or conflict, so we discuss. We try to think about ways to change things. I can talk to my colleagues I can tell them things like I wouldn't have done it this way I would have done it other ways, they accept it. They accept that they are doing things differently and when we make mistakes we accept criticism. We take responsibility.

The Pragmatist

Nancy Tofil

Do what you can, with what you have, where you are. (Theodore Roosevelt)

The pragmatist's attributes include being honest and realistic; diligent; emotionally somewhat detached in order to have the capacity for all patients in the ICU; resilient; and having a poor memory for bad events, so they can move forward.

Being honest, yet realistic, is a cornerstone of the pragmatist. Telling someone the truth (e.g. that they are going to die or that a treatment is not likely to work) is a trait of the pragmatist. After seeing complex patients with multisystem organ failure again and again, the pragmatist learns to brace themselves for failure.

I think you have to recognise that death and life are part of the same journey. And your mission in life cannot be to extinguish one and welcome the other. You have to find a balance and practice towards both goals.

So to me, that role of the physician as a 'healer' is to recognise when it's my job to guide and hold your hand and when it's my job to put a breathing tube into you and give you everything I have in the hospital. You are the person who can guide that family toward living or toward death. A death with dignity is a gift; a resuscitation leading to ongoing life is a gift. To do them both well is our job. So you need to be able to recognise when to mode switch.

With experience, the intensivist has either been burned by prior bad events or learned from colleagues about these events. This leads to diligence.

You plan for the worst-case scenarios.

These may not occur, but intensivists fear that if they don't share this with younger colleagues something may be missed. This diligence also consists of constantly striving for improvement. The pragmatist tries to look at the "big picture" of managing a large busy ICU. Their emotional capacity must be divided amongst all patients and cannot be so involved with one that they lose focus of others. This can be seen by others as emotional detachment.

You have to learn to be emotive and empathic, without being debilitated by it. Meaning, the intensivist to whom everything is just raw emotion - they will fall apart; they won't make it in the field. But the intensivist who sort of doesn't give anything of themselves, doesn't care, also I think will struggle. So, taking that side of yourself and not hiding it, bringing it out. Bringing your empathic self to the table.

However, empathy must accommodate resiliency. Resiliency is an important aspect of the pragmatist. Having a growth mindset, as described by Dweck [2] in 2006, can be critical. Taking on challenges as they occur and learning from each event. Realising you never have all the information to make a perfect decision but that no decision can be worse. Constantly increasing your abilities and experience.

I think from a medical perspective you have to teach people not to be risk adverse. Because stasis is death. ... So the goal is not to be stable, the goal is to be constantly pushing the envelope. What does this patient not need today? What can we get away with removing or stopping? And don't just assume that they can't, prove it. And if you don't constantly push that, you lose patients, you kill people. Because you add days to the ICU care; you add days on the ventilator; you add days to that toxic medicine; you add days to central IV access. If you're waiting for that certainty, you're killing patients.

Although less than 3% of children and about 10% of adults die in the PICU, over the years this emotional toll on the intensivist adds up. For whatever reason, there are some patients one never forgets and, in order for the pragmatist to move on, they have to have a short memory for the vast majority of patients. Otherwise, they fear not being able to care for the rest of the critically ill patients and stay vigilant for complications while constantly trying to move each patient forward towards the ultimate goal of leaving the ICU and, one day, going home.

References

1. Teaching Conflict Resolution in Medicine: Lessons from Business, Diplomacy, and Theatre Adam D. Wolfe, MD, PhD*, Kim B. Hoang, MD, Sarah F. Denniston, MD.
2. Dweck CS. Mindset: the new psychology of success. New York, NY: Random House; 2006.

Rahul Khanna is a practicing psychiatrist at the Austin Health's Psychological Trauma Recovery Service and serves as Director of Innovation & Medical Governance at Phoenix Australia—Centre for Post-traumatic Mental Health, based in Melbourne, Australia. He is a senior lecturer at the University of Melbourne and has a deep clinical and research interest in psychological trauma, particularly in leveraging novel technologies to enhance our understanding and treatment of trauma-related mental health conditions. Further background and contact details are available on https://rahul.au.

Michael Ruppe is board certified in paediatrics, internal medicine, and paediatric critical care, and is an attending physician in Paediatric Cardiac Critical Care at Norton Children's Hospital, Louisville, Kentucky, USA. He completed medical school at the University of Toledo College of Medicine followed by a combined internal medicine and paediatrics residency at the University Hospital of Cleveland/Rainbow Babies and Children's Hospital. He then completed a paediatric critical care fellowship at the Children's Hospital of Philadelphia. During this time his interests translated into research and publications in end-of-life decision making and medical ethics. In 2009 he moved to Louisville, Kentucky, and is active in quality improvement, point-of-care ultrasonography, international health, and paediatric cardiac critical care.

Marc Romain completed his undergraduate medical studies and speciality in internal medicine in South Africa before moving to Israel, where he currently resides and works. He is a specialist in internal medicine, general intensive care, and nephrology. He is a senior physician in the medical ICU and the head of the Critical Care Nephrology and Nutrition Unit at the Hadassah Medical Centers, Jerusalem. His interests include multi-organ support therapies (CRRT, hemoperfusion, ECMO), aviation medicine, and educating the next generation of doctors, nurses, and intensivists.

Caleb Fisher is an intensive care physician at Austin Health, Melbourne, Australia. He has completed dual overseas fellowships in liver disease and extra-corporeal support systems. Outside of work, he is the father of two highly active children, who indulge in his passion for the outdoors.

Peter Vernon van Heerden qualified as an anaesthetist and intensive care specialist and has practiced in South Africa, the UK, Australia, and Israel. He is the Director of the General Intensive Care Unit, Dept. of Anesthesiology, Critical Care and Pain Medicine, Faculty of Medicine, Hadassah Hospital and Hebrew University of Jerusalem, Israel.

Bradley Wibrow is an intensivist and emergency physician in Perth, Western Australia, and works in a neurological, cardiac, and liver specialist intensive care unit as well as a small peripheral emergency department. He is passionate about ensuring equal access to critical care for all Australians, ultrasound, research and finding ways to maintain morale in a high stress workplace. His research interests include management of delirium, post-ICU care, and finding ways to aid recovery for our patients and families as they deal with one of the worst times of their lives. In his other life he is a father to four children, attempts to run regularly, and gets down to the ocean whenever possible.

Katherine Potter joined the faculty of the University of Louisville School of Medicine in 2007 and since has served as the Fellowship Program Director and a clinician teacher in the paediatric ICU and paediatric cardiac ICU. She has written and revised curricula for the fellowship program including a clinical curriculum; a non-clinical curriculum discussing topics such as billing/coding, teaching methods, grant writing, clinical research, and quality improvement; and collaboratively created a simulation boot camp for incoming PCCM and emergency medicine fellows that includes physiologic simulation and training regarding difficult conversations. She has presented educational research at the regional and national level.

Nancy Tofil is a professor of paediatrics and the Division Director of Paediatric Critical Care. She is the Medical Director of the Paediatric Simulation Center at Children's of Alabama/University of Alabama at Birmingham (UAB). The Simulation Center has trained over 85,000 learners in almost 13 years. Our centre has a focus on interdisciplinary learning and parent education. Professor Tofil is the Senior Associate Program Director for the Paediatric Residency Training Program. She obtained her medical degree from The Ohio State University College of Medicine and her Master of Education from UAB. She completed her paediatric residency and fellowship training at UAB.

Chapter 14
Through the Looking Glass

Sacha Schweikert

> *The funny thing about truth, everyone seems to have their own version.*
>
> —Carlos Wallace

As we have seen, the ICU is a very specialised place in a hospital, where only the sickest patients get treated. Patients are on all sorts of life supports, including ventilators, dialysis machines, extracorporeal circuits, amongst others. Resources are scarce, and this holds true for various aspects including time, personnel, bedspace, and equipment. The stakes are high and decisions need to be made quickly, keeping the patient's wishes with regards to quality of life at heart. It certainly is not an environment for everyone to work in and it takes certain personal traits to fit in, get enjoyment, and work fulfilment ultimately leading to good patient outcomes.

> *I personally feel that mainly it is a toughness. We are supposed to be tough. We are supposed to be these tough doctors. We can see anything, cope with everything and it doesn't matter what's going on.*

Whilst Chapter 13 focused on the self-perceived attributes that defined the intensivist, the following chapter is an exploration into the intensivist's projected perception of others "looking in at them". The attributes which intensivists considered and how they were perceived by others outside of the ICU could be broadly categorised into three distinct entities. The superhero, the naysayer, and the dictator.

S. Schweikert (✉)
Department of Intensive Care, Sir Charles Gairdner Hospital, Perth, WA, Australia
e-mail: Sacha.Schweikert@health.wa.gov.au

121

The Superhero

It is easy to see why intensivists could be viewed as superheroes. The intensivist's understanding of human physiology and anatomy must be intricate and span the full breadth of systems. They also need to understand diverse disease processes and have an ability to rapidly form and update a differential diagnosis and systematically exclude or diagnose life threats whilst concurrently resuscitating the patient. They are expected to pounce with no warning and save a patient from an immediate life threat or a colleague from a potential misadventure. In the process, they need to remain level-headed and authoritative and be able to navigate difficult conversations with other specialists, peers, and families.

Clearly this is ultimately very challenging and quite possibly unachievable and could be viewed as an unreasonable expectation.

> *I think that the overall perception is that we are the super-humans that can handle anything and that is something that needs to change. We are all human beings who feel emotions and get burnt out from feeling emotions too much, and we need avenues to express that.*

> *That we are control freaks a little bit; like, want to manage everything; and I think sometimes, for us we try to take over everyone else's part; and I think that hurts sometimes the relationships [we have] with people, because we are seen as just swooping in...*

This fallacy and its limitations came through during the interviews. Burn-out amongst intensivists is a well-documented issue [1], and it would seem that exactly such projected superhuman personas and the expectations that come with them might at least in part be responsible for it.

The Naysayer

Intensivists admit multiple patients with a very grim prognosis to their unit daily. In conjunction with the treating specialist and surrogate decision-makers, they try and form goals of care in the patient's best interest. Nevertheless, there are patients in very dire situations who get admitted "to give them a go" or "for a trial of therapy", which tends to be time-limited depending on responsiveness to therapy.

Unfortunately, the majority of such dire admissions will in fact end up perishing from their disease, either during the immediate ICU stay or the same hospital stay. It is only logical that over time, a seasoned intensivist will form a pragmatic and realistic view and relate the same early on to family and peers in order to manage expectations.

It is exactly such pragmatic approaches, shaped by years of experience and to some degree recurring disappointment in treating certain conditions, that will be viewed as a Naysayer persona by others.

> *I think almost certainly they would see us as being pessimists. And that... because too often the only serious discussion... One of the serious discussions is about end-of-life or direc-*

tions of care. You know, they've invested a lot, they know the patients better than us, and for someone to be told that we think that they're actually dying, and that to pursue these things is probably not in the patient's best interest... would be quite confronting.

Oh I'm sure they see us as arrogant, dismissive, and many of us as being 'Doctor No's'. We say, "nah". Thanks for coming... nah". That's what I think.

The emotional detachment and poor memory for bad events described by participants and emblematic of the pragmatic persona are likely mechanisms of self-preservation. To some degree it may well be protective for the intensivist to be able to continue in their profession until retirement. Those same attributes would be seen as cold and harsh by others.

I think it's probably changing, fairly rapidly. I think the old one would be like they're the people who say "No" a lot. They say "No, you can't come to a unit"; "No, you can't do that operation"; "No, you can't share our scarce resources". But, I think even that's probably changing.

Worldwide, intensive care units are under immense constraints imposed by limited resources, and various guidelines for admission to the ICU have been proposed [1]. Updated and increasingly sophisticated scoring systems, such as APACHE and ANZROD can also help in the decision-making process [2]. Of course, such guidelines are open to interpretation and subjectivity [3].

At least anecdotally, it would seem that today's intensivist is more inclined to "give a patient a go", if their treating specialist thinks it might be worthwhile. Doing so will probably lead to a decrease in that Naysayer persona and will foster interdepartmental collaboration and relationships, but at the expense of further pressure on an already stretched healthcare system. Paradoxically it might also lead to further strengthening the pessimism amongst ICU personnel, medical, and others, through continued validation of negative connotations and little success from patients poorly selected for likely post-ICU recovery.

The Dictator

With the need to think quickly and make decisions fast, with little time to listen to everyone and incorporate all suggestions, comes the risk to come across as authoritarian and abrupt.

You know, to me what seems to be egregious behaviour among peers...judging each other, or being/acting better than your peers, more 'know-it-all' or having a heavy-handed method to resolve conflict, a little bit of arrogance. As a group, I think we are viewed in that way. We are viewed as a little bit intense and often a bit judgemental.

The exact personal attributes that are so important for a good intensivist to be the "fixer in difficult circumstances" as well as the "negotiator and diplomat" are also the ones that have likely led to the Dictator persona seen by others. It is all just a matter of perspective.

I think that's the perception, right? The idea of a 'resting bitch face' if you are female. Right, because you're not walking in telling people great news; we often don't give great news; we are the givers of bad news; people call us to do that. So it requires a certain sense of decorum and seriousness to do so.

I think most people perceive us as… There is a little bit of fear; and maybe some people think there is some arrogance.

Conclusion

The three personas constructed following traits described by study participants have been defined. The data reported here was collected in the same manner as for the self-perceived attributes from the intensivists themselves in Chapter 13. No data was collected from outsiders or allied health staff, so those perceptions were neither supported nor disconfirmed. Whilst this would have been interesting, it was beyond the scope of the work.

References

1. Burghi G, Lambert J, Chaize M, Goinheix K, Quiroga C, et al. Prevalence, risk factors and consequences of severe burnout syndrome in ICU. Intensive Care Med. 2014;40:1785–6.
2. Nates JL, Nunnally M, Kleinpell R, Blosser S, Goldner J, Birriel B, et al. ICU admission, discharge, and triage guidelines. Crit Care Med. 2016;44(8):1553–602.
3. Paul E, Bailey M, Kasza J, Pilcher D. The ANZROD model: better benchmarking of ICU outcomes and detection of outliers. Crit Care Resusc. 2016;18(1):25–36.PMID: 26947413.

Sacha Schweikert studied medicine in Switzerland before moving to Australia to pursue intensive care medicine training. He complemented training with a diploma in clinical ultrasound and undertook a Fellowship in Neurocritical Care at the University of Toronto before returning to Australia. He currently works as an intensive care specialist at Sir Charles Gairdner Hospital in Perth and has a special interest in all things neurocritical care.

Part IV:
Intensivists—Impervious or Vulnerable?

Foreword: It's Okay to Feel This Way

Rima Styra ⓘ

Today's burdens can strengthen you for tomorrow.
—Mark Twain

This introduction provides context for the emotions that intensivists experience related to their work in the ICU, and the emotional burdens that they often take on and carry to their own detriment. In describing these responses, we hope to both normalize them, and create an awareness of their impact on life outside of the workplace and their relationships. Although intensivists appear to sit at the top of the hierarchy of control in terms of healthcare delivery in the ICU, they should not presume that they carry the burdens of care in isolation or without an expectation of support for themselves. Lack of empathy and the negative effects of blame and accusation are highlighted by the comments of intensivists. Effective leadership in the ICU environment can play an essential role in building an environment of care and collaboration rather than attributing blame or guilt in stressful clinical scenarios.

We review how intensivists embody perfectionism and professionalism in their work which in the ecology of the ICU can lead to distressful feelings, such as anger and helplessness and without support, internalization of negative thoughts about oneself both as a professional and a person. Post-traumatic stress disorder symptoms involving recurrent intrusive symptoms, negative alternations in cognitions, avoidance, and alterations in arousal and reactivity are reviewed in the context of working as a front-line healthcare worker. Prolonged or repeated stress in the ICU environment can also result in exhaustion and burnout. We identify that this results not only in the emotional aspects of burnout but also cognitive and physical symptoms often leading to a low sense of personal accomplishment at work and overall low self-esteem. Lack of awareness of the frequent occurrence of these disorders in

R. Styra
Department of Psychiatry, University of Toronto, Toronto, ON, Canada

Center for Mental Health, University Health Network, Toronto, ON, Canada
e-mail: Rima.Styra@uhn.ca

ICU staff impacts inappropriate attribution of these symptoms to a weakness of the individual, and hampers or delays seeing appropriate assistance.

We discuss the relatability of the patient situation and cumulative life experience that can impact the intensivist, not solely the magnitude of the event. Coping by active distancing and compartmentalization are familiar strategies for intensivists, with the challenge being to maintain one's humanity and caring in the work. Imprinting of poor patient outcomes is discussed as not necessarily being negative as many of the intensivists recognized that there were educational benefits for the care of future patients.

Mitigating factors such as leadership, mentorship, and culture which can aid in stressful situations which may involve the occurrence of errors are explored. Intensivists often are required to deal with the stress of the dying patient or adverse clinical event and the need for sharing information in family conversations with empathy and honesty. Psychological recognition of the importance of patient care not only patient outcomes and family acknowledgement of the work of the treating team can have a positive impact on ICU staff and prevent burnout. Various approaches that are frequently undertaken to counteract the detrimental effect of the emotional overload common to the intensivist—emotional escapism, nonclinical professional activities, and rejuvenating philanthropy—are also reviewed. This part emphasizes how crucial it is to remember that the intensivist is not only a professional but a person with feelings working in a stressful environment who themselves may require support at times.

Rima Styra Dr Rima Styra is an Associate Professor of Psychiatry at the University of Toronto and works as a staff psychiatrist in the Medical Psychiatry Program at the Center for Mental Health at the University Health Network in Toronto, Canada. She is the Director of the Division of Consultation-Liaison Psychiatry at the University of Toronto. She is a member of the Toronto General Research Institute. She is a graduate of the Medical Faculty at the University of Toronto, where she completed her medical education and psychiatry residency training. She has a Master of Education from OISE and has been involved in numerous educational programs in particular in multidisciplinary areas. Dr Styra's research extends over several areas in the consultation-liaison field.

Chapter 15
Here Come Those Tears

Eileen Tay and Janice Sullivan

> *What lies behind you and what lies in front of you, pales in comparison to what lies inside of you.*
>
> —*Ralph Waldo Emerson*

Doctors in an ICU must use multiple skills simultaneously. Executive and cognitively demanding skills are essential with the need to make decisions in a timely and sometimes urgent manner in delivering care to the most acute and vulnerable patients. Emotional response or anticipatory skills, with the need to be empathic communicators to families in distress, is another essential skill set. All are clear recurring examples of demands on intensivists, the very human doctors working in this challenging yet also rewarding area of medicine, which contributes to a range of emotional responses from them. It is important to consider factors that may contribute to the "response in the moment" such as sleep deprivation due to shift work, personal stressors, and professional life stressors [1].

The demanding nature of the field means that intensivists must think quickly while feeling deeply enough to connect with the patients they are caring for, all while communicating effectively with each other and with other teams outside of the ICU. There is also the constant expectation of high levels of professionalism for

E. Tay (✉)
Faculty of Forensic Psychiatry, RANZCP, Melbourne, VIC, Australia

Faculty of Psychotherapy, RANZCP, Melbourne, VIC, Australia
e-mail: Eileen@hollywoodpsychiatry.com.au

J. Sullivan
Divisions of Pediatric Critical Care and Clinical and Translational Research, Department of Pediatrics, University of Louisville, Louisville, KY, USA

Norton Children's Research Institute, University of Louisville School of Medicine, Louisville, KY, USA

D. Dennis et al. (eds.), *Stories from ICU Doctors*,
https://doi.org/10.1007/978-3-031-32401-7_15

doctors, which can result in a reluctance to seek help when they are not coping or even recognise that they are not coping well. Coping mechanisms reported by intensivists are explored elsewhere in the book (Chap. 22).

The second aspect of examining why intensivists might experience the range of emotional responses that they reported would be to consider the ICU itself as a living, breathing organism with the staff within it being interdependent on each other and on the technologies that are vital to caring for patients in the ICU. How an ICU and its members interact with the wider hospital system also informs the health or the ecology of the ICU and its members. Multifaceted interprofessional relationships must be established and re-established as individual providers continuously rotate to and from the ICU and other medical services [2].

In this chapter, we use this ecology metaphor to explore intensivist emotional reactions in an effort to promote positive individual and institutional growth.

Types of Emotional Responses of Intensivists

It would be naive of us to imagine that any clinician or physician working in the ICU would not have some sort of emotional reaction based on the potential for errors related to the acuity of illness, complex needs, knowledge required for medications and new technologies, time demands, and factors related to communication [1]. Hence, the ecology model is relevant, as each physician and staff member's reaction impact on other team members as well as the patients' families. The wider systemic issues that impact how intensivist has to work are also consistent with an ecology model of understanding.

Emotional responses may be grouped into acute reactions and then more delayed reactions as well as a mixture of the two, in the specific context of stressful events usually with a bad outcome or death of the patient in the ICU. Near misses may trigger slightly different responses.

Acute and Delayed Reactions

> *I thought it took all of my emotional forces to deal with them. In the beginning I did not understand why they were so mad. I understood the situation was very stressful, but I couldn't understand why they were so mad. I had to breathe to remain calm myself a few times.*
>
> *We are very, very anxious about these things.*
>
> *Yes. I think part of it is a tendency to react a certain way to things that trigger sadness. Like I am a 'crier'…things that are heavy events …I think that in the intensive care setting we see all of that on fast forward, kind of all the time. So, I think I am probably …it's been a little more conditioned in this setting. But I think I came in with that tendency to react in the way that I do.*

I'm sure my eyes look close to having tears in them at times. Yeah, I think that's okay. I think that's okay, it's a bit uncomfortable for me but it's okay. It's okay. I'm even uncomfortable talking about it. But it's okay. It's a good thing and I've never come out of that thinking that was stupid or bad or I shouldn't have done that. I've always felt that in the end it was a positive thing and was okay. I think that's usually well received, and that's not fake.

These examples demonstrate acute reactions and a mixture of acute and delayed responses. Reactions may be due to the repeated exposure to stressful and distressing events in the ICU which trigger recall of past events as well as relating to pre-existing personality factors such as reacting by crying to emotional events. There might be other more personal reasons for their tendency to cry but it is also about the response of others around this doctor and within the ICU itself as to whether secondary emotional responses such as feelings of shame or embarrassment about showing emotions at work would arise, thereby adding to their "emotional baggage".

Medicine encompasses both the sciences and humanities, and it is definitely okay to cry as a sign of our own humanity, with or without the family, as per the last example. However, this participant had to reassure themselves repeatedly "that it was okay" which is a sign that permission to show human emotions in the face of a shared tragedy was somehow not there, which may have arisen from their personality structure, such as with the participant in the previous quote, or that it was not made explicit within the ICU that sharing a human emotion such as crying is appropriate and healthy. In other words, there are usually multiple reasons why certain types of emotional responses occur more frequently in these high acuity settings—or not—for the intensivists.

The need to stay calm in the face of overwhelming emotional reactions from others such as family members is a skill required not just of intensivists, as discussed in Chapter 13, but of doctors in general. However, what is specific to intensivists is expressed by the above quotations whereby participants reported being "very, very anxious" and then the fact that "we see all that on fast forward", meaning that the demand for the skill to remain calm is constant and expected. Remaining calm in the face of stressful events is important for containing anxiety in the rest of the team as well as for the family. It is considered a sign of professionalism. It is therefore not surprising that this specific skill takes its toll on the intensivists and hence may accounting for one participant stating:

I guess it was to some degree, maybe anger that it came to that. That I was …I felt responsible, and anger on my behalf, that I let it come to that.

However, feelings of anger and frustration may be entirely valid responses depending on the specific context of what happened in the ICU, who was involved, and so forth. Anger in the short term may be a supportive emotion for the intensivist, with the caveat that anger and frustration in the longer term would likely result in more prolonged emotional distress leading to other problems. Those doctors who continue to harbour anger and frustration may also possess other underlying personality factors that potentiate this. Feelings of anger may be a valid response, but a display of anger is not professional or acceptable. In the situation above, the intensivist felt responsible that they did not intervene earlier, and thus, the situation deteriorated, and they felt that responsibility. Anger can drive one to learn and avoid similar situations in the future.

Perfectionism

The personality trait of perfectionism is very commonly seen in doctors and featured in the data set of intensivist participants contributing to this book. While we have described the personas of the intensivist already (Chaps. 13 and 14), the subject of personality factors in doctors has been studied more broadly. In the book, *The Physician as Patient* [3], core features found in doctors were described, with "perfectionism" being especially prominent, to the extent that this specific trait is examined throughout this book. Perfectionism may be considered a desirable trait due to its association with high levels of conscientiousness and thoroughness—thus enabling medical school entry- but also seen as a positive attribute for completing their studies and progressing throughout their career. The fact that the wider societal culture tends to reward perfectionism (such as in competitive sports where perfect scores may be given) reinforces this in the culture of medicine.

However, as described in "The Physician as Patient" [3], the personal cost of maintaining perfectionism is that of increased levels of stress, anxiety, as well as depression, when high expectations are not able to be maintained. In addition, competition within the medical profession for placements, promotions, and other opportunities is usually fierce. This may become a source of cumulative stressors and compound the impact of perfectionism.

The Italian philosopher Voltaire was said to have reflected that "Perfect is the enemy of the good", meaning that perfectionism can rob the individual of enjoying more modest achievements. Perfectionism may also be used as a defence against criticism, rejection, and disapproval. The defensive function of perfectionism usually has origins related to the individual's developmental history; perfectionism can therefore be a double-edged sword:

> Interviewer: "So ...I hear that you are actually more vulnerable, because you are such a high achiever, a perfectionist, but no one's perfect, everybody is going to make mistakes, so you are actually more vulnerable with your personality because it's a bigger fall for you?"
>   Participant: Right, right.
>   Interviewer: You are up there, and you hold yourself up high ...
>   Participant: Right.
>   Interviewer: So, you see that vulnerability in yourself?
>   Participant: Yes. Yes.
>   Interviewer: But not just in medicine but in other things as well?
>   Participant: Right.

The above example would not be unique to intensivists but to many doctors; there is an inherent anxiety state associated with the need to "hold yourself up high…" and as per the example, it is perceived as a vulnerability, being "a high achiever" not just in medicine but in other things as well. The ICU ecological system is ever-changing with new treatments, devices, interventions, etc. which impacts even the more senior doctors who may face vulnerability in their leadership if they do not maintain the most current training and education related to new practices.

Interrelated Emotional Responses

Immediate-type emotional responses of humiliation, helplessness, blame, and anxiety are often interrelated which exemplifies the second aspect of why intensivists respond as they do to stressful events in the ICU, namely, the interdependence of the team.

> Helpless. Everybody felt helpless. It's a simple word. Everybody felt helpless because the attending senior felt helpless because her patient almost died because of something we did. I felt helpless because I couldn't have anticipated that the junior would make this mistake; the junior also felt helpless because he was doing what he thought the senior consultant was telling him to do. So, it was a …Because everybody felt helpless, this emotion of anger is coming to try and cover this helplessness.

There are many aspects to consider within this response to a complex scenario where the patient nearly died, but it clearly described what was referred to earlier as the ICU being an ecological system. This environment has interdependent parts composed of real people, who function well only when the basic assumptions of the group can be clarified, such as the expectations placed on the leader—usually the "senior" of the team. We have discussed leadership (Chapter 11) and teamwork (Chapter 9) in the ICU previously. In understanding group-based mentality, one approach based on psychoanalytic theory is to consider the nature of medical training, which is traditionally based on an apprenticeship model and creates dependency and power dynamics between the junior and senior doctors. Upon completing their training and becoming consultants, however, this hard-won status and newly found independence may result in defending this position [4]. What this means is that the inherent process of medical training may result in a senior or a consultant who operates from what is termed a counter-dependent state of mind, thereby rejecting the shared interdependency that defines teamwork (Chapter 9). This occurs at an unconscious level such that explicit and effective communications to the rest of the team do not occur. This unconscious process may explain the sorrowful cascade described in the example above, with anger as a resulting emotion used to cover up the helplessness generated by the lack of effective communication from leadership.

The medical hierarchy also means that it is often very confrontational to explicitly criticise the leader or the head of the department, even with structured supports in place, as there may also be an unconscious internalisation of "the organisation-in-the mind" which makes speaking out about how the team is not functioning as well as it could a very difficult process. Training in conflict resolution and the use of open disclosure teams in medical units are helpful, but addressing what the unconscious, internalised factors are and how these may be operating would contribute a to deeper understanding of dysfunction within teams [4].

More compellingly, there needs to be an examination of the simple assumptions of what the ICU is about, as ICUs serve a number of functions for the wider hospital system—from providing full life support and being life-saving, to being the technical experts at inserting a central line for other medical departments. For intensivists at the start of their careers, there may also be a need to acknowledge, as opposed to deny, anxieties about death and that when working in the ICU, the death of patients is a likely outcome.

It is important to acknowledge that feelings of helplessness and failure are to be expected, to be normalised, and must be exemplified from the top down so that responses such as the following need not arise:

> *And sometimes you ... I feel ...that there is a tendency to blame and accuse ... There's a tendency to be a bit harsh, a bit harsh. I think some people have a very good "retrospectoscope" and can not necessarily place themselves in your position at the time.*

The most difficult patient scenario is when there are acts of commission or omission which result in the death of a patient who was expected to "pull through", and perhaps that is when the judgemental "retrospectoscope" is most acutely and painfully applied to the emotional detriment of the entire team.

The other aspect of the example above alludes to the ecology model of interdependence when they described the inability of some people to "…place themselves in your position at the time". At one level this is an example of a lack of empathy for intensivists and, at another level, an example of the lack of appreciation of the emotional detriment of the blaming and accusing position taken against the intensivist or against the ICU itself. The mental, emotional, and psychological health and wellbeing of all doctors are an interdependent process. One of the first steps to a greater understanding of the interdependent nature of a wider hospital system, within which the ICU functions more or less autonomously, is to be able to place ones' self in the position of each other when decisions are made with respect to patient care and not just doing this as part of a debrief when there has been an adverse patient outcome.

Emotional Responses of Intensivists on Reflection

With the passage of time, some distance from the acute event, and on reflection of the event itself, some slightly different responses were prompted—with the emergence of grief, guilt, depression, detachment, and burnout as themes. These are not surprising responses and are consistent with the nature of the work in ICUs.

On guilt, one participant noted:

> *I think there is no... in medical school, nobody is preparing you for this guilt that you are going to feel when you cause mistakes that can cost this other person's life. And some of my mistakes did.*

Feeling guilty is not necessarily pathological, but normal, and in this case where a patient died, appropriate. Hopefully, guilt propels intensivists to examine their work and practices such that mistakes are not repeated. This was consistently reported during the interviews and is discussed at length in other chapters.

Grief has many facets to it. If the death was expected, such as from a serious illness in an aged and frail person, it may be easier to mourn and recover from this type of bereavement; but if it is sudden, as a result of violence such as homicide or a suicide victim, or from a road trauma, or a child, then it may have a much more profound impact on the families and doctors who tried to save these patients, and a more complicated bereavement ensues. If the intensivist and the team believed that they did all they could to save the person's life, but they died anyway, it may go some ways to assuage the grief. However, repeated losses will also compound the experience of grief and sadness. Over time, responses such as depression and detachment to burnout may emerge (these will be explored in the chapter that follows). These are not uncommon outcomes for doctors in the acute period, and there are, unfortunately, no successful "stress-inoculation" programmes to prevent some of these outcomes; but neither are these outcomes inevitable.

Healthcare institutions are now recognising the doctor as a "second victim" when medical errors occur, but the attention has not focused on how to frame post-event learning within a positive, rather than a "coping" or "surviving" framework [5]. Using these traumatic events for learning and professional growth, described as "posttraumatic growth" by Tedeschi and Calhoun, is essential [5]. A study by Plews-Ogan et al. concluded that the path forged by doctors who coped well with an error highlights ripe opportunities for developing infrastructure to facilitate posttraumatic growth and wisdom for clinicians and the organisation emphasising reflection, learning, and making positive changes [6].

Conclusion

A healthy ecology within the ICU would mean that emerging feelings are anticipated and not delayed until an adverse event occurs. Preparation of ICU doctors to acknowledge the emotional aspects of their training and preparation of them to function in the ICU ecological system is essential for the well-being of the intensivist, other team members, patients, and families. Monitoring of early warning signs regularly by all and for all so that early intervention and support are mobilised is essential. Traumatising experiences are inevitable in caring for critically ill patients. The counter-dependent culture which may be a by-product of medical training combined with the unconscious process of internalisation of role models and the wider organisational culture is a contributory factor to the range and depth of emotional responses in intensivists. Finally, there has to be space for a quietening of the minds and of the machines to allow for reflection on the privilege intensivists have of being the last possible barrier to death for some, but not all, of the patients that come through their ICUs.

References

1. Hawryluck L, Styra R. Coping with the psychological impact of medical errors: some practical strategies. ICU Manag Pract. 2022;22(1):1.
2. Hawryluck LA, Espin SL, Garwood KC, Evans CA, Lingard LA. Pulling together and pushing apart: tides of tension in the ICU team. Acad Med. 2002;77(10):S73–6.
3. Myers MF, Gabbard GO. The physician as patient; a clinical handbook for mental health professionals. Washington, DC: American Psychiatric Publishing; 2008.
4. Obholzer A, Roberts VZ, editors. The unconscious at work: individual and organisational stress in the human services. By the members of the Tavistock clinic consulting to institutions workshop. New York, NY: Brunner-Routledge; 2003.
5. Calhoun L, Tedeschi R, editors. Handbook of posttraumatic growth: research and practice. New York, NY: Lawrence Erlbaum Associates; 2006.
6. Plews-Ogan M, Nay N, Owens J, Ardelt M, Shapiro J, Bell S. Wisdom in Medicine: what helps physicians after a medical error? Acad Med. 2016;91(2):233–41.

Eileen Tay is a consultant psychiatrist in Perth, Australia. She is interested in developing further supervision skills for medical practitioners and is currently undertaking additional training in this field of work, as supervision is an increasingly recognised discipline in the helping professions. She has been involved in doctors' health for over 20 years as part of an advisory and treating clinician network. She is also developing comparative psychotherapy education modules for psychiatry trainees.

Janice Sullivan joined the Department of Pediatrics at the University of Louisville in July of 1995. She is a Professor of Paediatrics in the Divisions of Pediatric Critical Care and Clinical & Translational Research. She graduated from the University of Minnesota School of Medicine (1988), completed her Paediatric residency at Arkansas Children's Hospital in (1991), and a fellowship in Paediatric Critical Care and Clinical Pharmacology at Rainbow Babies and Children's Hospital in Cleveland, Ohio (1995). She is board certified in paediatrics, paediatric critical care, and clinical pharmacology. Currently she is the Vice Chair for Research in the Department of Pediatrics. In July 2021, she was appointed Assistant Chief Scientific Officer for Norton Children's Research Institute, the newly integrated paediatric clinical research enterprise between UofL and Norton Healthcare. She also is a co-investigator for the NIH-funded ECHO IDeA State Grant which is primarily dedicated to reaching rural and underserved populations for clinical trials in 5 specific focus areas related to environmental influences on child health. She has over 30 years of research experience which has primarily focused on clinical pharmacology trials for paediatric patients. Her current focus is faculty education and mentoring in clinical research to train the next generation of clinician scientists.

Chapter 16
Baggage and Burnout

Tracey Varker ⓘ**, Courtney Bowd, Rahul Khanna** ⓘ**, and Matthew Anstey** ⓘ

> *When we try to pick out anything by itself, we find it hitched to everything in the universe.*
>
> —*John Muir*

The role of the intensivist is complex and highly demanding. ICUs expose intensivists to a number of stressors than can be both traumatic and distressing. While the job can be exhilarating and rewarding, intensivists are often required to make difficult decisions in a fast-moving environment, manage large numbers of clinically complex patients, and regularly face high patient mortality. This chapter will extend on the previous one, focusing on how intensivists describe feelings of burnout, post-traumatic stress symptoms, and other emotional burdens in response to the stressors and traumas of the ICU, and the weight and emotional impact that these can cause.

T. Varker (✉) · C. Bowd · R. Khanna
Phoenix Australia—Centre for Post-traumatic Mental Health, Department of Psychiatry, University of Melbourne, Melbourne, VIC, Australia
e-mail: tvarker@unimelb.edu.au

M. Anstey
Sir Charles Gairdner Hospital, Perth, WA, Australia

School of Public Health, Curtin University, Perth, WA, Australia

School of Medicine, University of Western Australia, Perth, WA, Australia

Post-traumatic Stress Disorder (PTSD)

Intensivists working in the ICU repeatedly witness patient-related death and trauma and are exposed to the suffering of patients and families, while managing critical medical situations. As such, they are at risk of developing symptoms of post-traumatic stress disorder (PTSD) and burnout. PTSD is a psychiatric disorder which can occur in people who experience or witness a traumatic event [for a detailed explanation of the diagnostic criteria; see the Diagnostic and Statistical Manual of Mental Disorders Fifth Edition [1].

Burnout is a psychological syndrome that occurs in response to chronic stressors on the job. Symptoms of both PTSD and burnout can occur for those in the "helping professions" such as first responders and medical personnel, even though they are often thought of as being impervious to the challenges of their roles.

> *I think that the overall perception is that we are the super-humans that can handle anything and that is something that needs to change. We are all human beings who feel emotions and get burnt out from feeling emotions too much, and we need avenues to express that.*

To be diagnosed with PTSD, a person needs to experience disturbing thoughts and feelings related to the traumatic event, for more than 1 month after the event occurs. There will be many instances where intensivists experience PTSD-type symptoms, which dissipate within 1 month.

> *…I wanted my own therapeutic relationship, and found them [the therapist] to be very good at normalising my experience. I was having very intrusive visual memories. And I just wanted to be sure that I wasn't on the road to PTSD, are there things I should be doing? And I was reassured by my psychologist that totally normal, totally normal time frame, if things are persisting beyond this timeframe, or then, yes you will need further intervention, but a couple of visits and I was reassured that it was all fading away at the right tempo…*

The symptoms of PTSD fall into four categories. The first of these are intrusions, which can include intrusive memories, distressing dreams (or nightmares), or flashbacks of the traumatic event that the person experienced. Intensivists described experiencing such intrusive memories.

> *But went from 'well' to 'dying' very quickly, and left me with intrusive memories, and trips to the psychologist… and… in fact I only got the [official investigation] report a few months ago. And this was a case from four years ago.*

The second category of PTSD symptoms is avoidance, which involves avoiding reminders of traumatic events, such as people, places, or situations. For many intensivists, it is difficult to avoid and to continue doing their job effectively. However, for some, certain aspects of the job cause discomfort and are therefore avoided.

> *Yeah. That's a good question you ask. I couldn't do it. I couldn't do it…. Yes, since I've had my children I don't like it. So, I find… My first specialty was anaesthetics, and I avoid paediatric anaesthetics now as well. I don't like it. I just feel like… I feel like I'd come to work and upset kids and torture them, and see the look on their faces. Even when I walk through recovery with kids crying, I feel like… I feel… I don't like it… And then paediatric ICU, I could never do it. That's why I have deliberately chosen an adult hospital. If something happened in this hospital which needed my assistance, then of course I would help, but I*

generally avoid paediatrics - I don't like it. And more so since I've had my children, I don't like it. Yeah, emotionally I'd find it very upsetting.

The third category of PTSD symptoms is alterations in cognition and mood. These symptoms can include being unable to remember important parts of the traumatic event; negative thoughts or feelings; distorted thoughts about the cause or consequences of the events; feelings of fear, horror, anger, guilt, or shame; having much less interest in activities or people; and being unable to experience positive emotions. An example of negative thoughts or feelings and distorted thoughts about the consequences of events was provided by one intensivist.

I don't think I could change my... How could I change my... I mean that has affected me, and I don't...that's never gonna go, right? I'm not going to be able to cleanse myself or get over that event... There will always be questions about my management in my mind, no matter what other people or colleagues or my wife says, there will always be personal reflections... How do you live with that? You have to try to take, I have to try to take a... an educational experience from the event to improve my response next time.

The fourth category of PTSD symptoms is alterations in arousal and reactivity. This can include being more irritable than usual or having angry outbursts, being overly watchful of your surroundings, being easily startled, or having problems sleeping. Sometimes intensivists may notice some of these types of changes in colleagues.

I think the most... the sign that concerns me the most is that really subtle personality change. In that people who are reasonably friendly and laid back, get a bit short and snappy.

Many intensivists who are exposed to traumatic events experience symptoms similar to those that have been described above in the days that follow the event. However, for a person to be diagnosed with PTSD, the symptoms must last for more than a month and cause significant distress or difficulty with daily function. For some individuals, symptoms may appear a number of months after the traumatic event, and for some, the symptoms can persist for months or even years, particularly if left untreated.

Rumination can also commonly occur in the aftermath of a traumatic event. Rumination is when worrisome thoughts are thought about continuously. An intensivist spoke about having certain cases that stick with them, which they ruminated about, even though it had been some length of time since the traumatic event.

I still carry some of that from that person. I talk about rumination and feelings, so I still carry it. I still carry it.

Another intensivist described the physical feelings that can also occur, when ruminating about a previous case.

So, talking to you about this patient brought me that physical sensation that I get when I ruminate or feel badly about something...'.
Interviewer: 'So you do have some of these [cases] in your filing cabinet that are almost like PTSD events, in that you experience a physical feeling...'
Participant: 'Yes.'
Interviewer: 'Flashbacks? Do you get those?'

Participant: 'I wouldn't necessarily call it a flashback, but it's a physical feeling now, that like bringing that back up and talking about it... I will probably go home today because I'm tired, and ruminate on that case again ... I will probably start thinking about that patient for a couple more days, and then I will put it back in the filing cabinet.

Burnout

In addition to trauma reactions, it is also recognised that some intensivists also suffer from burnout. The International Classification of Diseases 11 [2] defines burnout as a syndrome which arises from chronic workplace stress, which has not been successfully managed.

It is characterised by feelings of energy depletion or exhaustion; increased mental distance from one's job, feelings of negativism, or cynicism related to one's job; and reduced professional efficacy. In the interviews, a number of intensivists recognised the signs of burnout in themselves.

I burnt out pretty bad a couple of years ago. And actually, it was affecting multiple phases of my professional performance...

Interviewer: 'So how did that manifest in that period, if you don't mind me asking?

Participant: 'My commitment, and my participation, my active participation in meetings and projects had diminished greatly; I looked like a depressed person...'

Interviewer: 'Did you see that in yourself, or did someone else see it?'

Participant: 'I do retrospectively. I don't think... I think a number of people were worried about it; no-one really said anything. I think it was because in general we're bad at identifying those things and don't really know how to manage it. I think it's because institutions say they have mechanisms for supporting those things, but our mechanisms were very rudimentary...and honestly, we didn't have the mechanisms.'

The intensivists also spoke about a lack of training and education on how to recognise the signs of PTSD or burnout in themselves, or a colleague.

I haven't had any training to recognise any signs of post-incident stressors. So there should probably be training around that, in how to actually recognise the signs of failure in that regard.

Some spoke about their perceived inability to identify if a colleague was struggling with their mental health more generally.

No. I think it's a very difficult diagnosis to make and I think these terms are often, how can I put it, often used as buzzwords, but we often miss the people who are in that situation. And I think over the years, I have seen people, 'spin out', where I had no idea, no idea and I mean no idea. Like people you'd been dealing with every day, and you think, "What???!" It's quite clear that I do not have the ability or the skills to identify that somebody may be in that zone at all, and the proof is in the pudding.

Despite the lack of training and education, several intensivists spoke about having innate skills for recognising colleagues in distress.

No, not sufficiently trained, no. I don't think there has been, in going through all of my training, and my fellowship trainings, I have not been aware of any training that I have done to recognise burnout or PTSD in myself or anybody else. Having said that, I've got reasonably acute skills, and I can see signs in people... who are...

Interviewer: 'Something else going on?'

Participant: 'Yeah.'

I definitely think that I can feel when somebody is in stress and because we know each other, and we are friends, I think it is a little bit like we are family. We definitely can find some people in stress... Maybe I'm missing people. Maybe some of them will burn out and that's why they are leaving. We don't have physicians leaving, but there are a lot of turnover of nurses. Each of them has their own reason why they want to leave, and why they don't want to come back. Maternity leave, working night shift, and weekends, that's generally the explanation but maybe there is also some burnout of emotions and stress that make them change to a more comfortable area of medicine.

I know it's something [burnout] that I always read about, and always looked into even years and years ago. I remember when the first articles started coming out 20 years ago. So, I think I can recognise it. I know it's there. I think I can see it in other people. I don't consider myself a psychological expert... I think I'm very sensitive to it.

There was also consideration given to ensuring that team members were safe, in regard to their mental health.

With my team, with a junior member, the first thing, I would make sure they are okay. And by that I mean that they've got adequate... that they're not going to do anything silly to themselves as a consequence. Whether that be start calling in sick, or even something worse than that. If we can act on that and try and recognise that in them I think that's number one.

Elaborating on the potentially devastating consequences that severe mental health issues can cause, several intensivists spoke about suicide or suicide attempts.

During my residency we had a resident that tried to commit suicide and another that had an inpatient psychiatric admission.

Another consequence of mental health issues may be the use of substances such as drugs, which was described by one intensivist.

On Facebook there is a physician Mom's group; it has doctors from all over the world; and they say 'Moms' but I think it's gone on to be mostly women physicians; and there was a woman about a year ago who committed suicide as a member of that group; and you know... There are physicians who have used drugs, you hear about that often, and it's normally a coping mechanism. People don't normally use drugs who are healthy...

Relatability

A critical fact that can impact the psychological effect of a traumatic event is the personal significance of what has occurred. Often it is not solely the magnitude of the event but the degree to which a person can relate to the situation, which can have a profound impact on a person's emotional reaction.

This theme was borne out by several intensivists, many of whom commented on the relatability of certain patients.

...she was mid-to-late 20s, attractive, reminded me a lot of my wife... And we worked on her for 12 hours continuously, and that was very.... visceral for me...I think because I sort of related to her as somebody that I knew and cared about, and she died, obviously.

She was my age, and the... I think that she had been lost in the system and mismanaged

Although the personal relatability exemplified above was raised often, the involvement of children was particularly salient. As the following highlights, this is not a moral question but merely a reality of our human nature.

Because you can put yourself in those shoes. It's not to say you can't put yourself or shouldn't, I don't want to say that it is easier to put myself in the shoes of somebody who looks like me, or who acts like me, or who reminds me of my sister; but it is probably true that it is easier to, sort of, relate to people who you think you will be friends with outside of here. For the children of the same age as my niece and nephew, and they look like them. It's harder. So, I can imagine having children and then taking care of a child who is the same age or the same gender as a child you know, and having something bad happen to them, even more challenging.

The relatability can be significant enough that it can potentially influence career decisions. This is particularly prominent in the choice between paediatric versus adult specialisations. Although this self-selection may be useful for those able to exercise it, there are likely others who are too late in their careers to switch easily. This was particularly problematic when the adverse outcome was very unexpected or involved a particularly strong rapport with the family members.

The child died...she was just very close in age to my daughter...almost like within a few days I think, and it was something quite random that she had. It literally was bad luck; anybody could have had it... And somehow, I thought, 'That could be me.' For some reason. I don't know why. The kid didn't look like my daughter or anything, [but]... We had a good rapport with the family, yes, and so sometimes it's something like that; it just triggers something, where you feel, 'Gosh, they're just like me', or 'This could have happened to my child, you know?'

Although most intensivists found parenthood to be a substantial factor in increasing the relatability and hence salience of traumatic events ("Being a parent threw everything for a loop"), there were also some benefits. For example, some found that it increased their empathy, and therefore capacity, as specialist doctors. Others found that having their own (healthy) children helped them cope and served as a distraction and comfort from the distress of work.

In a somewhat reciprocal relationship, the stress of work also made intensivists more grateful for the health of their own family.

I think it helped. I think it helped me to see how distressing it is for a parent to be in that situation. Especially when they're asking 8000 questions about... You know your six-month-old has bronchiolitis, they're gonna be fine in two days; you know, where they are coming from. And just understanding why kids act like they do. I mean we learn that in paediatric training but when you have your own...

I also need some real human contact. Like a hug. A lot of times for me, since I've had a child, it's that I need to go home and hold my child. I need, like, time. It's actually interesting because I'm getting a little bit emotional now just thinking about some of the deaths that I've had, and it's like, I just need to feel my child (emotional sounds).

I think mostly easier. Because I could go home and I knew that they were all healthy. And I just knew that they could snuggle up with me and not say anything...and it was a distraction from the horrible things that are going through your brain.

I'd say the number one most important part is appreciating health. Which has made me, I think, if I was in economics, you go home, and you're like, you know whatever, these are my kids. But I go home, and I see my healthy kids… It's that I see what it is to not have health on a very acute level each and every day. So, I also cherish my family.

Interestingly, the age and hence cumulative life experience of the intensivist often increased the discomfort associated with the practice. One spoke of their ability to remain more detached in their youth.

…When I was younger, I was very detached. You know if a patient died, I wouldn't sort of, I would feel sorry for them, but I wouldn't be upset by it. You know you could say, 'he was an old guy, it's a bit of bad luck'…since I've had my own children… I find myself getting really sad for some people sometimes…

In contrast, experience and age broadened the range of situations and people intensivists felt they could relate to and empathise with. For example:

I think again some of it is how you relate personally. I think sometimes I find it really quite emotional talking to the surviving partner of an old couple who have been together forever because I think how it was for my mother when my father died and she was kind of left. But then someone who's got a teenage child might relates to a situation when you're dealing with a teenager or someone who is just have a baby looking after that. So, I think a lot of it is how we relate to situations and how we put meaning on them from our own personal responses. It's not so much that you can't understand what it's like. I think the ones where you kind of feel more emotionally involved are ways where they trigger something in you and that usually come, again, like a debriefing example I gave, something that comes from within and from your own personal experiences.

Relatability was also a factor in how intensivists viewed their colleagues and the stressors of the ICU environment. When colleagues, whether local or those attracting media attention, faced adverse outcomes, their own vulnerability came to the fore. The case of Dr. Hadiza Bawa-Garba in the UK was specifically brought up as a chilling incident. In this case, a 6-year-old in the UK perished under the care of a trainee who, due to staffing gaps, was covering the job of two other doctors while her own rostered supervising consultant was out of town. The events, occurring in 2011, led to a criminal conviction in 2015 and caused shockwaves in the UK and internationally.

I think most people felt- well that could have been me. You know, that I could have been in that situation where you are working under pressure and you're trying to do the right thing for covering and keeping the system going, when someone is sick. But missing clear clinical signs and then not be able to prioritise properly and not checking results and not getting a chance to get back to doing all those things. So…a kind of horror and alarm that the system in the UK is such that people can potentially get a criminal conviction for that sort of thing.

One coping approach some participants cited was to actively distance themselves emotionally from the clinical encounters. This was a double-edged sword, and intensivists spoke of a spectrum of emotional involvement, hinting at a level of distance that may be counter-productive. Further, as much as this can be an active mitigation strategy, it can be forced by the nature of the environment.

I think there is a spectrum of how… how… emotionally involved you can be with your patients. You can be almost enmeshed in an unhealthy way; and then almost like robotic,

'I'm not gonna get to know this patient or family personally at all.' And I think ... there is for me, the right spot is somewhere in the middle, and there is probably sometimes where I'm probably a little bit more skewed towards the emotionally-protect-myself side and I don't think it compromises my care, but also I feel like if I... like it's influenced by a lot of things. If the unit gets really busy, there's just less time to sit down and talk to families beyond updating them about the medical situation. I try to make it a point to touch base with each family every day... It is not feasible to spend 30 minutes a day.

This distancing from the family can be particularly protective in one sense because it makes it easier to disconnect from the "healthy" version of the patient, reducing relatability.

...if I've never known the child as a healthy child, and I've only seen them on a ventilator, paralysed with pressors running, it is not so upsetting to me if that child dies, because in my mind, I never allowed myself to feel an attachment to that child. But once the family starts crying at the bedside, and their siblings come in and start crying at the bedside, it makes that child human again. That's when I really struggle.

The crux of the challenge then is to bring enough of one's humanity to the work to remain effective yet without getting so close as to get overwhelmed. Developing those parameters for each doctor is a unique and crucial journey and one that may change as one's own circumstances change.

...I think those kind of emotions – empathy, and the humanness of it... That can make you a good doctor, but if it's not in check... [without] having parameters around it, it can make you not a good doctor, because then you become too subjective. I think it's a fine balance of being very objective, looking very concretely at different things, yet having the human piece, and I think the same thing is true when there is a death that occurs. You deal with it, it's done, you have 20 other patients that you have to deal with, and your emotions are whatever it is, they cannot affect your judgement; they cannot affect your work.

Salience of Bad Outcomes

One of the challenges faced by intensivists is memories of traumatic events. This is unsurprising, as across a broad range of psychological processes, bad memories, events, and outcomes have been shown to be more powerful than their positive counterparts [3].

In some circumstances these memories of bad outcomes can be recalled with ease by intensivists and are often as part of a conscious choice to remember a particular patient or situation where clinically relevant to do so. However, as previously discussed intensivists can also experience these memories as intrusions, or "flashbacks" to past patients and situations. They may ruminate over decisions made in the past and reflect on moments where they feel they failed to act. In these situations, the memories have the potential to cause distress many years after the event itself.

But we all have a case that we remember that causes a lot of trauma....

When describing memories of bad outcomes, intensivists used various analogies, such that they stored these memories in a "filing cabinet" or a "room" that they could leave and come back to. This implied a sense of control, in terms of being able to actively recall memories of patients.

> *Participant: 'The filing cabinet is definitely there. You can say this, and I can open the drawer and I can tell you this person, and what room they were in, and who the nurse was; it's a very strange... I may not be able to remember something that you would think is simple.'*
>
> *Interviewer: 'So when you remember the name, the room number and the nurse... That suggests to me that you are visualising it? Do you actually have flashbacks to events, of exactly what it looked like?*
>
> *Participant: 'Yeah, I can see, even back to early in my training - like I was telling a nurse right before I walked over here - I remember the first day of my intern year; I was in room 19; and this was the nurse; this is what happened; the patient's name; the patient's diagnosis... '*
>
> *Interviewer: 'And this is your filing cabinet? This isn't a burden? '*
>
> *Participant: 'Yeah, this is my filing cabinet. There are very few that I think of as true burdens.'*

Compartmentalisation of emotion and thinking was a common theme:

> *But then I realised, no, it's that I compartmentalise, and I'm capable of visiting the room, and then leaving the room.*

Typically, these memories were seen as having educational value, which was often given as the reason why they stayed with the intensivist, so that if faced with similar circumstances they would recall these memories to make informed choices on the best course of action.

> *Participant: 'I mean there are things that stick with you, obviously. I don't think I look at it from the perspective of carrying it around with me as a burden per se. But I guess I do try to figure out, you know, this happened at this time with this, maybe if that exact same circumstance popped up again, I would look at it from a slightly different perspective. So I guess I use that bag or filing cabinet that you are talking about to see if I can change things going forward. I don't know if I ever really look at those things as a burden, or something I'm lugging around. I take it, I process it, and I use it going forward. I could probably pull those kinds of patients up for you, but I guess I don't go back and say, 'Look, if only...'*
>
> *Interviewer: 'If you could pull those patients up do they bring back emotion?'*
>
> *Participant: 'It's much more clinical for me.'.*

For some intensivists, this conceptualisation of bad memories in a "filing cabinet" for educational purposes extended to a list of patients they wish they had a second chance at treating, with the benefit of more years of experience and hindsight.

> *I mean I certainly have my list of patients that I typically remember the name, the bed number they were in, a lot of times the date, whenever something happened. Not all of them died, but whoever taught me something in a somewhat painful way, if you will. But something that stays with me. Certainly I do carry that. But the other group I would say, for me, I wouldn't call it a burden, but I have a short list of 'I wish I could have again to redo.' You know, 'I*

wish I could have a crack at these kids again, knowing what I know now.' It's not very long but I do have my 'I wish I could have another chance' list.

Not all intensivists, however, viewed the memories as being so easy to set aside. Some memories were seen as burdensome, and intensivists described these as ones they carried "in their bag", implying that even after many years they still held emotional weight and salience.

…she has a better prognosis, because I still have her [medical unit] number, and I'm looking at my computer, and I am watching her [progress], and it was something like two years ago, this event and she is still in treatment… But yes, I am carrying this. Emotionally, it is a bag that you carry on your shoulders.

… I think as I am going up in the hierarchy I am carrying a bigger bag… I carry the bags of the mistakes that my Fellows are doing. And if he does a mistake, I take it upon my responsibility, so it's a bigger bag I carry I think.

The passing of time appeared to have an impact, with memories of some bad outcomes being moved to the "filing cabinet" and becoming less burdensome as time passed, while more recent bad outcomes took their place in "the bag".

I think I have both of those. And then sometimes I think I have to empty out the bag and put them into the filing cabinet.
I think time sometimes heals, but new things get put into the bag for different reasons.
Sure. I think it's the same weight. Because I trade some heaviness… I might develop new heavy things but let go of some previous heavy things.

Under What Circumstances Do Bad Outcomes Imprint?

There are a number of different factors that appear to impact the likelihood of an intensivist remembering particular past patients and scenarios for which there was an adverse outcome. More broadly these factors can be thought of as factors external to the intensivist and factors related more directly to the individual. As previously discussed, relatability is a key factor in influencing whether an individual is emotionally impacted by a traumatic event.

I look back on my career and there are certain memorable patients that will forever be indwelled in my brain. And some of them because of the sort of lack of clarity about what happened; some of them because I feel like I had to do with the negative outcome; some of them because they were just utterly tragic.

When considering external factors, intensivists tended to describe situations that felt ambiguous or unexplained, where they feel as though they were let down by others or being placed in a situation where they were underprepared or resourced, as leading to memories imprinting or becoming more salient. Intensivists also spoke about the significant impact that witnessing the profound grief of the parent whose child had died.

I remember a 16-year-old who had been in an accident, a traffic accident, and died. And it wasn't the child's death that was so profoundly impactful, it was the mother's grief that was more impactful. It was her sobbing, you know 'How do I go on; what do I do; and where do I go?' And the days that she had been in the hospital, she confided in me, 'Am I going crazy? I wear his clothes; I want to smell his smell; I'm not going to ever change the linens on his bed' like all of these things… and that type of loss; recognising that the families are going home to laundry baskets, and to toys and to dreams that have just all of a sudden, been ended. That for me, has always been the saddest. It's not that children with chronic complex illnesses have deaths that are any worse, or not. It's just it's impacted me differently. I remember almost every child that's ever died on my watch. I have a recollection of the parent, or the event, or a part of the story.

The ability of intensivists to more clearly remember events that involved the death of a child can be further compounded when relatability is also high, with intensivists who are also parents reporting that these events are likely to stay with them when the child involved is a similar age to their own, or the situation causes them to reflect that as a parent they can potentially be placed in a similar circumstance due to an accident or illness.

One of them was not an adverse event or anything. The child died, but it was not because of error it was because of the degree of illness, not human failure, but she was just very close in age to my daughter. It literally was bad luck; anybody could have had it… And somehow I thought, 'That could be me.' For some reason. I don't know why. The kid didn't look like my daughter or anything, but there was something… I don't really know.

Another type of scenario that can be easily recalled by intensivists is when they felt they were let down by others or that they were placed in a difficult situation where patients experienced negative outcomes unnecessarily as a result. Exposure to such situations also has the potential to place intensivists at risk for moral injury. Moral injury is when one transgresses, or witnesses another transgress, deeply held morals or values and experiences enduring harms to psychological, social, and spiritual health as a result [4].

Participant: 'I remember two patients that I lost when I was a first-year fellow. Basically because I had no business taking care of these patients myself. I lost them; I couldn't save them; because I was vastly undertrained, vastly under supervised, vastly undereducated, and I should never have been asked to do that. Nowadays I could have saved both of them, and in the modern era I would not have been under-supervised.

Interviewer: 'You are obviously well down the line now… but those two cases are still easy to recall.'

Participant: 'Yes. It was unacceptable. Those patients didn't need to die. And those experiences make an impression'

There is a point at which, for some, imprinted memories can impact functioning and become more intrusive and burdensome. For example, memories of situations, where the patients' condition rapidly deteriorated, can result in PTSD symptoms such as intrusions.

Factors internal to the intensivist can also determine whether an adverse outcome is easily remembered. Where there are feelings of guilt surrounding their actions or inaction, this increases the salience of the memories.

I have a few patients that I still carry with me on my back. Because I felt guilty, including this patient. I don't have to look too much to remember him.

He died of sepsis that day. And I remember his name; I remember his family; I remember crying, and saying, 'I'm so sorry, this is all my fault'. I remember them saying, 'it's not your fault, it's not your fault'. But it was. It was my responsibility - it was the bacteria's fault. But it was my responsibility. And if I had managed his line better, he might be alive.

The amount of work experience an intensivist has had also appears to impact the ways in which they look upon these memories. With further experience, negative outcomes are often remembered from the perspective of wishing they had a second chance at the situation. However, it appears that there is a complex relationship between feelings of guilt and level of experience, often leading to rumination as to whether with further experience, or if the intensivists had known then what they know now, the outcomes would differ.

I have a couple of them. I didn't recognise something I should have recognised... And maybe that was some experience. Or I didn't get an intubation in on the patient and the patient died... Horrible it's just horrible and I'll never forget that... And I think like with a little bit more experience and a calmer head, maybe it would have been different, or I could have... I dunno...

The Impacts of Bad Outcomes Imprinted

When bad outcomes imprint, intensivists don't always perceive these memories as negative. In fact, the majority of those interviewed noted that there were educational benefits to remembering these particular patients, such as making them better doctors moving forward or that when presented with a similar situation in the future, they would make a more informed decision.

I feel like the ones where I felt like I could have done something different, hopefully I use those as a teaching experience for myself. In my life these days, I really tried to think about what I gain when I see tragedy in others, and a lot of times it's just gratitude for my own personal life. I don't know if you consider that a burden. I don't think I hold onto that in a way that holds me back. I don't think I think about so-and-so died and you know I'm not thinking now about the fact that so-and-so died and that was a terrible tragic incident. I don't think those things linger in my mind. I think the ones that linger are the ones where you sort of wish you could have done something differently, and then I hold them as a lesson.

It's a part of my experience and who I am. Because any death or survival story makes you better; it helps you grow; it helps with your experiences. If there is a bad outcome, and it's something you feel that you could have done differently, you can say, 'Well next time, I'll will do this differently for this next patient' because I don't want anybody's death that could have been prevented (to be) in vain. That's my thoughts on it. I don't really feel like it's a burden, because gosh, if it's a burden, then we've had a lot of bad outcomes and even the ones that are, it's unfortunate, but you have to reconcile it in some way, or you can't continue doing what you're doing. And it can't always be bad. Sometimes it's bad, 'Yes that was horrible, yes that sucked,' but did we do everything or not? And if we realise that we could have done something differently, we remember that, and we talk about those stories and we say, you know, 'There's that one time that this happened...' It changes your life; it changes the way you practice medicine.

Yep, so... Yeah there's a handful there. A few of those that are very impactful.

> *And I think… you know you can…so how do you deal with that? I guess I've had some very formative experiences where I've talked to other intensivists and said, 'What would you have done differently?' And those are important. I've had people say, 'You know, you're always going to remember this, but you always have to say, 'What can I learn from this, how can I be a better doctor?'*

For some, viewing these memories as educational was linked to the reason why these memories were imprinted. Others, however, found the memories difficult and often seemed to use the educational value of the memories as a coping mechanism to pull themselves from rumination or as an effort to look for a "silver lining" from the negative experience.

> *It's still… probably less so now, but for the first few years I remembered that case pretty vividly and kept… I've got his name on my computer still, if I need to go back and remind myself, you know to do things… In terms of trying to see that as somewhat of a positive thing. I guess I envisage one day even sending a message to his wife and saying like, 'I'm sorry that happened but these are some of the things that we are doing.'*

It was unclear, for the intensivists that were interviewed, whether the coping strategy of seeing difficult situations as a learning opportunity was taught or learned on the job. Increasingly, however, intensivists are being taught skills in dealing with such difficult situations as part of their training. For the intensivists that we interviewed, the ability to use memories of bad outcomes was seen as crucial for performing and succeeding in the role.

> *She one time said, 'I think I'd better see a counsellor, for all the dead kids I carry around with me every day,' which is a horribly morbid thing to say, but we shoulder responsibility, and we see children die every week of our lives. And that is a lot. You have to find ways to cope or you can't do this job well.*

For some intensivists, however, memories of previous bad outcomes had a detrimental impact causing the intensivist to second-guess their decision-making or causing feelings of emotional discomfort and strain many years after the event.

> *I think it's changed over the course of my… not terribly long career. I think that I had, within the span of a few years, had a handful of events that were definitely adverse patient events that I felt directly responsible for in some form or fashion… I was actually talking about this this past week with somebody… That sort of hangs over you, and they can be deleterious because it can sort of like… you can second-guess yourself … you don't want to make a mistake again…*

> *… 'This went poorly last time, I hope I don't screw this up again.' And they can be… it never got to the point where it was paralysing, but it definitely has a lot of emotional strain that comes back.*

As described earlier in this chapter, for some, these feelings of distress move to levels where they become symptoms of disorder and impair the intensivists' functioning.

Sharing Emotions

Intensive care clinicians are frequently faced with emotionally difficult situations: dealing with their own reactions to patients' illnesses, breaking news to grieving families, and navigating fractured family dynamics.

On the one hand, some intensivists describe this as:

a rewarding part of the job because you have the opportunity to meet people at this awful time for them and make a positive difference.

On the other hand, some intensivists may be cautious about the amount of emotional energy they give to their patients and the work that they do.

Because if one situation completely overwhelms you, you have nothing left for the next patient or the next shift or even worse, you have nothing left for your own family.

In our interviews, an emerging theme was the sharing of emotions and whether intensivists thought it acceptable to cry or be emotional with a patient or their family. It begs questions such as whether the intensivist is protecting themselves by not crying, whether they are protecting the patients and families, and what would be the "correct" response.

Emotional intelligence, the awareness of and ability to communicate emotions is a skill. In a way, emotions are a form of data to be observed, interpreted, and responded to. But they are liable to be misinterpreted, and there is no formula for the "right response". Sharing emotions may show families and patients that their doctor is caring for them.

I am not afraid to show my emotion. But at the same time, I do hold it in check in the sense that I am acutely aware that this is a moment that is for them; they are grieving; and if I feel the grief and I shed a tear, then I shed a tear.

In other circumstances it can be an instinctive personal response on the part of the intensivist, who is a caregiver and who is also intellectually and emotionally involved in the situation.

but I have [cried] many times… because it's personal for them but it's also personal for me, as their doctor I think in a way. Because I…. I put just as much into it, not just with my cognition, but also with my emotions.

Experiencing such emotion may cause the intensivists to feel self-aware, as if they are distracting from the "real" victims.

I'm cognizant that I don't want it to be like, 'Oh, they've got to take care of the doctor!' But I don't feel like it's like, 'Oh God, go hide your tears!'… I think it's important to show them.

Within such emotional reactions, distinctions can be made between empathy and caring. The focus of empathy is the specialist doctor's emotions, while caring can be considered the optimal emotional and behavioural response to the patient's needs [5]. Within this conceptualisation is the acknowledgement that it is not necessarily the outward emotional response that is defining the appropriate reaction to a grieving family or a difficult situation. Weiner and Auster [5] describe caring as a sustained, emotional investment in an individual's well-being, characterised by a desire to take actions that will benefit that person.

Our interviews revealed that paediatric intensivists appear to find themselves entangled in more emotional situations, with the rawness of the emotions of the parents and the fragility and innocence of the children involved.

> To this family the death of a child is new to them. You have been in that scenario 20 or 30 or 40 or 100 times. You cannot absolve yourself of the responsibility of (being) their guide. Which means you have to have a destination, and that means that in some way or another you have to guide them even as you read them. You could argue that that is inherently paternalistic. If you go into every encounter with no agenda, and no direction, and you are just like a passive guide for which the family is going to take you on, you are going to struggle, I tell you right now. You absolutely have to learn when and how that journey needs to be shaped, and not too much, and not too little, and it takes a lot of practice.

> If I'm delivering bad news for instance, I need to keep my emotions in check enough that I can deliver that news in a succinct way, that conveys information across, and allows them to have all of the information they need to make whatever decision they need to. But at the same time, I have to give them my... if they ask for it, what I feel from my experience having seen the spectrum of kids who have gone through it for instance... So, while I'm sad and I may shed a tear or two, it always has to be in check so that it is never to the point where I can't even talk because I'm too sad.

> They will have the memory of ... another Dad, another Mom. And then I think they definitely appreciate and are soothed by the compassion that a tear shows.

The intensivists are, however, aware and cautious about their own personal reactions.

> And I've actually felt guilty for doing that. And forcing parents to in a way, care for me. For them to see me suffering with them I think might be an emotional burden that I don't want to burden them even further.... I've never asked a parent if my emotions made them feel one way or another. But I would be curious to know actually.

As has been noted in the academic literature, caring for others is not without cost to the clinician.

The responses from the intensivists show a high degree of self-awareness and emotional burden. On the other hand, awareness of these situations can be a starting point for personal growth and engagement in self-care strategies for the intensivists.

Conclusion

As this chapter has highlighted, while there are many rewarding aspects to the role, intensivists also face significant occupational stressors and challenges. Our interviews have highlighted that symptoms of PTSD and burnout can be common and that there are some outcomes that are more likely to hold emotional weight than others. Overall, while these stressors and challenges may not always lead to a diagnosable mental health condition such as PTSD, there are clear impacts on the mental health and well-being of intensivists, highlighting the need for appropriate support for ICU professionals.

References

1. American Psychiatric Association. Diagnostic and statistical manual of mental disorders. DSM-5. Washington, DC. American Psychiatric Press; 2013.
2. World Health Organization. International classification of diseases for mortality and morbidity statistics (11th revision). 2018. https://www.who.int/standards/classifications/classification-of-diseases.
3. Baumeister RF, Bratslavsky E, Finkenauer C, Vohs KD. Bad is stronger than good. Rev Gen Psychol. 2001;5(4):323–70.
4. Litz BT, Stein N, Delaney E, et al. Moral injury and moral repair in war veterans: a preliminary model and intervention strategy. Clin Psychol Rev. 2009;29(8):695–706.
5. Weiner SJ, Auster S. From empathy to caring: defining the ideal approach to a healing relationship. Yale J Biol Med. 2007;80(3):123–30.

Tracey Varker is a senior research fellow in the Department of Psychiatry, University of Melbourne, and Phoenix Australia—Centre for Post-traumatic Mental Health. Dr Varker leads a team of researchers who focus on improving the lives of those affected by occupational trauma and stress. This includes emergency services and military personnel, healthcare professionals, and those working in heavy industry (e.g. mining and construction). Her research interests centre on improving the lives of those impacted by occupational trauma and stress; using evidence synthesis to promote the recovery of those affected by trauma; and improving our understanding of, and the treatment of, problematic anger.

Courtney Bowd completed her undergraduate degree at the University of Queensland and has recently completed the Master of Public and Social Policy at the Macquarie University, Sydney, Australia. She is currently a policy specialist at Phoenix Australia—Centre for Post-traumatic Mental Health in Melbourne, Australia, where she works across a range of knowledge translation, training, and policy review projects, with a particular focus on supporting disaster impacted communities, emergency service personnel, and the professionals who support them. Prior to joining Phoenix Australia, Courtney worked as a change management consultant for a professional services firm.

Rahul Khanna is a practicing psychiatrist at the Austin Health's Psychological Trauma Recovery Service and serves as Director, Innovation & Medical Governance, at Phoenix Australia—Centre for Post-traumatic Mental Health, based in Melbourne, Australia. He is a senior lecturer at the University of Melbourne and has a deep clinical and research interest in psychological trauma, particularly in leveraging novel technologies to enhance our understanding and treatment of trauma-related mental health conditions. Further background and contact details are available on https://rahul.au.

Matthew Anstey is an intensivist and researcher at Sir Charles Gairdner Hospital, Curtin University, and University of Western Australia in Perth. He has a Master of Public Health from Harvard University, and was the 2010-11 Harkness Fellow in Health Policy, based at Kaiser Permanente in California. He was the past chair of Choosing Wisely Australia advisory group. His research interests focus on improving outcomes for ICU survivors (and built the survivors website mylifeaftericu.com) and improving the quality of care received by patients.

Chapter 17
Making Things Better

Sigal Sviri, Mary Pinder, Z. Leah Harris, and Michael Ruppe

> *No one is useless in this world who lightens the burden of it to anyone else.*
>
> —*Charles Dickens*

In this chapter we describe some of the mitigating factors that can alleviate the stress and burden in the ICU environment. These factors relate to the cultural environment and leadership, to the personal and organizational approach to adverse events and errors, to the strength of the interprofessional team, to the impact of the interaction with patient relatives, and to the importance of developing non-clinical activities.

S. Sviri (✉)
Medical Intensive Care, Hadassah Medical Center and Faculty of Medicine, Hebrew University, Jerusalem, Israel
e-mail: Sigals1@hadassah.org.il

M. Pinder
Department of Intensive Care, Sir Charles Gairdner Hospital, Perth, WA, Australia

Z. L. Harris
The University of Texas at Austin and Dell Children's Medical Center, Austin, TX, USA

M. Ruppe
Division of Critical Care, Department of Pediatrics, University of Louisville, and Norton Children's Medical Group, Louisville, KY, USA

© The Author(s), under exclusive license to Springer Nature Switzerland AG 2023
D. Dennis et al. (eds.), *Stories from ICU Doctors*,
https://doi.org/10.1007/978-3-031-32401-7_17

151

Leadership, Mentorship, and Culture

As we have discussed in Chapter 11, in any stressful working environment, it is essential for the ICU team to have a leader: someone with a vision who creates a safe atmosphere. Leadership styles vary and are more like personality traits: different scenarios call for different approaches. Some scenarios may be more charismatic and self-empowering, and others may be more attentive and encourage collective decision-making. The leader teaches team members to strive to be better clinicians, encourages creativity, celebrates accomplishments, and supports the team through difficult times. Gone are the days where the leader was perceived as single handedly possessing all the abilities to lead all the time. As emphasized in Chapter 9, teams thrive when this responsibility is shared. As we moved towards shift work in the ICU, we recognized that the "leader" is usually the most senior intensivist in the unit at the time and that this role should be supported by a myriad of professionals including nurses, pharmacists, physiotherapists, social workers, chaplain, and security. The presence of visible or detectable leadership can thus mitigate the emotional stressors of team members:

> One of them was very charismatic, maybe egocentric, but the good thing was he was the leader. He wanted to make the unit a very good unit. He wanted it to be special. He wanted it to be the best. He brought in new things, and that taught me that you really have to believe that your unit is the best, and you have to make everybody else believe it, then they will follow you. They will want to work with you. They want to be with you. So that's one type of leader… its addictive, everyone wants to be like that.

> The other leaders were more holistic in the way they look to other people. They gave you respect and gave you place, and they were generous. He listened to what you thought. You weren't always wrong, and he wasn't always right, and there was a group discussion which was also important.

Mentoring is also an important aid to intensivists and nurses both clinically and academically. Mentorship can assist in improving productivity, job satisfaction, and reducing burden, and can also enhance academic development [1]. A mentor should be chosen for their ability to help a person develop one's career over time and should be someone that sees the potential for one's career development.

> You always need a mentor, like someone to go to when you don't know what to do in a stressful situation.

The culture of the workplace environment can influence the way intensivists experience failure and disappointment. A supportive culture is essential to mitigate frustration and negative experiences following untoward outcomes and mistakes. A safe and supportive culture acknowledges that we learn best from the times we fail to meet our ambition and that we all fail at something every day. Failure is not the opposite of success: the person who fails went into that experience wanting to succeed but didn't. Not even trying—mediocrity or indifference—is the opposite of success and will destroy an ICU culture quickly.

> *To me, so much comes down to the culture though. So, I'd like to think that as an everyday thing I try to contribute to a culture in which it is safe to work, that we are happy to speak to each other, that we strive to do the best we can, we also try to acknowledge and identify our own areas of weakness, and feel safe to talk to our colleagues and discuss things... The way I would like to contribute to the culture, is to be here, talk, to be open, to acknowledge my own mistakes, be sceptical of myself, be sceptical of others, but in a serious sort of way, so that we know we are fallible, we know we make mistakes, and we have to keep a constant eye out for ourselves and for our colleagues.*

Working as a group and not as individuals provides informal support, especially in times of crisis.

> *I think the culture of our ICU is very supportive in terms of the debriefing and in informally supporting each other. Like the group of Consultants. It is very usual for us to talk about cases and get second opinions in all sorts of scenarios, so I actually think that that environment provides informal support.*

Learning from Error

An important aspect of progress and professional development in the ICU is learning from mistakes and errors. This can be a personal process but more importantly should be a part of the teamwork culture, to enhance our understanding of what went wrong and how we can improve our practices. The ICU environment should be constructively critical and also encourage learning from mistakes, having joint open discussions, and internalizing conclusions for future improvement and prevention [2].

> *I think we try to learn from each other. You should not only think about what you did wrong, but also think about how you can fix it and how you can prevent it next time. We discuss it, we remember it, we raise it, once in a while, and we tell people about the mistakes, because they can also learn from others' experiences. I think that the fact that we are trying to learn helps us professionally. So, we try to change something in our practice that would make us feel that we learnt something from this event. Because if you don't learn anything from an event, it's like a disaster.*

> *The seniors had a meeting, I think it was once a month, to discuss all of the patients who had died and complications that had happened in the unit, to try to learn from them... And it was an in-house meeting, not pointing fingers, to try to learn from that. I think the most helpful thing is that the parties who were involved need to sit together, and discuss what happened, why it happened and come up with a solution as to how it's not going to happen again.... So, I think the point of stopping, and the parties involved need to sit down in a calm manner, discuss what happened and plan for the future.*

An essential part of learning from adverse events is not only the willingness to discuss them, but also being prepared to delve into the processes that led to these events and to find specific and systematic or organizational changes that can prevent the next error from happening. Implementing training programs for coping with adverse events and providing support for the team are also important [3].

We need to understand where the error was and what the event was, so that we can have a collective unified mental model of what the problem is and how to reverse it. If you know what the problem is, then you can devise a solution that's specific to that problem, which is high yielding.

In those situations, the child died, the IV infiltrated, or the child fell out of bed, 'What are you going to do to make sure this never happens to another child?' You hear that question from families over and over again. And I think one of the reasons why that's such a useful learning mechanism for my trainees, it's important that we tell them, 'You learn something from this', because if you can learn how to figure out what you're learning from something, you're going to be able to answer that question that families are going to ask you. 'What did you do?' …. 'What are you doing to make sure this doesn't happen again?' And you can only answer that question if you've learned something from the event.

Errors can sometimes act as catalysts for incorporating new technologies and improving standards, such as checklists and guidelines.

The analogy of singing off the same hymnbook of basics is very good for ensuring that the team has a basic team framework. Professionally, having seen a lot of clinical incidents, I think some teams are much more willing to implement and promote checklists and use them rather than making people feel like they're being talked down to. So that's been something that I have implemented and am more willingly engaged with rather than seeing it as an insult to my knowledge and confidence.

In seeking a profound understanding of the processes that led to our mistakes, allowing open and transparent discussions, and finding preventive measures for the future, we can turn mistakes into a positive experience and as a platform for professional growth, both personally and collectively.

Care over Outcome

It is also important to differentiate between patient outcome and level of care. Doctors and families usually strive for the best patient outcome, but the level of care is not less important. Knowing we have offered the best appropriate care available, even if the outcome is not as good as expected, can alleviate some of the burden for both healthcare intensivists and families.

I used to run the transport program. We have a very large community group that meets with transport quarterly. It's really the community because when the hospital was built it was the first heliport that was put into the center of the city… And so, the idea of having this whirly bird come down and make noise…. And one of the metrics they wanted to know, was how many transports we did. But then they also wanted to know how many of those children died… And I refused to tell them that. Because I said to them it doesn't matter if they live or die; it matters to their families; it matters to their caregivers; but you can do everything right, and use all of the resources; and be the right place for that child to have come; you can put them on dialysis; you can put them on ECMO; you can get them an organ; and you can do all of those things that make us so special; and still have the child die. I can't promise anybody an outcome. But I can promise you that the children in on my watch are going to get world-class care. That's a very different promise and commitment.

Patient Families: Grace and Privilege

Interaction with patients' families can be highly stressful and also immensely rewarding, contributing to job satisfaction. The stress often stems from the burden of relaying bad news about the patient's prognosis; the responsibility of open disclosure following adverse events; and the emotional toll of confronting a family's grief response which may take the form of anger and aggression towards the treating team. Study participants recognized that critical illness in a family member imposes a strain on family dynamics and this is exacerbated in families with pre-existing intra-familial relationship problems.

> *…dealing with families in adverse events is both enriching, and inspiring, and immensely frustrating and it depends on the family… I think you have extraordinarily caring, nurturing and reasonable families that you admire and deal with. And you think, 'Wow, this was a bunch of really united people caring for each other, working as a unit, and caring about the patient, wanting the best, and understanding the difficulties of what we do.' Or, you have a dysfunctional family who, well beyond whatever it is that you do or say, are already in full-blown intra-family conflict, where an adverse event then becomes actually a tool for enlarged and more aggressive intra-family conflict. But I have never been in a situation where a family member has been aggressive to me, because of a mistake or something that happened to the patient.*

The emotional burden of family interactions is mitigated by knowing that the family acknowledges and values the work of the treating team in caring for their family member. This also serves as feedback for the intensivist on their professionalism [4]. While a difficult family often makes communication more stressful, this is a family that requires overcommunication. Central to most difficulties is a lack of trust or sense that elements of care are being hidden. Avoiding conversations with difficult families only magnifies these issues. To mitigate stress in these situations, find someone that has a trusting relationship with the family and partner with them.

> *…when that process has gone well, and the family tells me it has gone well, whether it's because that's the way I perceive it, or the way others perceive it, it's very professionally satisfying, and personally satisfying. Because it makes me remember that if I didn't get the sense of personal satisfaction, it probably means that I've become a little bit too cold-hearted to be effective at doing this job.*

> *…people are usually appreciative of everything that you have done, because they have seen that you have been doing a lot of things, even if something went wrong. They've seen that you have been there, you have been doing a lot of things, you've been talking to them, and all those sorts of things so I think from a positive point of view, the families feel that you have contributed, you have helped in some way…We are used to talking to them and*

explaining things in a way that they can understand. So, I think that that is a rewarding thing, where you can helpfully explain what has gone on, even if it's not what everyone wanted...

It is nice that they recognise that we did our best. And that is... that makes some of these children that I carry probably easier. That you have that memory.

Study participants also reported on the positive impact of the sense of having managed a challenging situation well.

The communication with the family I usually do myself because I never know what the communication has been like with other physicians. 'What is the information that they transfer?' I prefer to take it on myself. It took a while before I became better at that. I think at the beginning I can remember some mistakes. But in the last few years I think I communicate well with the families. We usually end up being friends and hugging, but sometimes it's challenging, especially when the situation is not optimal.

Open disclosure relating to adverse events is particularly stressful but can be made a positive experience through helping families understand the process and come to terms with what has happened.

On a positive note, trying to either reassure them that we have identified that this has been a system error, that we are going to look at this, or even directing them towards a patient representative, or even saying that they ask really good questions, it's really important I think that if there are questions, you deserve an answer to. 'It may not be the right time now to get them, but maybe in a couple of months' time, once the dust settles down, you come back and you speak to us.' That type of thing, has generally been quite productive with the families in that I'll try to help them to get through this ... I've given them something positive...

It's not about me, it's trying to help them get over it. What things can be put in place, 'This has happened, we're really sorry it happened, and this is the reason why we think it's happened', and then putting things in place to help them come to terms with it. Because no one is ever expecting that conversation, when you sit down, and say, 'we've harmed your loved one'.

There was also appreciation and humility in recognizing that, as intensivists, we are sharing in an important moment of the patient's life, and that of their family, and seeing this as a privilege. This in turn gives value and meaning to our own lived experiences.

Trying to prepare the family; building rapport; demonstrating to them that I'm doing everything I can for their child; and helping them to see that, even with all of the things that we are doing for them, it may not be enough. You know it's such a privilege of our jobs to walk a family through the death of their child.

I think one of the great privileges of medicine for me has been... I think it's made me more humble and empathetic than I would have been had I been in a different profession. It's a privilege to be invited to be part of another person's narrative during a very stark time. And that has enhanced my appreciation for my own experiences in my own life. And who knows, it's a fool's game to say, Boy if I had been a journalist or a musician or something, I might have ended up the same person or I might have ended up kind of selfish. You think you have troubles, you want to see troubles? I can show you people's troubles!

...adult ICUs do a lot with just the individuals, where we [in the PICU] are really dealing with the whole family. And that changes your dynamics enormously. Because you get to think about, 'this is a terrible situation, but if I do this well, I leave the family with grace and dignity?' And I don't want anyone else to do that, but me, with them. So it's viewed more as an honour. This is a privilege; this is a privilege to serve.

The participants expressed astonishment at the graciousness of family members in showing their appreciation of the intensive care team even when their loved one had a poor health outcome.

The graciousness that families can offer to whole teams in thanking them... And that is more about when they have seen the best of care, and still have adverse outcomes, rather than an adverse event. It amazes me how gracious people can be even after terrible situations. I work in [organ and tissue] donation, where 100% of our patients are dead. Many of whom through their own misadventure, and many through iatrogenic or under-recognised things. The graciousness of families to think of others, is amazing.

The stress of dealing with dying patients and families is also eased by facilitating the patient's death with dignity and without pain, and in respecting their wishes.

We think about our lives as Intensivists as being focused on saving lives; sometimes it is; but - and I have learned this over the course of time - there is a part of us that needs to be a palliative care physician as well, because that is part of critical care.

He said 'I want to die, and I've had enough; this is enough for me'. And his family were all on board... but at the end of it, when you went through it all - when you sat down with him through it all - the outcome was that he died fairly quickly, but comfortably. And the family, after initially being quite upset, were very thankful and appreciated all of the help from the ICU and actually came back later just to say thank you.

Sharing information in family conversations with empathy and honesty is integral to the role of the intensivist. These conversations can be a source of significant stress, particularly in the setting of a dying patient or an adverse clinical event, and the emotional burden is alleviated by finding meaning in the experience, a key step in preventing burnout [5]. Mitigating strategies for stress include receiving words of thanks and appreciation from family members; facilitating "a good death" for the patient; and, importantly, feeling privileged and humbled to be sharing such an important moment in the lives of others, in turn giving value and a sense of purpose for our own.

Other Endeavours Outside of Usual Workspace

An intensivist's sustainability in the face of chronic high stress and high investment of emotional capital is a well-appreciated cause of career dissatisfaction and burnout. Adopting strategies to address this aspect of the career is therefore essential to sustain a successful career.

Three approaches are frequently taken to counteract the detrimental effect of the emotional overload common to the intensivist: emotional escapism, non-clinical professional activities, and rejuvenating philanthropy.

Escapism

Emotional escapism for the intensivist has characteristics that overlap with many other professions. Healthy as well as unhealthy "endeavours" can rebalance an intensivist's mind and provide emotional sustainability. This can manifest itself as a powerful need to exercise, indulge in vices such as shopping or alcohol use, or perpetually plan leisure activities such as exotic travel. While these activities are often controlled and can fit into the lifestyle that being an intensivist affords, they frequently become necessary crutches to support the emotional burden of the career.

Non-clinical Activity

Non-clinical professional activity is typically a huge piece of an intensivist's career and underappreciated for its value in balancing the emotional weight associated with clinical care. These activities can be categorized into several large groups including administrative roles, research, education, and clinical development [6].

Concurrent with a clinical career, intensivists can pursue a number of administrative responsibilities. Common examples of these positions include quality and safety officer, ICU medical director, division chief, transport team director, and simulation director. Intensivists are regularly members of hospital committees and serve vital roles in shaping policies and providing oversight for hospital-wide initiatives. It is the intensivists' understanding of hospital operations through their interactions with the emergency room, operating room, hospital wards, ICU floor, and outside hospitals that make them ideal hospital leaders.

Traditional examples of non-clinical activities include committees related to morbidity and mortality review, pharmacology and therapeutics, and infection prevention. Along with committee involvement, intensivists are often charged with collaborative work with nursing and allied health or therapist groups to develop clinical policies, create guidelines and protocols, review new therapeutics, or appraise clinical outcomes. These opportunities serve as a wonderful counterbalance for the intensivist to make professional contributions without adding an emotional component to the work.

An obvious exception to this would be the routine review of patient morbidities, mortalities, and medical errors. The need to comprehensively review complications is a fundamental aspect of critical care and an inevitability in this complex environment. Both the reviewing committee and the involved individuals can experience emotional strain from this potentially punitive process [7]. Fundamental to this work, and often difficult to manifest, is the importance of emphasizing processes rather than people, without compromising the honest reality of the event.

Traditional medical training has rarely emphasized the importance of self and social awareness while interacting with colleagues in emotionally charged situations. A lack of this "emotional intelligence" can have the unintended consequence of exacerbating tense clinical reviews, leading to a massive emotional burden on the intensivist, as rifts between individuals can create a divisive and often hostile environment [8].

The best way we can honour that child and this incredible profession that we are part of, is to be as honest... as brutally honest as possible

Many intensivists are often deeply involved in an educational mission throughout their career. This can be evident from activities such as the routine teaching of bedside nurses, creating a critical care ultrasound training curriculum, or becoming a program director for ICU fellowship training. In the United States, most large paediatric ICUs are affiliated with undergraduate universities and medical schools.

Intensivists are regularly granted faculty professorships to teach medical students, train residents and fellows, and mentor other paediatric/adult intensivists. Educational experiences such as delivering "grand rounds", creating training curricula, or leading a multidisciplinary session with trainees, nurses, and therapists can also reinvigorate the intensivist and reaffirm their passion for the profession.

"Walking alongside" a patient and family's journey during the strain of an ICU stay is an honour and privilege. Training and inspiring future generations to carry this torch can in turn serve to mitigate the emotional burden of the intensivist.

Research functions as another outlet for the intensivist to have professional satisfaction with minimal emotional cost. Away from the bedside, many intensivists are engaged in scientific discovery. Projects are often aligned with the individual's interests and can range from federally funded bench research to translational studies and from quality improvement trials within a hospital to multicentre (and often multi-national) collaborative projects. This can provide expansive benefits to the intensivist from financial funding to networking and travel. These projects can give an intensivist a sense of contributing to the field on a "macro" level and are often considered the most enduring aspects of the career as an intensivist reflects on their journey once retired.

The burden develops when there are competing time interests that pit research time against clinical time and when salary is tied to clinical time and the researcher feels "punished" for their engagement in activities outside the ICU.

Philanthropy

Finally, intensivists can recharge their "emotional batteries" by pursuing philanthropic activities. International medical groups commonly seek intensivists to support their missions. These opportunities draw like-minded individuals from all corners of the world with a shared mission. It epitomizes the purity of the career of a healer: helping others in need. While profoundly emotional for the intensivist, these activities can have a renewing effect and remind the intensivist of the beauty and importance of their career.

> *It's much more visceral. It's much more emotionally heightened because you are in an environment that is so energetic, because it's so different to you. The bonding of the team is through the roof and the shared passion is palpable.*

> *If people didn't do that, the kids wouldn't get heart surgery, so it's really good for them. I get to work with all the doctors there, which I've done that for 16 years, so I have a good relationship with them, and I've been to Africa a few times as well doing the same thing. I mean to get to go to Africa, it's amazing, so it's just a great opportunity to see something and it's interesting and you do a lot of teaching and training and that sort of thing… you see what's available here and compare the two. Yeah, it's great. I really love it and made a lot of good friends, going on the trips and it's sort of a group from all around so it's good contacts…*

> *…allowed me to have this huge bolus of career satisfaction and personal satisfaction whenever I want, for free.*

Conclusion

The intensivist, as a member of a continuously improving interprofessional team, has constant reminders to continue driving towards balancing the art and science, along with the rational and emotional aspects, of local, and global, critical care clinical practice. A holistic approach as a person, professional, and team member is important in working on ways to bring the best of the intensivist, and the best of a health system, to the right patient, at the right time, for the right purpose.

References

1. McKenna AM, Straus SE. Charting a professional course: a review of mentorship in medicine. J Am Coll Radiol. 2011;8(2):109–12. https://doi.org/10.1016/j.jacr.2010.07.005.
2. Malinowska-Lipień I, Micek A, Gabryś T, Kózka M, Gajda K, Gniadek A, Brzostek T, Squires A. Nurses and physicians attitudes towards factors related to hospitalized patient safety. PLoS One. 2021;16(12):e0260926.
3. Liukka M, Steven A, Vizcaya Moreno MF, Sara-Aho AM, Khakurel J, Pearson P, Turunen H, Tella S. Action after adverse events in healthcare: an integrative literature review. Int J Environ Res Public Health. 2020;17:4717. https://doi.org/10.3390/ijerph17134717.
4. Herbland A, Goldberg M, Garric N, Lesieur O. Thank you letters from patients in an intensive care unit: from the expression of gratitude to an applied ethic of care. Intensive Crit Care Nurs. 2017;43:47–54. https://doi.org/10.1016/j.iccn.2017.05.007.
5. Brindley PG. Psychological burnout and the intensive care practitioner: a practical and candid review for those who care. J Intensive Care Soc. 2017;18(4):270–5. https://doi.org/10.1177/1751143717713088.
6. Norvell JG, Baker AM, Carlberg DJ, et al. Does academic practice protect emergency physicians against burnout? J Am Coll Emerg Physicians Open. 2020;2(1):e12329.
7. Jansson PS, Schuur JD, Baker O, Hagan SC, Nadel ES, Aaronson EL. 2019. Anonymity decreases the punitive nature of a departmental morbidity and mortality conference. J Patient Saf. 2019;15(4):e86–9. https://doi.org/10.1097/PTS.0000000000000555.
8. Psilopanagioti A, Anagnostopoulos F, Mourtou E, Niakas D. Emotional intelligence, emotional labor, and job satisfaction among physicians in Greece. BMC Health Serv Res. 2012;12(1):463–74. https://doi.org/10.1186/1472-6963-12-463.

Sigal Sviri is a specialist in internal medicine and critical care. She is the Director of the Medical ICU at the Hadassah Medical Center, Jerusalem, Israel, and was in charge of the COVID-19 ICU during the COVID-19 pandemic. She has served as the Secretary of the Israeli Society of Critical Care and the Director of the Israeli Board of Eexaminations committee in critical care. Her interests include mechanical ventilation, prognostication in the ICU, ethics, and end-of-life decision making. She is part of the VIP Group (very elderly patients in the ICU) which studies prognostic factors, decision making, and outcomes in critically ill elderly patients.

Mary Pinder is an intensive care specialist and Director of Clinical Training based at Sir Charles Gairdner Hospital in Perth, Western Australia. She trained in intensive care in the UK and South Africa as well as Australia. She is on the Board of the College of Intensive Care Medicine and roles with CICM have included Chair of the Second Part Exam Committee, Chair of the Assessments Committee, and College President.

Z. Leah Harris currently serves as Professor and Chair of the Department of Paediatrics for the Dell Medical School at The University of Texas at Austin, Director of the Dell Paediatric Research Institute, and Physician-in-Chief at Dell Children's Medical Center. She is a proud practicing paediatric critical care medicine physician, lifelong learner, and multidisciplinary supporter.

Michael Ruppe is board certified in paediatrics, internal medicine, and paediatric critical care and is an attending physician in Paediatric Cardiac Critical Care at Norton Children's Hospital, Louisville, Kentucky, USA. He completed medical school at the University of Toledo College of Medicine followed by a combined internal medicine and pediatrics residency at the University Hospital of Cleveland/Rainbow Babies and Children's Hospital. He then completed a pediatric critical care fellowship at the Children's Hospital of Philadelphia. During this time his interests translated into research and publications in end-of-life decision making and medical ethics. In 2009 he moved to Louisville, Kentucky, and is active in quality improvement, point-of-care ultrasonography, international health, and paediatric cardiac critical care.

Part V:
Actions and Reactions

Foreword: The Route to Resilience Is Through Action

Jennifer Wild

That physician will hardly be thought very careful of the health of others who neglects his own.
    —Galen

There are many ways to save a life. Keeping intensive care workers healthy and able to manage their stress well might be one of them. This chapter uncovers how intensivists cope with the daily grind of their work. Like elite athletes, intensivists must make split second decisions which will have lasting consequences, sometimes highly detrimental. How do they deal with this sort of pressure? We discover that intensivists are human. They dwell over and struggle with the outcomes of their patients' surgical and drug interventions. They might blame themselves or the system they are a part of when a patient doesn't make it, especially when an error has been made. Intensivists make use of a range of healthy coping strategies like exercising, cycling to interrupt rumination, yoga, taking space to escape stressful thinking with an upbeat movie and talking with other colleagues or friends, who share similar kinds of work.

Intensivists like many people in high pressured jobs can struggle to find time to sleep and when they do sleep it is often for fewer hours than what most would manage in a night. Some turn to alcohol and drugs to cope or gambling for a dopamine hit, a high-risk distraction that gives instant escape. We learn that paediatric intensivists experience unique stressors linked to working with children. The unexpected death of a child is tough to bear as is the reality that compared to adults, few if any children have a role in the diseases or conditions that put then in an ICU.

Taking space to reflect on the course of events is helpful. A hospital that encourages staff to report mistakes, focusing on systems in place to support reporting, makes it safer for staff to note potential errors and learn from them. We discover that

J. Wild
Phoenix Australia-Centre for Post-traumatic Mental Health, Melbourne, Australia
e-mail: j.wild@unimelb.edu.au

like other professions, social cohesion is highly protective and that intensivists benefit from supporting each other with their challenges and joys. One intensivist reported how helpful storytelling is as a tool to learn from mistakes.

The final two chapters of this part focus on how intensivists may help themselves. We learn about strategies that are common in the aftermath of a traumatic incident for those who stay well or who thrive, such as reframing the event, accepting what happened, and perspective taking. We also discover the strategies, such as suppression, that predict a poor response to stressor events, which is aligned with research demonstrating the harmful role of suppression in the aftermath of trauma [1]. We learn that connecting with family can be important for an intensivist as well as their capacity for insight into their own strengths and struggles. It's tough to deal with death. An intensivist who has a hard time moving forward with loss is going to struggle in the ICU environment.

Finally, professional support may be unhelpful for some intensivists. Given the medical conditions that put people in ICU, the ups and downs of their daily work are unlikely to change. But hospital management can be forthright in valuing the work of intensivists and how they manage their stressors recognising there is no one size approach for all.

References

1. Clohessy S, Ehlers A. PTSD symptoms, response to intrusive memories and coping in ambulance service workers. Br J Clin Psychol. 1999;38(3):251–65. https://doi.org/10.1348/014466599162836.

Jennifer Wild Professor Wild is an Associate Professor in Experimental Psychology and Consultant Clinical Psychologist. Her research focuses on three areas: memory and cognitive processes linked to post-traumatic stress disorder (PTSD) and social anxiety, treatment development and evaluation, and how best to achieve clinician competency in evidence-based interventions for psychological disorders. Her PTSD research primarily focuses on why people over-remember what they most wish to forget. She has a special interest in how traumatic memories are formed and how they drive symptoms of PTSD. She is studying how factors such as poor sleep and rumination may affect how unwanted memories develop and how they then become intrusive and easily triggered.

Chapter 18
As a Human

Bradley Wibrow ⓘ **and Sigal Sviri** ⓘ

> *A champion is someone who gets up when he can't.*
>
> —*Jack Dempsey*

Intensivists have different cultural, spiritual, social, and geographical backgrounds, and unsurprisingly they report a variety of personal behaviours to mitigate against stressors of ICU.

So it is a lot of emotional stress that we carry. A lot of the time we take it home.

Prior research has outlined common strategies that healthcare professionals employ including: prioritising, seeking support from colleagues, keeping perspective, and being active. [1] This chapter will focus on the personal coping strategies of intensivists.

Hitting the Pavement and Clearing the Mind

One would hope highly trained medical professionals are aware of the benefits of exercise. Several intensivists reported exercise to be their favoured 'treatment' for stress management and a way to 'clear the head'.

B. Wibrow (✉)
Department of Intensive Care, Sir Charles Gairdner Hospital, Perth, WA, Australia
e-mail: Bradley.Wibrow@health.wa.gov.au

S. Sviri
Medical Intensive Care, Hadassah Medical Center and Faculty of Medicine, Hebrew University of Jerusalem, Jerusalem, Israel

One of the ways of dealing with stress is I try to ride to work as often as possible... sometimes you do ruminate too when you are riding bikes and so you need to be a bit careful

A large part of an intense job is the ability to 'compartmentalise' by separating aspects of mental or emotional processes to allow continued job or social function. This allows an individual to manage stressors that adversely affect good decision-making; allowing reflection and trying to keep a clear mind, thus leading to better patient care; and at the same time allowing one to be present in other aspects of life:

I don't run with music, I run with my thoughts. I find the endorphin rush very positive. It's a clear mind I think, moving my body which really helps.

Recognising in myself ... something has occurred and troubled me. And then saying 'right, this is the time I need to go for a run'. This is the time to do this. Rather than just getting grumpy with my kids or my wife.

There is some evidence yoga and mindfulness help in dealing with workplace stress, both in patients and staff. Studies have reported improvements in self-reported mood measures, burnout questionnaires, increased life purpose, and greater self-confidence in stressful situations [2–4].

I started yoga. You do breathing exercises and meditation or relaxation or mindfulness or whatever you like to call it. It's amazing how powerful it is in joining your brain and your reflexes to your inside. Things come out during this exercise that are very clear but are not obvious. You can call it your subconscious, but I don't call it just my subconscious. It's who I really am.

Just spending some time to enjoy the simple things in life cannot be underestimated. Sometimes intensivists just need a way to switch off their minds and not have to think:

Sometimes after a really difficult day, me and my husband go the cinema and watch a really stupid movie and that helps.

And then there is food… There is a reason Maslow put physiological needs at the bottom of the 'needs pyramid'. Sometimes just some space, a cup of tea, and a biscuit or two are enough to get one's mind back on track:

Personal needs... Umm... Sweet food, cups of tea, space, acknowledgement of the challenges that the individual and teams have gone through.

Let's Talk About It

Intensivists are no doubt aware of the benefits of counselling and psychological support. However, the responders consistently see the stress as 'part and parcel' of the job and see barriers in debriefing with non-medical people, largely in part due to the lack of shared experiences.

I do some social interactions with my non-medical friends. But I wouldn't usually talk to them about the details. Because there is not going to be that degree of familiarity or understanding, and I don't know if it would add anything.

Perhaps a better pathway to debrief the general everyday ICU work, rather than just high-stress resuscitation events and adverse outcomes would have meaningful long-term benefits.

Sleep

Sleep is restorative. In fact, a lot of ICU research in the past decade has focused on the sleep environment in ICU and the ways to optimise patient sleep. Problems often seem imminently more solveable once some time has elapsed.

Sleeping tonight would be difficult. Once I got to sleep and woke up the next day, rested, I would be able to reframe it in a more logical way.

Several intensivists reported the impact that stress and stressful events have on their sleep.

When I wasn't actually present, I sort of wrestled with myself for quite some time, lost a bit of sleep...

...it made me stressed for more than a week. I almost didn't sleep at night... my appetite was really low... influencing my energy and my ability to relate to my family... waking with nightmares.

It is also interesting to hear that intensivists recognise and understand the importance of sleep but continue to starve themselves of something so essential.

Participant: 'Sleep is a huge issue.'
  Interviewer: 'How many hours to you sleep a night?'
  Participant: 'Probably 5-6 on average, It's not very good; I realise that... I have a lot of committees and stuff, so it is not uncommon for me to get here at 12 or 1 o'clock in the afternoon, work a day and night on call and then be here with meetings until 8 or 10 or noon the next day.'

Alcohol, Drugs, and Negative Behaviours

Doctors are at high risk of drug and alcohol use due to accessibility. A 2013 study of 55 doctors under monitoring for substance-related impairment reported that the top five reasons for misusing drugs were pain; emotional and psychiatric stress; managing stressful situations; recreational; and managing drug withdrawal [5].

Intensivists would be expected to be more aware of the harmful effects of negative behaviours and, in fact, regularly see the consequences of negative behaviours in the patients within their units. However, despite this, several mentioned they employ some negative behaviours, while being aware they may not always be healthy.

It's okay to wallow a bit; okay to go home and have one too many scotches... to do that once... it's not okay to do that every night of the week.

It is interesting to hear an intensivist explain the physiological response of a typically considered negative behaviour like gambling, but still utilise it to de-stress:

I like to play poker on my phone; and 1130 at night when you've gotta be up at six, the last thing you should do is gamble on your phone. And you gamble because it's the win/loss dopamine-releasing sort of trigger that gamblers have... you recognise that they are negatives, but you have something bad happen, you are stressed out... I go to my phone and play a game of poker.

There Must Be a Lot of Death

As well as the stress of the workplace, intensivists regularly deal with death. It is often an expected patient outcome and sometimes can be the right outcome for the patient and their family, if managed well. However, it can also be very difficult and unexpected, particularly with young patients, and a mix of healthy and not-so-healthy behaviours are utilised:

Commiserating with the gang ... where someone has died, I'll say 'let's go to the bar and get a drink'. For me it involves going home, having a drink and a cigarette on the back porch; and just breathing...

Is the Constant Pressure to Achieve Worth It?

Intensivists are often hard workers, thriving on constantly achieving and striving for excellence. However, career expectations do change over time, as well as recognition that other aspects of life are just as important.

I trained at a reasonably aggressive, top-tier program, always had a very good work ethic and ran marathons and had a beautiful wife and kids and each and every year it was 'push yourself; do better; shoot for the stars'. And I was capable of that.

Is it just, you know, 'you need to be more efficient'. Is it you need to have less distraction? Is it... Are you shooting for things that are unreasonably ambitious? And so if you are shifting the pendulum towards ... you're failing to meet what you desire more and more.

Do the Hospitals Have an Obligation?

In today's world, in order to foster success in their organisations, employers need to be leaders themselves in creating proactive systems and company policies that identify and mitigate workplace stress and provide support pathways [6], as well as stress-reducing activities.

Interestingly, none of the intensivists mentioned any expectation of their employers or hospitals to assist in dealing with stress. All intensivists appeared to see dealing with stress as their own responsibility and just part of the job. Perhaps this should be a focus for the current and future generation of health professionals—shifting the responsibility away from the individual and changing the institutional culture to normalise support for workers with high stress and burnout and to improve their well-being, as well as the well-being of patients and the institution as a whole.

Conclusion

As the World Health Organization has recognised with the 11th Revision of the International Classification of Diseases (ICD-11), burnout (QD85) is a 'syndrome conceptualized as resulting from chronic workplace stress that has not been successfully managed' [7]. Mental and physical well-being in the intensive care unit requires constant vigilance and curation for the intensivist. When these self-preservation and care mechanisms are overwhelmed, occupational health in hospitals and systematic redesign of intensive care work is a future frontier for intensivist well-being.

References

1. Teasdale EL. Workplace stress. Psychiatry. 2006;5(7):251–4. https://doi.org/10.1053/j. mppsy.2006.04.006.
2. Gilstrap CM, Bernier D. Dealing with the demands: strategies healthcare communication professionals use to cope with workplace stress. Qual Res Rep Commun. 2017;18(1):73–81. https://doi.org/10.1080/17459435.2017.1330277.
3. Köhn M, Persson Lundholm U, Bryngelsson IL, Anderzén-Carlsson A, Westerdahl E. Medical yoga for patients with stress-related symptoms and diagnoses in primary health care: a randomized controlled trial. Evid Based Complement Alternat Med. 2013;2013:215348. https://doi. org/10.1155/2013/215348.
4. Mandal S, Misra P, Sharma G, et al. Effect of structured yoga program on stress and professional quality of life among nursing staff in a Tertiary Care Hospital of Delhi—a small scale phase-II trial. J Evid-Based Integr Med. 2021;26:2515690X21991998. https://doi.org/10.117 7/2515690X21991998.
5. Merlo LJ, Singhakant S, Cummings SM, Cottler LB. Reasons for misuse of prescription medication among physicians undergoing monitoring by a physician health program. J Addict Med. 2013;7(5):349–53. https://doi.org/10.1097/ADM.0b013e31829da074.
6. Chu C, Dwyer S. Employer role in integrative workplace health management. Dis Manag Health Outcomes. 2002;10(3):175–86. https://doi.org/10.2165/00115677-200210030-00005.
7. World Health Organisation. ICD-11 for mortality and morbidity statistics (Version 02/2022). https://icd.who.int/browse11/l-m/en. Accessed 6 Nov 2022.

Bradley Wibrow is an intensivist and emergency physician in Perth, Western Australia, and works in a neuro, cardiac, and liver specialist intensive care unit as well as at a small peripheral Emergency Department. He is passionate about ensuring equal access to critical care for all Australians, ultrasound, research and finding ways to maintain morale in a high stress workplace. His research interests include management of delirium, post-ICU care, and finding ways to aid recovery for our patients and families as they deal with one of the worst times of their lives. In his other life he is a father to four children, attempts to run regularly, and gets down to the ocean whenever possible.

Sigal Sviri is a specialist in Internal Medicine and Critical Care. She is the Director of the Medical ICU at the Hadassah Medical Center, Jerusalem, Israel, and was in charge of one of the COVID-19 ICU's at Hadassah Hospital during the COVID-19 pandemic. She has served as the Secretary of the Israeli Society of Critical Care and the Director of the Israeli Board examinations committee in Critical Care. Her interests include mechanical ventilation, prognostication in the ICU, ethics, and end-of-life decision making. She is part of the VIP Group (very elderly patients in the ICU) which studies prognostic factors, decision making, and outcomes in critically ill elderly patients.

Chapter 19
As a Professional

Chrystal Rutledge ⓘ **and Nancy Tofil**

> *Your work is going to fill a large part of your life, and the only*
> *way to be truly satisfied is to do what you believe is great work.*
> *And the only way to do great work is to love what you do. If you*
> *haven't found it yet, keep looking. Don't settle. As with all*
> *matters of the heart, you'll know when you find it.*
>
> —*Steve Jobs*

To succeed, intensivists must professional behavioural responses to workplace stressors. Adaptive and positive responses are helpful to their well-being. At other times maladaptive responses lead to burnout and depersonalisation [1, 2]. Most of the current literature that exists in the area has explored responses of those working in the adult ICU; there remains little data pertaining to the paediatric intensivist.

It is normal to have negative feelings when a bad outcome occurs, but especially when this occurs in a child. One of the most common things intensivists do is attempt to make sense of the events through self-reflection:

I mean firstly I think I probably just want some space or time where I'm not necessarily required to talk about it, or whatever. Like, I think I just like some thinking time. And I'm not even sure how long that is.

I need a little bit of immediate venting first-aid, then I need contemplative time, then I usually choose peer-based debriefing. So, peers that would understand. I am lucky enough to

C. Rutledge (✉)
Division of Paediatric Critical Care, Department of Paediatrics,, University of Alabama at Birmingham Heersink School of Medicine, Birmingham, AL, USA

Simulation Center at Children's of Alabama, Birmingham, AL, USA
e-mail: clrutledge@uabmc.edu

N. Tofil
Division of Paediatric Critical Care and Paediatric Simulation Center, Children's of Alabama, University of Alabama at Birmingham, Birmingham, AL, USA

© The Author(s), under exclusive license to Springer Nature   171
Switzerland AG 2023
D. Dennis et al. (eds.), *Stories from ICU Doctors*,
https://doi.org/10.1007/978-3-031-32401-7_19

be married to a nurse, who at least understands the mechanics, as well as the emotional reactions.

Taking time for sense-making is a very prevalent behaviour. Another often-mentioned behaviour was mentally rewinding and replaying the negative event and wondering how it might have played out differently if other things had occurred.

The 'if's' are there all the time. I question, 'If I would have done that, you know?' 'If I would have done it another way, the outcome may have been different?' You never know. But the fact is, that you are doing something, for the benefit of the child, but at the end, because what you have done, the outcome is very poor.

What led to the sequence of events that happened... Firstly that it happened. It shouldn't have happened. It shouldn't have been that way. Then, yes, I didn't communicate with the family well: They were at one point, and I was at another. We didn't understand each other. Also, the discussion was very emotional. When I understood what happened we all relaxed. I was also very stressed I did not understand the situation well. Only after I understood it all I relaxed a little bit. It was challenging to speak with them. It took days for them to relax. I understand that of course.

The personality of the intensivist likely plays a role in when and how they discuss the case with others. Extroverts likely talk with many people early in their processing of the negative outcome.

I talked it through with a lot of the staff that were affected, because we had all spent months. I think it's tough because they were young.

Whereas introverts often need more time to process and work through the details themselves.

Introverts try and make sense of it, and then only present it in a space when they feel safe and have processed it and packaged it to some extent, so we have a different way of dealing with it and I think we understand that. But we have a different philosophy as well, it's deeper than that, but we have a different way of dealing with those things, so there's a bit of that too.

Another interesting response is the degree of 'expectedness' of the clinical event. For example, some children die very sadly after an event, such as a prolonged cardiopulmonary arrest from a trauma or a drowning. Experienced intensivists begin to mentally and emotionally process this outcome the moment they get the referral call from the outside facility. They are preparing themselves for the very likely event of this child dying. Less-experienced intensivists and trainees however may not have the same mental model. This likely leads to a team disconnect when the child does die.

The team leader is potentially days ahead in emotional processing than the rest of the team. The intensivist may even come off as cold or not caring. Moral distress or moral injury may be experienced by other members of the intensive care team with closer bedside care proximity, less authority, or less control over clinical decision-making.

However, for deaths that are unexpected, the whole team feels the tragedy in a similar and dramatic way.

There's sort of like, the kid who dies who you're not surprised died, but you wonder if he would have died or the same thing would have happened if another…. people were saying 'Maybe we could have done this more than we did', and I wonder if that was an outcome that could have made a difference for this particular patient. That's more expected. I remember when that patient died, I didn't think much of it in that regard until I had more time to look back and think about it, and talk with other people and hear what other people had to say about it. And then that's hard!

The kid that you left thinking was fine, and you come in the next morning, and the teams like 'so-and-so exploded and this and this and this happened… And you didn't see it coming?

Most experienced intensivists commented on the importance of seeking solitude and taking time. This action is often not part of the intensive care training curriculum but instead modelled by older intensivists (mentors) to younger learners (mentees).

To deal with an adverse event I probably rely most around giving myself time and space to do so. I find that very useful, so that's what I do. It's not internalising, but that's just leaving me to my own devices to work through something and think about it.

…It's my internal root cause analysis of what happened.

…and then just taking a bit of time out and trying to focus on other aspects of my life - spending time with the kids

I usually need some time to… I still cry every time a child dies. And I need some time and space to do that. And many times, that's after whatever shift has ended for the day.

Transparency and open disclosure are important for excellent patient care and quality improvement. This area has changed in a good way over the last few decades. Timely, candid and honest disclosure of errors to patients and their families is important. It also can help the intensivist deal with knowing about an error, but not sharing it. It should be done honestly, focusing on facts and not judgements. Sharing with the family and patient what we do know and being honest about things that we do not know.

Most families find this helpful and often want to know what can be done in the future to prevent similar errors. They want to know steps are being taken to keep patients safer.

'Despite the treatment we gave to your child, there was a significant deterioration, and we did CPR, and we will figure out what happened, and we will come and tell you exactly what we think'. We are trying to be completely open to the families in every case. And generally, you can avoid after that, the anger of the family against the team. By being open. We do make mistakes and when you act you make a mistake also. But it is my opinion that we need to be open with the family and tell them all of the truths that we know.

I encourage honesty and openness to the behaviour of open disclosure. If bad things happen, I think it's very important, it's what I'm trying to teach… I mean I'm teaching that to my kids as well. Do not try and brush things under the table and I'd much rather be open. That is very important, to have open disclosure… lead by example

I think that when I was a younger, I would try to hide it. Try to - if I did a mistake - try to say that it maybe there was not a very bad mistake, or it's not my mistake. I think today, I know that the opposite is true: You should expose it, and the light, the sunlight is the best disinfectant.

More robust quality reporting systems and more engagement with risk management early in the adverse event process help protect the team and bring closure to the family. When errors are investigated with a focus on systems, and not individuals, more systematised learning can occur. People are less defensive and more likely to share 'near misses'. These near misses, when used for learning purposes, can help prevent future errors from ever reaching a patient. Recently, a prospective study in a large university paediatric ICU [3] identified 236 unique latent safety events in 188 h of observation time. Most of these events were attributed to system factors, with only 14% being attributed to an individual's error. In addition, there were zero events labelled as illegal—that is, with disregard for standard policies and protocols.

I'm very happy with the quality of reporting systems here. I teach here and elsewhere around open disclosure. So, I sort of understand the theory and practice behind that, and from what I see, the mechanics here… I mean I participate in the Deteriorating Patient Committee and that is gratifying being part of the governance structure to see the more immediate closed loops out of risk events and adverse events.

So, the culture changed over the years. And then risk management started to be, to infiltrate, the clinical aspect of medical care. Whereas before it was like a side arm, where the legal cases went to where they discussed it among themselves. Now they are more incorporated, they do courses, they do workshops, we have to send them reports every month or so about near mishaps or about clear mistakes and it's becoming more of the culture to discuss this within ourselves and with the patients and families.

Unfortunately, transparency does not always happen. This can be very difficult for an intensivist, as their patients' care journeys intersect many parts of the hospital, including the emergency room and operating room and often have multiple clinicians involved. When not everyone is being transparent with this collective approach to system improvement, the task is made more challenging.

But in some places around the hospital it doesn't happen. We had some fairly frosty conversations with outside specialists who don't think an error has been made, when we think they should be talking to the patient.

I think that at the end of the day, my feeling is that it is my responsibility is to be honest to the patients and their families. And I suppose that's how I rationalise my actions to myself, in that I am, in some ways, an advocate for safety and quality within the hospital for the patients, and not for, necessarily, my colleagues. And so, I'm not, like, pointing fingers in those situations, but explaining that this is what happened, these are the things that everybody tried to do, but this is unfortunate…

Improving the education and training of the entire critical care team is important for both better care of patients, as well as the team knowing what actions to take in a complex, time-limited, critically ill clinical crisis. This may be a situation where peer and or group upskilling would be beneficial. This can be done in traditional courses as well as using simulation-based education, especially with standardised patients in an interdisciplinary learning environment. It is vital that this training includes at least some basic information on delivering bad news, counselling, and debriefing, as there is very little of this training in more traditional medical education.

There is a course ... for all of the medical students on how to deliver bad news with simulations using actors, etc... We try to involve the resident whenever we have serious discussions with the families.

In addition to group training, personal upskilling is also an important and common behavioural response of intensivists. Learning lessons from a tragic event helps healthcare professionals move forward.

That's something that also helps me, is to kind of come away with a lesson from it, if you will. It actually helps in a way if you can learn something from it. Even though it's terrible, and sometimes the price is steep. It seems like that might be one way to make that whole experience worth something, if you can come away with something that you learned from it.

'How do you live with that?' You have to try to take, I have to try to take a… an educational experience from the event to improve my response next time. That's what I would like to feel that I should do or have done…. Because as I pointed out, I personally feel I can get over things better if I can take something away from it. Some education out of it that will help me in the future.

So, we try to change something in our practice that would make us feel that we learned something from this event. Because if you don't learn anything from an event, it's like a disaster.

Finally, it is crucial to improve training in self-care. This may be a good situation to bring in professions who are trained in counselling. When continuing intense stressors are not dealt with, higher rates of mental illness and burnout can occur. Sadly, many intensivists do not access counselling regularly or proactively.

Well, I think the training itself in critical care - the professional training gives skills… and then just experience. The area gives you some skills, but I think the College itself can and should offer, just like they do for communication skills, which is one way to prevent things, is also being able to identify when you are not coping and having coping strategies, so all of this resilience side of things is the flipside.

…Whether that was taught to me specifically? Probably not that much. Other than a degree of self-directed learning – talking to others, et cetera. But I guess we don't have a… Well, we probably do, it's probably on the Intranet or something… I don't think we have a direct "this is what you must do, these are the steps you must take". We certainly got a critical incident notification system. But it's hard to sit down and go through a twenty-page intranet thing, with things going on, perhaps someone crying, the family upset, et cetera.

I haven't had any training to recognise any signs of post-incident stressors. So, there should probably be training around that, in how to actually recognise the signs of failure in that regard. And then also specific coping mechanisms and coping strategies to have in place. … How exactly that would be done I'm not sure. Maybe through help with… and seminars with psychologists, I guess they would have to deal with that a lot, there might be room for even psychiatrists?

No training at all. Really, no training at all.

So, I would certainly be a proponent of people making sure that they have done some sort of resilience training, and never feeling like, just the intrinsic skills that we have in life are all we can have.

I think learning in real-time with real events is the best way to learn. Given that you can't create that same experience for everybody because it's depending on who you happen to see over the course of your Fellowship, what kind of experiences you have, I think simulation is the next best alternative. So, I think that a combination of both, making sure that you're taking all of the opportunities in real-time that exist, as well as using simulation to fill in the gaps, and making sure that there is some sort of consistency in what people are exposed to.

There are some obvious differences between the stressors experienced by practitioners of adult and paediatric intensive care. These included the differences in the relationships with staff and family, differences in patient features, and biases of individual intensivists. Also, patients' perceived responsibility for their illness may vary between adults and children. Paediatric intensivists mostly view their patients as innocent, whereas adult intensivists often view their patients as having had life factors leading to their illnesses.

Conclusion

Paediatric and adult intensivists reported very similar behavioural responses to the stressors of the ICU. Utilising reflective learning as well as learning from mistakes helps intensivists move forward from tragic events. Having better self-care skills and utilising professional counsellors more may help overall well-being.

References

1. Suttle ML, Chase MA, Sasser WC 3rd, Moore-Clingenpeel M, Maa T, Werner JA, Bone MF, Boyer DL, Marcdante KJ, Mason KE, McCabe ME, Mink RB, Su F, Turner DA, Education in Pediatric Intensive Care (E.P.I.C.) Investigators. Burnout in paediatric critical care fellows. Crit Care Med. 2020;48(6):872–80.
2. Yazıcı MU, Teksam O, Agın H, Erkek N, Arslankoylu AE, Akca H, Esen F, Derinoz O, Yener N, Kılınc MA, Yılmaz R, Koksoy Ö, Kendirli T, Anıl AB, Yıldızdas D, Ozturk N, Tekerek N, Duyu M, Kalkan G, Emeksiz S, Kurt F, Alakaya M, Goktug A, Ceylan G, Bayrakcı B. The burden of burnout syndrome in paediatric intensive care unit and paediatric emergency department: a multicentre evaluation. Pediatr Emerg Care. 2021;37(120):e955–61.
3. Trbovich PL, Tomasi JN, Kolodzey L, Pinkney SJ, Guerguerian A, Hubbert J, Kirsch R, Laussen PC. Human factor analysis of latent safety threats in a pediatric critical care unit. Pediat Crit Care Med. 2022;23(3):151–9.

Chrystal Rutledge is an Associate Professor of Paediatrics in the Division of Paediatric Critical Care. She is Vice Chair of Diversity, Equity and Inclusion (DEI) for Paediatrics and Co-Director of the Simulation Center at Children's of Alabama. She is also Assistant Program Director for the Paediatrics Residency program. She is a graduate of the University of Alabama at Birmingham (UAB) Heersink School of Medicine. She completed her paediatric residency at the University of North Carolina—Chapel Hill and her paediatric critical care medicine fellowship at UAB. Her non-clinical interests focus on improving equitable healthcare through simulation, DEI initiatives, and community outreach.

Nancy Tofil is a Professor of Paediatrics and the Division Director of Paediatric Critical Care. She is the Medical Director of the Paediatric Simulation Center at Children's of Alabama/ University of Alabama at Birmingham (UAB). The Simulation Center has trained over 85,000 learners in almost 13 years. Our centre has a focus on interdisciplinary learning and parent education. Professor Tofil is the Senior Associate Program Director for the Paediatric Residency Training Program. She obtained her medical degree from The Ohio State University College of Medicine and her Master of Education from UAB. She completed her paediatric residency and fellowship training at UAB.

Chapter 20
How Can I Help?

Denise Goodman (ID)**, Caleb Fisher, and Chrystal Rutledge** (ID)

Life's most persistent and urgent question is: what are you doing for others?

—Martin Luther King, Jr

As detailed throughout this book, the ICU is an environment rich in the breadth of human emotion, from elation and success to grief and trauma. Some of the reasons are obvious, including the nature of critical illness, the burden of unexpected events, and the humanity of identifying with patients and families. We are part of the most important and intimate health events in the lives of patients and their families, balancing knowledge, responsibility, and the realization that some events are beyond our control: work relationships and conflict and the necessary scrutiny of our work add to the stress.

An intrinsic part of critical care practice is the team approach as discussed in Chapter 9. Numerous disciplines come together with their individual expertise and collective focus, and within each of these, there may be a hierarchy of experience

D. Goodman (✉)
Division of Pediatric Critical Care, Department of Pediatrics, Ann & Robert H. Lurie Children's Hospital of Chicago and Northwestern University Feinberg School of Medicine, Chicago, IL, USA
e-mail: dgoodman@luriechildrens.org

C. Fisher
Department of Intensive Care, Austin Health, Heidelberg, VIC, Australia

Department of Critical Care, The University of Melbourne, Melbourne, VIC, Australia

C. Rutledge
Division of Paediatric Critical Care, Department of Paediatrics, University of Alabama at Birmingham Heersink School of Medicine, Birmingham, AL, USA

Simulation Center at Children's of Alabama, Birmingham, AL, USA

[1]. It is natural for team members to support each other as they work through both the challenges and joys of everyday practice.

> *Personally, I feel responsibility for everybody that is around or who is involved. So, the way I am trying to deal with an error or a clinical event that is bringing stress to myself and to the team is to check around and discuss it with everybody. And to see if anybody is in any abnormal or pathological stress. I mean, stress is normal in those events. So, then I look to help them... Personally, when there is a stressful event, I try to involve all the people from the social work to the cleaners to make sure they are feeling okay.*

> *And I felt that as the clinical leader, it was my job to at least make sure that everyone went home with the facts of the matter. It's not my job to counsel, and nor am I qualified to do so, but I think it's important that we all go home with the same set of facts. We're all going to handle it differently emotionally...*

> *... And we didn't really do a great deal of, 'Here's how I'm feeling', or 'How must you all be feeling', but just said many of us may need help, there are help avenues available; the professional avenues are these; look after each other... So that was the team first-aid...*

> *And that was helpful to me. It's like in the first instance at a cardiac arrest, take your own pulse. 'What do I need to do? Okay, I need to lead my team. I need to lead my team in psychological first aid. Then I need to think about my own self-care afterwards.'*

> *Everyone was working a lot of extra shifts and it was quite stressful... But we were all kind of mutually supportive. And then we did some things to make the staff feel valued. We got some meals catered, massages and things like that for them.*

Although inextricably linked as a team, there are still challenges to identifying needs between each other. Some of these are differences in roles, such as intensivist versus nurse. Some challenges are related to differences in development and professional maturity, so the response of an intensivist to a trainee may differ from that of peer intensivists. Depending on those relationships, and one's own comfort level, it may become easy to delegate responsibility or to assume it is being handled by someone else. While not intrinsically wrong, each team member does owe it to self and others to be present and aware of the struggles of coworkers.

> *So I mean we've certainly been situations where junior staff members have been very stressed or tearful and I guess one of the problems is that when the job gets really busy, it's very easy to be focused on what needs to be done and not kind of notice how everyone else is travelling. Often the nursing staff will pick up things and then come to me.*

> *...So, with a peer I'll probably go more for a beer or a coffee. Whereas a junior doctor, I would more have a corridor conversation, debrief, check in with them early on and then check in with them again a couple of days' time to make sure that they are coping and can concentrate at work, and see that anything asked that I can do. Or that we can do from institutional point of view. If we actually need to organise work placement or time off or annual leave.*

> *... and even though I have very good relations with all of the nurses in our ICU, if they did a mistake I would not do any, say, 'authorised' meeting with them, I will let the head nurse do it. But if it was one of the residents, I would take responsibility for them.*

> *...Occasionally we have someone coming through who is struggling with the stress of the job and often they have other outside stresses in their lives that are having an impact. I guess that's difficult too, because you may have someone who is just in your unit for a short*

period of time because of rosters and you may not get that much exposure to them. You don't want to pry into everyone's personal life, so it can be difficult.

There is also the issue of logistics and time management, finding time in a busy unit where the needs of the other patients don't change in the wake of a critical event, difficult conversations, or the death of a patient. In addition, if the event is near a shift change or a team member has the next several days off, regrouping may be difficult. When delayed, the raw emotion of the acute event may have dissipated, yet temporal distance may also permit a more clear-eyed examination of both events and responses.

If you have the opportunity - and you don't always have this in critical care - try and get the team back together. Everyone who was there, within like, an hour. And that can be difficult because even in that short amount of time, that you've been getting the patient settled, people have moved on.

When there is an adverse event and some of the nurses are involved [you may be] not sure how many nurses there are and that they may not be a shift for some time is difficult.

You've got to have enough time for immediate dust to settle and emotional decompression. But you do need a bit of recency and immediacy for people to still have the facts and feelings clear.

How should we be supporting our colleagues? Formal processes, such as critical incident debriefing and multidisciplinary case reviews, which are linked to system improvement, are important, particularly where everyone has a chance to examine the facts of the events, their own reactions, and those of others [2]. Equally important is taking the time to check in with someone, to listen, and to be present [3].

...I was told about it, and I wasn't present, but I came up and checked that she was okay. And just talked to her. When she was so upset, as you might imagine... I think that's an important part of intensive care, and it should be a part of medicine generally, but I think it's a particularly important part of intensive care because we have such a close relationship with the nursing staff and with allied health. We work very closely together on the same patient at the same time sometimes, and that the bond is unique. It's one of the things that attracted me to the ICU, but also a responsibility from my point of view, is more than from the medical point of view, it could be the person cleaning for floor, it could be the registrar, the nurse, the physio, you know... So the first thing is just to make contact with them, and quickly establish whether they are okay. The way you do that depends on your relationship. How well you know them; whether you can have a conversation. Get away from it, go and have a chat somewhere else or a coffee or something like that, just get away from that. Rather than asking 'Are you okay?' at the bedside. That's probably not the best place to do it. Because [they will say] 'Of course I'm okay!' And just listen. Invite them to say as much as they feel comfortable, but just listen. Don't judge.

Peers? I'd certainly... just find the right time to tap them on the shoulder. Perhaps when they're in their office on their own, perhaps take them down for a coffee, and have a chat and see how they are going. And give them the opportunity to open up rather than try to drag something out of them.

I think the first way to support a peer is presence. Just to be there. And to let them have the chance to either say something, or to say nothing at all. And that's when you can gauge whether or not they need a debrief of what happened, or a coffee, and a talk about something completely different. Because I think everyone's needs are very different and it depends on the situation and the person. It's too easy to try to do something rather than let the situation guide itself. So, I think the first thing is just to be there.

The need is equally important whether you are the intensivist lead or a brief participant in a critical event, as there can be "secondary victims" of witnessed traumatic events, even among those bearing the emotional burden of positional authority [4, 5].

Sometimes you're not noticing who the staff are most affected, because it is not always the person who gave the wrong drug, it's not always the person in front of you, it might be the person in the corner - the student, or the patient care assistant or the orderly who has just walked in and seen something bad.

And you haven't, in that time, you haven't given anything to your staff that you want to give to them in some way... often in these events, the nursing managers often jump in and say to the nurses, you know, 'All these things are offered'. But it is not common from the doctor's side for people to come in and say, 'Look, you got these people, we're going to refer to these people, or this is what you're going to need.' The doctors are supposed to lead the response to coping with these critical incidents and then they are the ones that are potentially forgotten in that. You're the one looking after everybody else, but who's looking after you? ...

I think whether you want to have that responsibility or not, you have it. When you are on for the unit, you are the person that everybody comes to for the questions, so whether or not you want the responsibility, ...I think you do have some responsibility.

I recommend counselling to all of our Fellows - I personally do. Just because I think, our world, talking about the boxes, and compartmentalising.... It has the potential to hurt your personal life; and who you are in your soul; you know it could... Watching people's kids die is not a normal activity! And the fact that we do that, for years and years and years; and that's your job; you get paid for it; it's an honour; but it's also a burden. And if you don't take care of yourself, you're not going to be good at that either.

Decompression more than reflection. Just to breathe. Most of us drink some sort of coffee, or hot chocolate... just do that.

They remember stories... So, if you want to get people to become reflective clinicians, and think about these skills that they might want to apply to their profession, storytelling, to me is the most powerful way to do it ... It's something in the human mind. We sit around the fire and tell stories and we make up narratives. It's the dominant form of communication in human beings.

Conclusion

In working at the extremes of the human condition these participants exemplify the king who is the protagonist of the short story *The Three Questions* by Leo Tolstoy. The king seeks wisdom and insight to answer the three questions he feels most important: When are we to do things? Who are we to do it with? What are we to do? He disguises himself and visits a wise hermit, and through a series of events, he discovers the answer: The right time is now. The most important person is the one you are with. The most important thing is to give them whatever they need.

Sharing emotional and psychological burdens within the team through informal, formal, personal, and collective processes to maintain team function are features of an intensive care unit culture. Making space and time for explicit teaching and learning best-practice techniques is part of the "hidden curriculum" of the intensivist.

References

1. Denham D, Grandey AA. The emotional labor of being a leader. Brighton, MA: Harvard Business Review; 2022. https://hbr.org/2022/11/the-emotional-labor-of-being-a-leader. Accessed 7 Nov 2022.
2. Australian New Zealand College of Anaesthetists. Critical Incident Debriefing. Online published 21 October 2022. https://www.anzca.edu.au/about-us/doctors-health-and-wellbeing/critical-incident-debriefing. Accessed 7 November 2022.
3. Austen L. Increasing emotional support for healthcare workers can rebalance clinical detachment and empathy. Br J Gen Pract. 2016;66(648):376–7. https://doi.org/10.3399/bjgp16X685957. PMID: 27364670; PMCID: PMC4917040.
4. Wilson SN. How supportive leaders approach emotional conversations. Harvard business review Mar 1, 2022. Accessed 28 Nov 2022. https://hbr.org/2022/03/how-supportive-leaders-approach-emotional-conversations.
5. Kumar RDC. Leadership in healthcare. Clin Integr Care. 2022;10:100080.

Denise Goodman   trained in pediatrics at Cincinnati Children's Hospital Medical Center and pediatric critical care at Children's Hospital of Pittsburgh. Prior to this she had undertaken a BS(Physics) at Niagara University, her MD at the State University of NY at Buffalo (now Jacobs School of Medicine at University at Buffalo), and her MS (Epidemiology) at Harvard T.H. Chan School of Public Health. She spent 2012-2013 academic year as the Morris Fishbein Fellow in Medical Editing at JAMA. Her interests include delivery of care, outcomes, care of children with medical complexity, and medical editing. She considers it a privilege to accompany children and their families through some of the most difficult experiences in their lives, and to share both their joys and challenges.

Caleb Fisher   is an intensive care physician at Austin Health, Melbourne, Australia. He has completed dual overseas fellowships in liver disease and extra-corporeal support systems. Outside of work, he is the father of two highly active children, who indulge in his passion for the outdoors.

Chrystal Rutledge   is an Associate Professor of Pediatrics in the Division of Pediatric Critical Care. She is Vice Chair of Diversity, Equity and Inclusion (DEI) for Pediatrics and Co-Director of the Simulation Center at Children's of Alabama. She is also Assistant Program Director for the Pediatrics Residency program. She is a graduate of the University of Alabama at Birmingham (UAB) Heersink School of Medicine. She completed her pediatric residency at the University of North Carolina—Chapel Hill and her pediatric critical care medicine fellowship at UAB. Her non-clinical interests focus on improving equitable healthcare through simulation, DEI initiatives, and community outreach.

Chapter 21
How Do I Help Myself?

Greg Roebuck, Aaron Calhoun ⓘ**, Efrat Orenbuch-Harroch,
and Rahul Khanna** ⓘ

> *Not knowing how he lost himself, or how he recovered himself,
> he may never feel certain of not losing himself again.*
>
> —Charles Dickens, A Tale of Two Cities

Coping strategies are thoughts and behaviours used to manage stressful situations. Problem-focused strategies involve acting on the environment to remove the stressor or 'fix the problem' [1]. Emotion-focused strategies involve regulating the emotional response to a stressor. A third type of coping strategy is relationship-focused coping, in which support is sought from other people. Coping strategies can also be categorised according to whether they are oriented towards or away from stressors [2]. Approach-oriented coping strategies include cognitive reappraisal, in which the meaning of a stressor is reinterpreted so that the emotional response to the stressor is reduced or altered in some way. Avoidance-oriented strategies include escape, denial, and distraction.

G. Roebuck (✉) · R. Khanna
Phoenix Australia—Centre for Post-traumatic Mental Health, Department of Psychiatry, University of Melbourne, Melbourne, VIC, Australia
e-mail: greg.roebuck@unimelb.edu.au

A. Calhoun
Division of Critical Care, Department of Pediatrics, University of Louisville, and Norton Children's Medical Group, Louisville, KY, USA

E. Orenbuch-Harroch
Medical Intensive Care Unit, Hadassah University Medical Center, Jerusalem, Israel

D. Dennis et al. (eds.), *Stories from ICU Doctors*,
https://doi.org/10.1007/978-3-031-32401-7_21

Coping is a dynamic process, and different strategies can be used at different stages of the response to a stressor. Although strategies are sometimes described as generically 'adaptive' or 'maladaptive', it is likely that the usefulness of a particular strategy depends on the person using it and the specific stressor they are experiencing. For example, emotion-focused strategies may be more useful than problem-focused strategies for dealing with stressors that cannot readily be changed. Similarly, the effectiveness of relationship-focused strategies will depend on a person's interpersonal skills and the social resources available to them. A key aspect of psychological resilience may therefore be 'regulatory flexibility' or the ability to utilise a diverse range of coping strategies and to apply these flexibly, as the circumstances demand [3].

Intensive care unit (ICU) practitioners manage severely ill patients who are at high risk of death and other adverse outcomes. They are often required to make difficult clinical decisions under time pressures and in ethically complex situations. They also perform stressful and emotionally draining tasks such as delivering bad news to family members. Many practitioners work long hours with heavy patient loads. Perhaps unsurprisingly, rates of psychological stress and burnout among intensivists are very high [4].

The question of how ICU practitioners manage the stressors that they experience at work is therefore of vital importance. This chapter will outline the coping strategies that participants reported using to manage the demands of their work.

Normalising

A common coping strategy seen in intensivists interviewed was to normalise stressful situations. Practitioners described a need to share their experiences with colleagues and to have colleagues tell them that these experiences were in some sense normal.

> *Acknowledge. Normalize. Share war stories. 'Gosh, something similar happened to me, and here is how I felt, and this is what I did for a few days, and that's what next…'*

> *It's something in particular that I need a person to tell me, 'it happens, this is what we are going to learn from it'. … it's very important for me to share the situations I have been in and not keep it to myself, as may be some people can do, I find it very important for me to discuss with somebody else, to normalize the situation and not just make it my issue.*

Practitioners found it particularly helpful to hear that their colleagues had previously had similar experiences themselves.

> *I think probably like hearing … I think hearing other people's perspective on the event, or hearing that other people have experienced similar things?*

> *Certainly, talking and hearing other people say 'Well, you know, that's happened to us as well', or 'I've seen that before', or 'I completely understand how that happened.'*

Many intensivists reported telling colleagues who had dealt with a difficult clinical situation that they would have managed the situation similarly. In this way, normalisation appears to overlap with reassurance about an intensivist's clinical competence.

… most of us here would sort of say, reassure them that we all think that they are good, that they practise to a high standard. I would usually say something like you know 'If it was me, I would have done the same thing'. Or, 'I would have done something very little different'; 'You couldn't have known'; those sort of things. That's usually the way I sort of go. I don't like … I'm usually very sort of 'soft' about it.

Several intensivists commented on the importance of a 'soft' approach when providing feedback to colleagues. They felt that medical practitioners tend to engage in harsh self-judgements and that a more critical approach would only serve to reinforce these judgements.

Support a peer? I think that I try to be objective about it and give feedback. That feedback is always gently given. If, look to be honest, if somebody asked me for feedback about something, I would always err on the side of saying, 'Well, look, I would have either done the same thing,' or in the case we've just had, 'Look, you've done more than I would have done'. I don't… [pause] … I don't see the … Most of the time I feel, if I've done something wrong or badly wrong, or actually if I put… if someone else has done something wrong, most of the time they will actually know that they've done something wrong. They don't need to be told by me, so for me to go and tell them, it just makes it worse. So, most of the time, I'll be honest, but generally I will be very soft about it. I don't see … I would always be objective, but I will be very fair, and err on the side of being very gentle. I don't like being critical of other people because I know for myself, if I've done something wrong, I don't need to be told …

Perspective-Taking

A related coping strategy was to put the stressful event in perspective. The experiences of patients and their family members provided a reference point for this perspective-taking.

… yesterday was a pretty tough day. We had two people who became brain-dead and talking to the families is always quite tough. When I went home, I thought yes, a glass of red would be really nice. But I think as well, you have to be aware that however bad the day is for you, it's a million times worse for the patients and their families, I think. If I've had a bad day, I get to go home, I get to hand over to someone else. It's nothing like what the patients and their families are going through. I don't know. Some of that brings a whole lot of other stresses that are different. I think for me the work thing always comes back to it's way more stressful for the patient and their family, and that always puts it into perspective for me.

Sometimes, perspective-taking involved putting a clinical error into context and reassuring a colleague that it was unlikely to cause serious harm to the patient. Practitioners noted the importance of acknowledging the distress that a clinician can feel after making a clinical error and not 'trivialising' the incident.

I guess I probably talk to them first. I'd say talk to them and share some experiences. Be able to reassure them. Everything seems worse when it has just happened. Being able to take a bit of time to break things down and think about the steps and, you know, how we can look at things. You don't want to trivialise things, you know. Residents can, if they have written the wrong dose of metoprolol down, they can get quite upset, and think that they have done something to hurt the patient, you know we have other drugs that can do the opposite of that to fix it, so a lot of the time it's about saying don't worry about it. But at the same time, you don't want to trivialise their worry and say you don't need to worry about it, just crack on. It's recognising those signs that it's important for that person. And doing something, to take the time.

Other forms of perspective-taking involved practitioners consciously directing their attention towards positive things about themselves or their contributions to patient care. One participant made reference to the rigorous selection criteria required to become an intensivist.

You have to recognise that if you admit you're imperfect, it's not like an imposter syndrome where you will be found out or have failed. Everybody who gets here was at the top of the class at some point in their schooling. No 'D' students got to this point.

Another commented on the importance of taking credit for good patient outcomes.

There was some event that happened, and like most of us, she would beat herself up about it, and her Mom said, 'Do you take credit when they get better?', And she said, 'No, we give them the medicine and they get better - they're supposed to get better' ... And she was like, 'So how come you give yourself so much credit for their death?' And I said, 'Yeah, you know, we are there to help to the best we can, we're not perfect, nobody is perfect. We don't know what's going to happen tomorrow. If we did, we'd be a whole lot better with this.' And so by sort of saying, you need to take as much credit, which is usually not a whole lot for their survival as you do for the death, they need to be equal, and don't beat yourself up for some little thing you did wrong, when you don't give yourself credit for the millions of good things you do.

This tendency to accept responsibility for negative events but disavow responsibility for positive outcomes resonates strongly with the authors' experiences of critical care practice and may represent a fundamental miscalibration of expectation that could be addressed as a way of improving practitioner resilience.

Compartmentalisation

Another frequently used coping strategy was compartmentalisation. This strategy involved psychologically separating practitioners' work lives from their personal lives.

I think with the stuff, I definitely compartmentalize my life. I don't let things here affect my home life. I walk off happily after work and I don't think about what's happened. I do review it to myself, and think next time how to do better, but I never let it upset me, and I rationalise it. ... If you are taking this stuff home, then that's really bad. And I think detrimental to psychiatric health probably.

... I think that if you are going to work in an area of acute medicine then, I think, you have to appreciate and be rational about it. Compartmentalizing things a bit, and not letting things that happen at work affect your life outside of work. You have to let go of it. I think that surgeons are very good at it. They can be a bit... they can be a bit unemotional. Which I think is good in many ways.

And then just taking a bit of time out and trying to focus on other aspects of my life - spending time with the kids and so forth.

So, I think if you are taking your ... what you see here at work home, I think you know, you are torturing yourself, I think. So, you have to dissociate yourself from it.

Some intensivists found it challenging to compartmentalise, commenting that they had difficulty abruptly 'switching off' after a day of working in the ICU.

I probably ponder over it, and I would find myself certainly in a situation where I am at home, I'm off, I should just go and play with the kids in the evening, when I just come home from work, I might be there physically, but not really mentally. It would be my wife that would alert me to that, and I would think, 'Hmm, yeah, that's what I'm doing'. I think [if] I'm aware of it at the time, then I'm able to turn off and really focus on what I'm doing, but it certainly has happened on several occasions that I find myself in this situation. That's not necessarily with regards to critical incidents, it's with regards to any distressing intensive care unit day. It's not every day, it's mostly business as usual, but then if I have a distressing day, it's hard to just come home and switch off.

I've been doing this so long, I'm so used to not extricating myself, and taking it home! I take it home, I complain a little bit to my wife, we talk about it. But I've gotten – I guess, I think, this is part of it – I've got quite tainted by it. These things just don't drive me into the ground anymore. They just don't. I get upset about it; I talk about it a little; and then just move on. If every incident like that got me to the point where I couldn't work, I would have stopped working a long time ago.

It is possible that the ability to compartmentalise is a learned skill that develops over time. At least one practitioner noted that their ability to separate their work and home lives had improved over the course of their career.

I think over the years I have been getting better at switching off and keeping personal life and professional life separate ... So, you have to be able to detach yourself from it. A bit. And I think some people can do that very well, and some people can't stop. And I've seen colleagues in other specialties, like cry in family meetings, and I think that's nice in some ways, but you're just torturing yourself, because it's not personal, it's professional.

Compartmentalisation was also used during the working day to circumscribe the emotional responses to specific stressors encountered in the ICU. Multiple participants commented on the need to limit their responses to these stressors in order to care for 'the next patient'.

I think the day you stop feeling is the day you should completely give up clinical work. So, you don't want to decompensate, you don't want to get burnt out, you don't want to have nothing left to give to the next person, and I think that's what I meant when I said that I compartmentalise. I can have a family conversation and be quite you know, in tears with them, but then I can leave them and step into the next room and go and deal with something else. And I think you need to do that. Because if one situation completely overwhelms you, you have nothing left for the next patient, or the next shift, or even worse, you have nothing left for your own family.

Suppression and Dissociative Amnesia

A large number of practitioners reported having a limited recollection of stressful or difficult experiences in the ICU.

I think one of the coping mechanisms that a lot of us have is poor memory for bad events.

I do have this memory problem whereby I forget and whether that's a subconscious coping thing, I may blot out bad things that happen. I guess again, not something I can comment on, but I think it might be a bit like childbirth where people forget the bad bits.

My memory is so bad, I think that is part of my coping mechanism, that I just like, flush it. I mean, I really do. I just block it out, the stuff that is bad. Like, I have to be reminded; someone has to give me some context clues, and I'm like, 'Oh, yeah, okay, now I get it. Now I remember that patient or that thing.'

For some intensivists, this limited recall extended to a patient's name and face or recent clinical events involving the patient. Some participants reported being unable to remember patients when they visited the ICU after recovering from their acute illness.

… I do forget. Like I remember the medicine, but I forget the person. Like somebody will say to me, 'Oh remember six months ago, Joe Smith …' And I'm like, 'No, I don't remember Joe Smith.' Like I don't remember names; I'm mean there are certainly very, very distinct memories about some patients that were really outside of the normal experience; but for the most part, I don't really remember that much of the people.

No, I have a poor working memory. The other day one of my colleagues was preparing the Mortality and Morbidity meeting asked me about this patient. And this was only from three weeks ago. And I asked her to call me to discuss because I couldn't recall the patient. When she called, and briefly reconstructed the story for me, I remembered what the problems were. But otherwise, I had completely forgotten. I could only recall it if provoked …

The tendency not to recall difficult experiences was universally regarded as adaptive within the environment of the ICU.

I have a lifelong challenge that 'I can't remember yesterday, I can't plan for tomorrow, so I live in the present.' It's a terrible skill in the outside world, it's a reasonably useful skill [or] adaptation in the ICU.

Some practitioners described their limited memories of difficult experiences as due to an 'active' process of 'trying to forget'. This recalls the psychoanalytic defence mechanism of suppression, in which conscious attempts are made to forget unpleasant experiences.

I really think that that is one of my defence mechanisms is … I try to forget about them. Clearly, I haven't forgotten about all of the bad outcomes that I would like to; but I really actively try to … When everything is done, they're gone. If I run into them and they remember me, that's fine; but I don't try and remember anything that happened before today.

Other practitioners characterised the process underlying their poor memories of these experiences as 'subconscious' or 'not volitional'.

I relatively quickly let things go or can't remember the details. Actually, it's not a question of letting things go. Letting things go sounds like an active sort of process. For me it's more of a complete crowding out of memory and a focus on the present. And so, I don't tend to hang on to some of these events. Not so much errors. Errors are probably a different thing. But bad events such as a patient death for example, I don't find those experience to be as injurious as some of my colleagues do. It doesn't stay with me in the same way.

The references to a 'focus on the present' and 'complete crowding out of memory' suggest that intensivists may experience a form of mild dissociation while managing stressful situations in the ICU. If this is the case, their limited recollection of these situations may represent a type of dissociative amnesia. In contrast with the severe memory deficits that trauma victims can experience as a result of profound dissociation, this kind of mild dissociative amnesia may well be adaptive in the special environment of the ICU.

Acceptance

Some practitioners also reported developing a sense of acceptance regarding adverse clinical outcomes and other stressful experiences in the ICU.

For us it becomes more and more routine to see bad stuff day by day, and I just accept that as part of intensive care.

I have sort of accepted it and moved on. And it's not that it doesn't… I mean it's not that it still doesn't make me sad for them and their family. I don't mean it that way in not having emotion attached to it, but I don't feel like the same pain with time. With time, I stop feeling the same personal responsibility. Which also sounds terrible, I can still be responsible, but it doesn't hurt; it doesn't weigh on me in the same way that it did when it first happened. And that somehow, I have processed it, such that I have accepted it, and then I do think it helps to feel as though … that this is what I will remember from that case and hopefully apply it to my future practice.

Acceptance can be viewed as related to normalisation. Both strategies involve reinterpreting stressors encountered in the ICU as normal or ordinary in that environment. In normalisation, this reinterpretation is usually proposed by a colleague while in acceptance, it is initiated by the individual themselves.

An interesting divergence of opinion arose regarding the use of acceptance to deal with clinical errors. Some participants felt that it was hard for intensivists to accept that they had made an error or allowed an error to occur.

… the margin for error is not very great sometimes; I think we all know that errors are going to occur; I don't know that any of us can accept that. I think it's very hard for an Intensivist to accept that we can allow an error to occur, and we are pretty focused on error prevention.

Other participants viewed acceptance of the potential for errors as a necessary condition for having a successful career in the ICU.

Yeah, you go back and say, 'Did you set out to do it?' 'No.' 'What was your error? Where were the problems starting?' Things happen that you're going to have to be able to accept. Medicine is not perfect in any way shape or form, things happen. You have to at least be able to live with that… If not, you're going to have a problem long-term career-wise, because there is no way you can always be 100% right in everything you do, no matter what your situation is.

Another perspective on errors was to reframe them as opportunities for growth and development.

> *To me, it's summed up in what my Dean said to us when we graduated. [He said], 'You will kill people, just don't kill them the same way twice.' Which obviously makes grandmothers reel in horror at graduation, but it's almost like, that 'Shit happens, but you're part of the solution.' So adverse events will happen because of you; adverse events will happen around you; adverse events will happen to you. And that's normal. You're not less of a human being because of it.*

Demonstrating Empathy

Some practitioners emphasised the importance of displaying empathy for patients' families. They noted that making efforts to support and connect with family members helped them to build positive relationships with families. These relationships, in turn, led to reciprocal support for the intensivist that assisted them to cope with the demands of their work.

> *I think that at the bottom of it, we have to give empathy to receive empathy. If we don't give empathy and we don't receive empathy, then we are left in a very cold and hostile environment. If you bridge and connect with people – if you look at them. You know we have people that come and die with us. And the family say that you smiled. It helps. It gives you strength. So, I didn't kill the patient. The patient died despite what I tried to do, but I supported the family, and the family gave me back empathy, love, respect for what I did. And we have to use up a lot of our internal power and resources to work on relationships with our families. Families because it is ICU, and patients because it makes up our worth and our whole as a human being, not as a technocrat who makes mistakes. And I think that when you have a good relationship with the family … it makes everything much more compatible with life. But we have to work at it, because it takes energy from you. But you give, and you get back.*

Reconnecting with Own Family

Another crucial coping strategy used by ICU practitioners was to seek support from their own immediate families. During their recollections of traumatic events, family meetings, and disclosures of difficult information within the ICU environment, many participants directly referenced family support as key source of their emotional resilience.

> *I have my family. They help. I go home and hug my kids and my husband and that helps. Sometimes after a really difficult day me and my husband go to the cinema and watch a really stupid movie and that helps.*

> *Recognition that either I'm in the midst of an event that is having an impact, or has the potential to have an impact, or … I mean even today, knowing the meeting I was going to have today, it was, take my time, enjoy my family, have a big hug with my daughter.*

One intensivist noted that family support was particularly valuable in a case where the patient's children were of a similar age to their own children.

I think part of the issue with him, was that his kids were the same age as my kids. So, getting home and getting somewhat away and seeing your own children probably helps somewhat.

Despite the overall sense of comfort derived from family members, some practitioners expressed concern regarding their behaviour towards their families after stressful experiences at work.

Personally? I think I hug my kids a little bit more. I try to be more patient with them. I'm not sure I always managed to do that.

This suggests that while family can be a source of support, the presence of ongoing emotional stress can place strain on those relationships as well, potentially creating additional internal distress for the practitioner.

Re-evaluating Career Choice

Some intensivists responded to the stress of working in the ICU by considering a change of career.

I go through phases of questioning my career. I presume everybody does ... We talk about stigma ... I suspect that if I was to abandon medicine and retrain [in] a different domain that that would be seen as ... I think that there would be stigma associated with that.

In some cases, such thoughts arose at times of acute emotional overload.

Yes. Like I've had colleagues call me from here, junior colleagues that have rung me up in the middle of the night and said, 'I can't do this anymore, I think I'm, I'm second-guessing myself, I don't know what's going on.' So, I'll say, 'Okay, let's run through it. Do you want me to come in?' 'No, no it's okay' 'Alright' ... And follow up again the next day and then some months later as well. 'How's that sentiment going, has that passed? Or is that behind you or is that still there? Are we looking after you well enough?'

Leaving a profession like medicine is a complex decision. The path involved in professional training is long and tedious and involves an investment of time and resources. Leaving the field may lead to a feeling of guilt for the waste of time and resources. In addition, this intensive training does not always make it possible to delve into other fields and therefore retraining may require learning a new skill set from scratch, which is not always possible in the late phases of a career.

A change of professional direction nevertheless arises as a possibility in several situations. One such situation is when the person realises that he or she does not fit the nature of the work in intensive care. Dealing with death and suffering on a daily basis can be extremely difficult and is not suitable for everyone.

Participant... we had a trainee who had to leave actually ... they're not doing intensive care anymore. They were a fine doctor - that was not the problem. The problem was, they could not handle anybody dying. Ever. Now that's a problem. You're going to have people die, unfortunately.

> *Interviewer: 'So, it is interesting to me that they were able to identify that and leave though. My sense is that people find it difficult to leave, even though they recognise difficulties?*
> *Participant:'Yeah, it took a few years … but it was admirable; that's admirable …'*
> *Interviewer: 'That they left?'*
> *Participant:'Yes. That they had the insight, first of all, to recognise that this was a problem. And then they had the courage to say, 'I'm going to make a change.*

Another factor that may contribute to thoughts of changing careers is the amount of time spent engaging in activities and tasks that are not considered meaningful by the individual. Dealing with technical and bureaucratic issues, instead of clinical or academic work, can increase frustration levels and lead to a desire to change careers. The amount of time spent working on non-meaningful tasks is a strong risk factor for burnout in intensivists [5].

The atmosphere in the intensive care department and the way things are handled and managed by colleagues can also lead to dissatisfaction and a desire for change.

> *You know I think there are certainly jobs that I went through as a trainee that I knew I wouldn't seek work there because of the way certain adverse clinical events were handled. I was like, 'Nah, I'm not going to work there.'*

Finally, the demanding hours worked by practitioners may lead to a suboptimal work-life balance and difficulty meeting family responsibilities, which can also prompt practitioners to re-evaluate their career choice.

Natural Resilience

Some ICU practitioners had difficulty describing specific coping strategies that they used. Many of these practitioners expressed the belief that they possessed a 'natural resilience' that enabled them to cope with their work.

> *… I mean I can't really comment on how other people cope or their coping strategies, but I think for me the things that I have is that I'm probably naturally quite resilient. When things happen, I kind of just accept it and get on with it. As best I can and move through it. And that's been the case for dramatic events in my own life. I think also that was the way I was brought up. You know, you didn't kinda … You didn't dwell on it, you got on with things. Things were a lot worse for other people and you know, you just cope.*

> *… I think for me personally, I think I probably do have natural resilience.*

One intensivist noted that a certain amount of psychological resilience was necessary to work in ICU.

> *I think it takes all sorts. I think you do need to be able to function under pressure, I guess. Or have … or be resilient and have coping mechanisms of some description.*

Some practitioners appeared to suggest that they did not generally experience their work as stressful or difficult.

… I've never had an incident bad enough where maybe [psychological support] was warranted. If there was something on offer, I don't know if I would take that up, probably not.

Usually, we just feel strong and put it in the subconscious.

These comments are interesting given intensivists' frequent exposure to potentially traumatic events such as suffering and death. It is possible that they reflect the extensive use of avoidance-oriented coping strategies such as repression and denial. Some of these strategies may be unconsciously employed and may serve to prevent intensivists from becoming consciously aware of the emotional significance of the stressors that they encounter in the ICU. The use of avoidance-oriented strategies may be reinforced by the culture of the medical profession, which has strong norms of stoicism, self-sacrifice, and invulnerability and continues to stigmatise doctors who experience psychological distress and mental health difficulties [6].

Alternatively, intensivists who feel minimally affected by their work may genuinely have reduced emotional responses to these stressors. This may reflect their underlying personality or be an acquired trait resulting from their medical training or experiences working in the ICU. One practitioner suggested that there were positive aspects to preserving some emotional reactivity to stressors in the ICU.

I wouldn't say that I'm too prone to being too psychologically impacted, but I think every now and again there is the exception to that rule. Which in some ways is a good thing.

Another practitioner questioned the resilience of intensivists who loudly proclaimed their own hardiness or invulnerability.

I like to think I'm resilient, but I fear saying that out loud because oftentimes the people who are least resilient are the ones who say that they are.

It can be challenging for practitioners to know whether they are truly resilient to stressors or alternatively are placing excessive and unhealthy reliance on avoidance-based coping strategies. Engaging with a mental health professional can help practitioners to understand the patterns in how they respond to stressors and the helpfulness or otherwise of these patterns.

Personal Support

The final coping strategy that practitioners reported using was to seek support from other people. The most common person that they sought support from was their spouse or partner.

One of the things that helps me is to talk about it. I discuss with my wife quite often.

If I really need to talk about things or de-stress … . I know once I came home after a bad day where it was in another hospital but this trache had gone very badly and ended up being sorted out but it was just really awful at the time. I went home and I went, you know 'this is awful, this is what happened and this is what happened and this is awful' and [my partner] just looked at me and said 'you deal in a high-risk specialty, shit is going to happen, deal with it, move on, glass of red'. And that was the kind of … That was all I needed …

Sometimes it really bothers me, and I discuss it with my wife. She is one of my supporters.

... [my partner] was trying to give me some support. It was difficult. She is not in the field, but she felt that I am very, very, very stressed toward the talk about breaking bad news with this patient. She is a support for me, because she is helping me to clarify things and maybe giving suggestions how to deal with that.

In a number of cases, practitioners' partners had worked, or continued to work, in healthcare themselves. Some practitioners felt that this helped their partners to understand their experiences in the ICU.

I am lucky enough to be married to a former nurse, who at least understands the mechanics, as well as the emotional reactions ... She is an emotional confidante, and with a lovely minimum amount of phrasing, I can say, 'Look, I've had a bit of a shit day today.'

And at that point I probably talk to my wife about it. She's a nurse, and sort of understands the health-system-related issues.

Other practitioners commented that there were advantages to their life partner not being a healthcare worker. One advantage was that they could provide calibration from the perspective of a 'lay person' regarding difficult situations.

This is strange, in that I actually think ... you know, the people that talk about debriefing are probably right, but the scenario for me is trying to do that with someone who is non-medical ... which is my wife, usually ... she has this good sort of crosscheck of what is acceptable standard versus ... Also as a non-medical, knowing nothing about medicine: 'Sounds like you did the right thing, you communicated the right way, sounds like you gave everything you could.' So for me to talk to her and to get that sort of crosscheck, is actually really helpful.

Another perceived advantage was that it reduced the potential for competition between the intensivist and their partner.

... having someone not in the field, firstly he admires me because I know things he doesn't know. And I admire him for knowing things I do not know. Second of all, there is less competition in terms of professionalism. But he does not understand what I'm going through. He doesn't know what I'm going through. He doesn't realise what I'm going through. I don't think you can, unless you are there.

Some practitioners tended to focus on technical clinical issues when seeking support from their partners.

I also unfortunately debrief to my wife a lot... So she is, so there is ... that's a debrief. And I guess my debriefs are usually quite clinical and dry. So that's a sounding board. So that's, in many ways she is an extension of my time and space in that she's a wall to bounce things off.

Others felt that the main purpose of debriefing was to express and share their emotional responses to difficult situations.

Interviewer: '... do you think it is sharing the emotions that you are feeling or is sharing the technical side of how we could have done this, this or this? What do you think?'
Participant: 'I think both. Mainly the emotional. Well, the technical, if this happened it may be, well, I think this should have happened, or could have been done in another way. Those are the technical issues. I think that the main thing is to bring out the emotions. And

to share the emotions. Like in any psychological treatment. To feel that somebody is sharing with you the distress.'

Partners may not instinctively know how to respond when intensivists share their experiences of stressful situations in the ICU. One participant commented that they had had to 'educate' their partner about how they wanted him to respond when they shared an experience with him.

Participant: '... Oh. After probably a couple of times when I got frustrated with the way that my husband kind of, listened when I need to tell him about stuff at work, we ended up talking quite a lot about what I needed him to do. That was probably the biggest thing, I think. It doesn't sound very big but...'
Interviewer: 'Educating your husband, about your needs?'
Participant: 'Yep.'

Some practitioners also debriefed their colleagues about difficult experiences. These interactions presumably prompted the use of coping strategies discussed earlier such as normalisation.

So probably my most common coping mechanism is personal reflection and then discussion with my wife. ... Not always the wife, colleagues as well. But usually my wife.

... I can't say I have a certain way to try to get over that. It's mainly sharing the stress with other people even within the team or at home and to talk it out.

Interestingly, not all practitioners reported seeking support from their spouses or partners regarding stressful experiences.

I don't talk about work at home. I never talk about work at home. My wife still doesn't really know what I do! (Laughs) ... I just don't... I just don't talk about work.

Obviously there are a small number of cases that just are so different and maybe interesting that you talk about at home, but I don't tend to take work home.

My wife would complain that I don't say enough. She is a nurse. So, her complaint and just one, is that I probably would not say enough. That I probably go home and just ruminate. And might go through it, and go through it, and then I just get to a point where I have to say something. It's a personal failing, I think. She would be ... I would be better if I went home and more easily ... [talked]

The tendency to seek support from spouses or partners is likely to reflect in part an intensivist's personality structure. Personality traits such as extraversion are associated with an increased likelihood of using relationship-focused coping strategies [7].

The widespread use of this coping strategy raises the question of its effects on intensivists' relationships with their spouses and partners. One participant commented on the importance of not overburdening their partner. They felt that they needed to be selective in what they shared.

Yes, but just on that, I've been very careful to think ... to be careful about using the sound-board of my beautiful wife. You know, because it's very, very ... it would be very easy to overload her, you know, just dump on her frequently, particularly with all the crap that goes on inside ICU. I think, so the other change, I guess, would be to, you know, choose the important things, not just the 'any' things that happen, I think that's almost like a grading system of things that you use a sounding board on, so that a sounding board doesn't get broken …

This quote suggests that there may be limits on the emotional support that an intensivist can seek from their spouse or partner without placing the relationship under strain. This highlights the potential importance of external professional support such as mental health professionals.

Conclusion

Intensive care practitioners use a range of coping strategies to deal with the stressors that they encounter at work. One group of strategies involves cognitive reappraisal. Strategies in this group are aimed at reinterpreting stressors in the ICU as normal, manageable relative to other problems, or acceptable. They include normalisation, perspective-taking, and acceptance. Another group of strategies involves psychologically separating stressful experiences in the ICU from experiences in other domains of life. These strategies include compartmentalisation and suppression or dissociative amnesia. The final group of strategies involves seeking support from others, including partners, family members, and colleagues. Practitioners' spouses or partners are particularly likely to be used as a 'sounding board'.

Some practitioners had difficulty describing the coping strategies that they used and tended to describe themselves as 'naturally resilient'. It is unclear whether these comments reflect true resilience or are indicative of the use of avoidance-oriented coping strategies such as repression and denial. Engagement with outside sources of support, particularly mental health professionals, can aid practitioners to process the stressful and difficult events they experience in the ICU.

References

1. Lazarus R, Folkman S. Stress, appraisal, and coping. In: Stress, appraisal and coping. Cham: Springer; 1984. https://books.google.com/books/about/Stress_Appraisal_and_Coping.html?id=i-ySQQuUpr8C.
2. Roth S, Cohen LJ. Approach, avoidance, and coping with stress. Am Psychol. 1986;41(7):813–9. https://doi.org/10.1037/0003-066X.41.7.813.
3. Bonanno GA, Burton CL. Regulatory flexibility: an individual differences perspective on coping and emotion regulation. Perspect Psychol Sci. 2013;8(6):591–612. https://doi.org/10.1177/1745691613504116.
4. Kerlin MP, McPeake J, Mikkelsen ME. Burnout and joy in the profession of critical care medicine. Crit Care. 2020;24(1):1–6. https://doi.org/10.1186/S13054-020-2784-Z/FIGURES/1.
5. Shanafelt TD, West CP, Sloan JA, Novotny PJ, Poland GA, Menaker R, Rummans TA, Dyrbye LN. Career fit and burnout among academic faculty. Arch Intern Med. 2009;169(10):990–5. https://doi.org/10.1001/ARCHINTERNMED.2009.70.

6. Shanafelt TD, Schein E, Minor LB, Trockel M, Schein P, Kirch D. Healing the professional culture of medicine. Mayo Clin Proc. 2019;94(8):1556–66. https://doi.org/10.1016/J.MAYOCP.2019.03.026.
7. Connor-Smith JK, Flachsbart C. Relations between personality and coping: a meta-analysis. J Pers Soc Psychol. 2007;93(6):1080–107. https://doi.org/10.1037/0022-3514.93.6.1080.

Greg Roebuck   is a consultant psychiatrist and researcher at Phoenix Australia and the Institute for Mental and Physical Health and Clinical Translation at Deakin University. He has diverse research interests and has authored articles in the fields of traumatology, mood disorders, anxiety disorders, psychophysiology, pain science, and sports psychology.

Aaron Calhoun   is a tenured professor in the Department of Pediatrics, Division of Pediatric Critical Care at the University of Louisville, and is an attending physician in the Just for Kids Critical Care Center at Norton Children's Hospital. He received his MD from Johns Hopkins University School of Medicine in 2001, completed general pediatrics residency at Children's Memorial Hospital/Northwestern University Feinberg School of Medicine in 2004, and completed pediatric critical care fellowship at Children's Hospital of Boston/Harvard School of Medicine in 2007. Dr Calhoun is the Associate Division Chief of Pediatric Critical Care and has numerous publications in the field of simulation and medical education.

Efrat Orenbuch-Harroch   completed her training in internal medicine, intensive care, and infectious diseases and works as an intensivist at the medical intensive care unit and as infectious diseases consultant at Hadassah Hebrew University Medical Center, Jerusalem, Israel. She is currently doing a clinical fellowship in transplant infectious diseases at the University of Alberta hospital in Edmonton, Canada, and plans to combine the knowledge she acquired in order to provide accurate care to transplant patients in the intensive care unit.

Rahul Khanna   is a practicing psychiatrist at Austin Health's Psychological Trauma Recovery Service and serves as Director, Innovation & Medical Governance, at Phoenix Australia—Centre for Post-traumatic Mental Health, based in Melbourne, Australia. He is a senior lecturer at the University of Melbourne and has a deep clinical and research interest in psychological trauma, particularly in leveraging novel technologies to enhance our understanding and treatment of trauma-related mental health conditions. Further background and contact details are available on https://rahul.au.

Chapter 22
Where Do I Go?

Efrat Orenbuch-Harroch, Courtney Bowd, and Sacha Schweikert

> *In times of stress, the best thing we can do for each other is to listen with our ears and our hearts and to be assured that our questions are just as important as our answers.*
>
> —Mister Rogers

Intensivists are exposed to a variety of patient and environmental stressors in their work and may experience emotional distress that can lead to disadvantageous outcomes for the intensivists themselves, as well as their patients. Intensivists experience higher rates of burnout [1, 2] which, when not properly managed, may lead to maladaptive coping mechanisms, mental health disturbances, and increased risk of self-harm and suicidal ideation. In addition, intensivist distress influences performance which can result in more medical errors and the displaying of less empathy, both of which can influence patient outcomes [3].

A common response amongst intensivists to mitigate the stressors of the ICU is to seek emotional support from colleagues. However, there are numerous barriers to support seeking, such as a lack of awareness of the problem, time constraints, and stigma, which may interfere with seeking professional and nonprofessional emotional support.

E. Orenbuch-Harroch (✉)
Medical Intensive Care Unit, Hadassah University Medical Center, Jerusalem, Israel

C. Bowd
Phoenix Australia—Centre for Post-traumatic Mental Health, Melbourne, VIC, Australia

S. Schweikert
Department of Intensive Care, Sir Charles Gairdner Hospital, Perth, WA, Australia

© The Author(s), under exclusive license to Springer Nature
Switzerland AG 2023
D. Dennis et al. (eds.), *Stories from ICU Doctors*,
https://doi.org/10.1007/978-3-031-32401-7_22

201

Do Intensivists Seek Emotional Support?

Awareness of the need for emotional support may be aroused by the individuals themselves or by the surroundings, when the intensity and magnitude of the stressful events are exceptional, or when 'red flags' indicate poor coping.

My wife has said to me, "You should think about seeing a psychologist…" I was like, "What do you mean?"

I had one really bad one when I was a Fellow, and I went several nights without sleeping well, and finally my partner, he said, "Maybe you should go and see a therapist?" And it was actually one of the best recommendations.

It is well documented that in general, intensivists are poor at engaging in self-care, failing to follow basic health recommendations as routine preventive screening [4]. Amongst the high workload and pressures of the ICU, many intensivists admit that there should be more emphasis placed on seeking emotional support; however, those who do seek support show a preference for seeking support informally through colleagues and partners. These experiences align with previous research findings; in a study that evaluated rates of support seeking amongst intensivists, intensivist colleagues were the most commonly endorsed source of potential support (88%) [3].

Probably the one person that I have spoken to is [Doctor's name]. I spoke about what was going on and I started to feel that something wasn't right, and identified that it was burnout. But I think that it is something that we don't talk about enough.

We don't know how to help ourselves. I didn't have anyone who could help me, really.

I would always see your colleagues as a first step. And anybody that you have a mentoring-type relationship with. Rather than a formal consult with a… psychology- type.

In terms of support or help, I think really, we've got quite a tight knit group and we tend to talk with each other over something that like that.

I suppose what we're talking about there is not debriefing, but more de-griefing, right? When we say debriefing we normally mean de-griefing – we usually mean a forum for everybody to vent their emotions around what has happened, rather than a true, sort of functional, actionable debrief.

It's nice to have a confidante in one's wife, but even talking to say a personal trainer, poor buggers - it must be, like hairdressers, they are probably defacto psychologists! So they are, wrong place, wrong time, but that's a helpful outlet as well.

Support seeking from colleagues typically tends to focus on the details of the case, allowing the intensivist to objectively discuss the patient, events that occurred and the decisions made. However, seeking collegiate support regarding the more technical details of events or patients appeared to build a sense of support and provide opportunity to discuss any emotional impacts as well.

But I guess I find it relatively easy to… not easy, but I feel okay talking to people, both in terms of seeing how other people are going and also if I had to do that myself, but yeah, I'm trying to think… I don't know if I have spoken to anyone about burnout. But more-so worrying or upsetting situations, from other senior registrars and things along the way…

Then I think you can… feel negatively affected. How do I deal with it? Usually by talking through everything with your colleagues. I think it can be very useful to have senior colleagues who either know the case or don't, but who are just around. It's natural to focus on the technical aspects of what happened rather than on the emotional aspects, and that would be sufficient for most cases I would think. I wouldn't say that I'm too prone to being too psychologically impacted, but I think every now and again there is the exception to that rule. Which in some ways is a good thing.

It is very usual for us to talk about cases and get second opinions in all sorts of scenarios, so I actually think that that environment provides, informal support.

I speak to my boss particularly, and through that, I try and debrief the situation, get all of the weight off me and at least bounce the ideas off others.

I think I do have a sort of a "want to be right"…a perfectionist streak to me, so I do then want to crosscheck my practice with my colleagues. So I will then informally sit down and ask them, "these are the things that I did, what do you think?" and I think this is helpful for me personally, because I think allaying the stress comes from believing that you have done what is acceptable. I think the difficulty is, I imagine one day, and I'm sure it happens to everybody in their career, they do something that they think "actually I think that I made a mistake." and having to deal with that I think will be the harder one, is to understand, "look actually I made a decision there" or, you know it not from any, you know, malice or anything, but people make mistakes and I think it is, I suppose it… I suppose it depends on your degree of self-reflection and self-acceptance of those things.

In several situations it seemed that there was a preference from the intensivists to seek emotional support from colleagues, as there was a perception that someone from outside would not be able to completely understand the complexity of the distress related to the nature of work in the ICU. While a professional therapist may support the emotions raised by situations, there was a perception that they would not understand completely the magnitude or the stress that can arise from daily ICU work. Intensivists cope with emotions relating to delivering bad news to families, sadness, blame, and grief that are often directed at them from patients, in addition to heavy workload and bureaucratic obstacles, and this combination was thought to be difficult to perceive from the outside.

I'm definitely aware that I want an opportunity to sort of talk and debrief afterwards. I think that the challenge then, is that it seems to be particularly effective talking or debriefing to someone who actually understands.

They need to understand technically what I'm talking about, and then but also, I mean, I can think of any number of intensive care doctors who would technically understand and yet have zero capacity to empathize with that. So they will need to have both the capacity for empathy as well as a technical understanding of what's happened.

I remember thinking, "You literally have no idea what it's like to feel like, responsible for someone's death, or something, because that is typically not something that would occur to you in your job". And particularly to hear that at a time when you were feeling vulnerable, which is like well, less than useless.

I think, the best forum I think is amongst your colleagues who you've known for a while and who know you. I find sometimes when people from... when external people come, they can be a little bit... they probably don't understand the situation and our workplace practice...

But I would feel that it would be very difficult for someone who doesn't work in this environment to really understand all of the nuances of a particular event.

Nonprofessional support may not always be constructive. Exposing the emotions in front of colleagues may have a deleterious effect if the response is offensive or not supportive. Additionally, such collegiate support is likely to be 'in the moment', focusing on technicalities and importantly will likely suffer from time constraints and lack of follow-up with the individual concerned. Demonstrating vulnerability may not be appropriate for every work environment and in several situations could lead to further emotional distress. Then again, strong emotions are considered an appropriate response in the face of experienced stressors and not necessarily pathological and as such do not always raise the need for assistance.

We don't have, really, a supporting group where we speak about emotional stress and things like this. It could be a good idea, I don't know how to do it, but because you know bringing in different people within the hierarchy and have them starting to talk about the emotion is something that is not... something easy. It could have the opposite effect. Instead of ventilating, it might feel like the opposite person is attacking you, that you didn't do so well.

You don't always feel like talking to your colleagues about it. And, umm... I guess that's either because there's this kind of perception that you might be... well, either the colleagues have been involved in the incident and therefore might have their own bias, and then... or, they haven't been involved, in which case you feel like you might be judged, that you've just been incompetent or something.

No. I feel like I function reasonably well and that if you didn't have any emotional response you'd be in one form of trouble. And I've had two big emotional responses, but I feel like it's okay to have some response, and you don't need to seek help just because you have... emotions.

Hierarchical considerations may also affect the provider's reluctance to share their distress in a professional environment. The intensivist, being the team leader, is considered the supporting element in the team, and sometimes does not feel comfortable exposing vulnerability in front of junior colleagues and being left without a suitable source of support.

Some intensivists reported that they did not seek support, as they were aware of the warning signs and had not experienced them to this point. They did however not exclude the possibility of seeking it should the need appear. Such willingness to seek support may be increased by specific stressful events, such as medical errors or adverse patient outcomes. Although a substantial proportion of intensivists indicated that they were willing to seek help, or were aware of the need, practically they rarely did so.

> *I think at the moment, that it's working because I love coming back to work, I don't have any anxiety or stress about coming back to work. I actually get excited before I have a week of clinical coming on, so yes... but that's a very good point.*

> *Even though I can't exactly switch off, straight away, I don't have sleepless nights over it, and after a couple of hours I can certainly turn off so I think so I have the thought that generally I am coping mentally reasonably well with that and would not have thought of, looking for, and getting professional help.*

> *I think it would be very beneficial, a reflection back on what my coping skills are like, and my management of these skills are like. I've thought about it, but I've never acted on it.*

Barriers in Seeking Emotional Support

A variety of emotional and practical barriers stand in the way of an intensivist who is interested in seeking support. Even when the awareness of the need exists, emotional support is sometimes difficult to obtain.

Lack of Awareness

Given the heavy workload in intensive care units, it is not intuitive that an individual will take a pause to reflect on their emotions and coping mechanisms. After a stressful experience, it is easier just to move on to the next patient.

> *...I sort of cope and support by "doing".*

> *I don't find that people stop enough to analyse the event enough. We say, okay this is what happened, maybe I should have done it, maybe he should have done it, or whatever, and we move on.*

> *The awareness of 'if you are struggling or not' partially depends on your openness as a person to admit it, and it partially depends on the astuteness of whoever is senior to you, whether it's your faculty buddy or your division head. They have to notice.*

> *I think I do not see it as a necessity until some situations happen. Sometimes I think we really need something like that, but then a regular day comes and then it goes away.*

Time Constraints

The process of addressing psychological support is energy- and time-consuming and requires bureaucratic processes, and the busy intensivist may not find the time or energy to get into it. It is also difficult to commit to a course of treatments in a job that includes shifts and inconsistent working hours.

> *I do not have time for that actually. If it would be something in our unit, something that we would organise I would be happy to be involved because I think it's very important.*

> *I think the problem in ICU is that we are so busy, and we move from one fire to the next that we sometimes don't have that time to stop.*

Availability of Services

A repeated argument was that there was a perception that psychological services were not available or accessible enough, and the worn-out provider, even when reaching for help, does not know where to go to seek professional emotional support. Similarly, in a group debrief environment combining medical and nursing staff, the intensivist would be looked at as the leader and able to support everyone else. It would be highly unusual for a senior intensivist to share his emotions effectively in such a forum and benefit from it emotionally.

> *In terms of, is there support? I think it's a blank space. I don't think it's either positive or negative. It's not obvious where to access that support should you desire to. I don't think it's obstructive. I just think it's a blank space.*

> *I don't know who to go to.*

> *To my feeling, there is no way in this hospital that the staff are followed or helped on a regular basis, or having a service that you can really easily go and ask for some help, or to share emotional issues.*

> *In terms of staff after-care... Certainly for medical, that's close to non-existent. I don't think our ICU is unique in our hospital for that.*

> *We don't have, really, a supporting group where we speak about emotional stress and things like this.*

> *There is no organized, proactive group therapy or person who is dedicated, or whose job is to help medical workers in dealing with things like that. There is no support system. There is none.*

While some intensivists identified that support systems did exist, they also commented on the need for services to be more proactive in taking care of worker's well-being and tailored to the unique needs of the role so that they are easily accessible given the time constraints.

I remember at the time at a Consultant level, we talked about it, a psychiatrist came and offered us support, but that's all it sort of was. And I don't think anybody actually took it up, and whilst I thought it was good for a psychiatrist to come in and offer that support, it doesn't happen all the time, I'm not sure that it was proactive enough. It seemed still too hard for junior and, really, Consultant staff as well... I think it's been too easy to avoid it, but it's too easy not to go and seek the help that maybe some of us could have needed at the time. The steps required are quite proactive ... you would need to call the psychiatrist, make an appointment... and then it's a psychiatrist. You don't really want to talk to a psychiatrist necessarily. So I think there probably could be more on offer that is more readily available. And less structured, so you don't feel like you are talking to a shrink.

The only help that we really got was from the head of the psychiatric department who called me and said, "Okay if you need something, call me." But nobody really made an active... And I think in those incidents, you get a little bit of, depression I would say. And you are not looking around for, actively for, help. That help is not coming. Somebody who would come to the unit and say, "Is everybody okay?"; talk to me; talk to the nurses; and maybe engage in a conversation with the team more actively. And that was never done.

Where services do not already exist, there was a desire for more formal well-being policies and routine supports to be made available.

...I think I'd like to see... maybe even a policy within the ICU that says that, "If this happens you need to come and see the head of department or talk to one of the senior members in the department, and, come and just have a chat." And make sure that it's available in a completely non-threatening and confidential environment, so that somebody can feel free to come and talk... Just making sure that people know that they can come. And again, in professional development review session, so as an annual event, you can always reiterate that you know, 'We've noticed this or that we haven't noticed that you must almost feel free to come and talk about this'...

I think it would be reasonable for every program to have the residents meet with a psychologist speak to the residents every few months. Or even on the intensivist level you know, to see. You can't force people, but clearly, I think there should be a lot more availability for psychological support for the staff, because I think there is a tremendous amount of stuff that goes on.

Stigma

The literature identifies multiple dimensions or types of mental health-related stigma, including self-stigma, public stigma, professional stigma, and institutional stigma. All types have been related to poor outcomes, such as failure to access treatment, disempowerment, reduced self-efficacy, and decreased quality of life [5]. Implicit self-stigma is manifested by the perception of failure when admitting the

need for help. Concerns about confidentiality, documentation, fear of legal consequences, or negative impact on career have also been reported by intensivists as
influencing the decision whether to seek support or not. Most interviewees asserted
that there was still a degree of stigma surrounding seeking emotional support and
that they would prefer no one to know about their support-seeking behaviours, as it
would make them seem vulnerable and not capable.

> *I think that there is something in there about, that by doing that, you are sort of admitting
> failure or fault in some way.*

> *You won't be seen to be a capable person", but you have also got to manage these stresses.*

> *I do know that my peers have done that, and peers that I think are amazing and incredibly
> respected. But I would not let other people know if I chose to go down that path.*

> *I guess it would need to be very confidential I think.*

However, stigma is strongly influenced by cultural and contextual value systems
that differ over time. The growing awareness today related to mental health and
well-being in the general population and medical doctors alike will likely alleviate
the stigma associated with seeking emotional support. This was confirmed in the
interview process with several responders expressing hope, that it may not be a
significant obstacle amongst junior teams.

> *The concerns about practitioner mental health and compulsory reporting I think are becom-
> ing less. I think they're still there, probably in our older generational colleagues rather than
> in the younger ones.*

> *I think that probably would have had some stigma at some point in time, but I think we've
> changed enough to realise that's probably not the best way to tackle it. So I think it is less
> of an issue at this point in time, right now.*

> *So our intern group in the residency program is probably 30 interns. Every one of those 30
> interns in their first year have to meet with her (mental health professional), and they found
> that it actually was... The feedback that we got from the interns was tremendous.*

> *It may be that being brought up and being able to express your feelings or share might be
> more helpful to them than preceding generations who kind of "toughed it out" and bottled
> it all up inside.*

Conclusion

In summary, despite continued exposure to stressful experiences as part of their
daily work, intensivists are often reluctant to seek emotional support. Barriers to
obtaining support are numerous and include time constraints, lack of availability of
the services, and the fear of the stigma related to mental health diseases. When
intensivists do seek help, they will often prefer to talk to their colleagues rather than
mental health professionals, feeling that someone from outside could not understand the complexity of the situations they encounter. A supportive work

environment was repeatedly considered as a beneficial factor in the provider's well-being, but there is still a need of creating an organised, proactive, available, and well-championed supporting system.

References

1. Kerlin MP, McPeake J, Mikkelsen ME. Burnout and joy in the profession of critical care medicine. Crit Care. 2020;24(1):98.
2. Sanfilippo F, Palumbo GJ, Noto A, et al. Prevalence of burnout among intensive care physicians: a systematic review. Rev Bras Ter Intensiva. 2020;32(3):458–67.
3. Hu Y-Y, Fix ML, Hevelone ND, et al. Physicians' needs in coping with emotional stressors: the case for peer support. Arch Surg. 2012;147(3):212–7.
4. Gross CP, Mead LA, Ford DE, et al. Physician, heal thyself? Regular source of care and use of preventive health services among physicians. Arch Intern Med. 2000;160(21):3209–14.
5. Subu MA, Wati DF, Netrida N, et al. Types of stigma experienced by patients with mental illness and mental health nurses in Indonesia: a qualitative content analysis. Int J Ment Heal Syst. 2021;15(1):1–12.

Efrat Orenbuch-Harroch completed her training in internal medicine, intensive care, and infectious diseases and works as an intensivist at the medical intensive care unit and as an infectious diseases consultant at Hadassah Hebrew University Medical Center, Jerusalem, Israel. She is currently doing a clinical fellowship in transplant infectious diseases at the University of Alberta hospital in Edmonton, Canada, and plans to utilize the knowledge she acquired in order to provide accurate care to transplant patients in the intensive care unit.

Courtney Bowd completed her undergraduate degree at the University of Queensland and has recently completed the Master of Public and Social Policy at the Macquarie University, Sydney, Australia. She is currently a policy specialist at Phoenix Australia—Centre for Post-traumatic Mental Health in Melbourne, Australia, where she works across a range of knowledge translation, training, and policy review projects, with a particular focus on supporting disaster impacted communities, emergency service personnel, and the professionals who support them. Prior to joining Phoenix Australia, Courtney worked as a change management consultant for a professional services firm.

Sacha Schweikert studied medicine in Switzerland before moving to Australia to pursue intensive care medicine training. He complemented training with a diploma in clinical ultrasound and undertook a Fellowship in neurocritical care at the University of Toronto before returning to Australia. He currently works as an intensive care specialist at Sir Charles Gairdner Hospital in Perth and has a special interest in all things neurocritical care.

Part VI:
On Being Part of the Solution

Foreword: Those Who Are There; Those Who Have Been There

Laura Hawryluck ⓘ

A pessimist sees the difficulty in every opportunity; an optimist sees the opportunity in every difficulty.
    —*Sir Winston Churchill*

Intensivists are highly trained to recognize serious and life-threatening illnesses, to anticipate acute deteriorations, and to rescue those in need of resuscitation. To do this, they need to apply an obsessive attention to detail, frequent reassessments, monitoring of symptoms, physical exam findings and lab work, and use a collaborative team approach to care—for no one can be everywhere at any given moment in time. Once signs of trouble are recognized, a plan to rescue must be developed, one that reflects the urgency of the situation, one that escalates the care being provided, one that is comprehensive enough to get someone through a life-threatening event. Often our role is to respond to the failures of others to both recognize and rescue. Often, it's to respond to error events on hospital wards; the ICU and its Rapid Response teams being the last stronghold to save someone from harm, to correct a significant wrong. In most hospitals, the intensivist and ICU team play an important role in identifying risks to patient safety and in advocating for solutions. Yet what if you, as the intensivist, played a role in the error event? What if it happened in the ICU? What if you couldn't mitigate its impact? What if you can't fix it and your patient is then forever altered or… dies?

All healthcare professionals are human, and all are highly likely at some point in their career to be involved in an error event. Yet, for intensivists, error events can feel like a primeval existential crisis, an event that cuts deep and makes them question their abilities as a physician and their sense of self as a person. Not because they have a hero complex but because a *rescuer*, a professional with the ultimate responsibility to care, is who they are and what they do.

L. Hawryluck
Toronto Western Hospital, University of Toronto, Toronto, ON, Canada
e-mail: Laura.Hawryluck@uhn.ca

The ICU is a very challenging and increasingly complex environment with new and evolving technologies and practices. Every ICU team is composed of ever-changing healthcare professionals with different levels of skill, knowledge, and experience, different areas of professional and personal strengths. The nature of life-threatening illnesses means the stakes are high and the need is great to make sure nothing in treatment plans goes wrong. ICUs are busy, sometimes crazily so, and frequently multiple patients need to be admitted simultaneously. All these factors create significant risks for error events with serious consequences. Yet very few intensivists have ever received training on dealing with such events or even know who to turn to for help. How do you deal with feelings of failure, anxiety, profound distress? What are our normal reactions and their pitfalls? What strategies can help us cope enough to carry on and still provide care? What can we do to prevent error events from happening again? Can you *be* an intensivist when you finally understand that such events will in all likelihood recur? For far too long, these questions have not been openly discussed. Coping, often in silence, has been seen as an expectation and yet another obligation. Guidance can be very difficult to find.

This part of the book will provide much needed advice *for intensivists from intensivists,* those who have experienced and "survived" error events in their own clinical practice. Their insights, support, and calm, practical leadership are invaluable no matter the stage of your career. For who better to listen to, than those who *are* there, or who *have been* there.

Laura Hawryluck Professor Hawryluck is a Professor of Critical Care Medicine in the Inter-Departmental Critical Care Medicine Program (IDDCM) at the University of Toronto, Canada. She is the Physician Lead of Critical Care Rapid Response Team at Toronto Western Hospital and was Corporate Chair of the Acute Resuscitation Committee at University Health Network, Toronto, for over a decade until May 2021. She is a past President of the Medico-Legal Society of Toronto (MLST). Her international work aims to develop and promote education and training in critical care medicine, end-of-life decision-making and care, medico-legal issues, policy and quality improvement initiatives. She was awarded the Queen's Golden Jubilee Medal for contributions to Canada for improving end-of-life care for Canadians, the MLST award for contributions to law and medicine, and the IDDCM's Humanitarian award. She has authored and co-edited *The Law of Acute Care Medicine* (Thomson Reuters) and three books of poetry *An ICU Doctor's Reflections, Words that Matter, and ICU Pandemic Diary* (Olympia Publishers (UK)).

Chapter 23
Preparing Oneself

Marc Romain ⓘ, **Denise Goodman** ⓘ, **and Tracey Varker** ⓘ

> *A day that I don't learn something new is a wasted day*
>
> *—B.B. King*

The first piece of advice is that critical care practice requires intensive preparation. The knowledge needed is broad, requiring painstaking study and practice, with a commitment to being a lifelong learner. Every person the intensivist encounters will teach him/her something new, but medical knowledge is only part of the preparation. Equally important, we must be fully aware of the emotional impact, and this in turn requires us to know ourselves as highly trained and caring, but fallible human beings.

> *I think just the first thing is just having any sort of appreciation of the personal, not so much the professional impact, but the personal impact of these events. In truth, I don't know if I would have believed my former self. Accepting that they do have a big impact. That you are going to feel very stressed and upset, somewhat being forewarned is forearmed, that while this has happened, you know this is going to have this impact on me. I think that in itself is helpful.*

The question remains, how can we adequately prepare ourselves as individuals for this practice?

M. Romain (✉)
Department of Medical Intensive Care, Hadassah Medical Center, Faculty of Medicine, Hebrew University of Jerusalem, Jerusalem, Israel
e-mail: marcro@hadassah.org.il

D. Goodman
Lurie Children's Hospital, Chicago, IL, USA

T. Varker
Department of Psychiatry, Centre for Post-traumatic Mental Health, University of Melbourne, and Phoenix Australia, Melbourne, VIC, Australia

I think you never are fully prepared for it. Like as a Resident, you see people doing these things, but you don't appreciate ... And even as a Fellow, you don't appreciate the burden of doing it until you're doing it. But as a Resident when I was trying to make the decision, I knew I was going to be doing sick things, I knew I would be in stressful situations; I don't think I appreciated the burden. And I still talk people into doing critical care. The medicine and the ... Yes, we do a lot of hard things, but there are so many good things. Like I can tell you, for every bad story, I can tell you three good ones.

One of the important steps is recognizing, as an individual, what coping mechanisms you can develop and implement to maintain your own mental health and well-being:

... you have to figure out what it is that's going to make you able to cope [or] able to process the bad things that we see; that you can come back and keep doing this job and do it well.

I think the advice I would give is that you do need coping strategies. If you don't naturally have some, or they don't kind of inadvertently fall into your life then I think you need to think about what would work for you, and work on building these up. I think everyone is different.

A foundational step is to realize that we are human beings with a full spectrum of emotions. We are not invincible, and we may fail. The stakes are very high in ICU as the patient remains suspended between life and death. Every decision becomes critical. The intensivist also needs to believe in themself, yet at the same time understand that they are fallible [1].

... perhaps just being a bit more self-aware; being a bit more self-aware that you are fallible; that you will make mistakes. I mentioned the word hubris before, and I think it's real. Particularly if you've done intensive care for a while. You think you've seen most things; you think you can anticipate most things; you think you've got a handle on most things; and that you can read most things and you find yourself in that sort of space. And yes, there is truth to that. With experience, you've got some very good mechanisms, you know? But you can too easily think you are infallible. You know, 'It won't happen to me, it happens to them, that's not me, there's always been shortcuts and it won't happen to me.' And I think probably the most important thing I've learned is fallibility and being aware of it.

Acknowledging that a part of fallibility is to acknowledge that not every patient can be saved, particularly in the intensive care unit, is critical:

Interviewer: 'You were one of those doctors who thought you could save everyone?'
  Participant: 'Absolutely, right? That you can do everything; you should know everything; Now, I realise I don't know everything, and I probably never will know everything, but I can always know more today than I did the day before; and I can keep working on it; and it's a process; and I don't control everything.'

The important thing is to not just "show up" for work every day but to give everything you can on any given day or night:

You don't have the option of having a bad day; when I come to work, I can't give 50% today because I'm tired, or because I don't feel like it; because if this were my child, I want a person who is giving 100%.' And so, I always give 100%, and so clinically, I feel like I'm making a concerted effort to always do a good job when I'm taking care of the patients and to do good.

The internal conflict that exists for the individual between accepting fallibility whilst maintaining the expection of close to zero error, needs to be resolved (at least partially):

> *... the margin for error is not very great sometimes; I think we all know that errors are going to occur; I don't know that any of us can accept that. I think it's very hard for an Intensivist to accept that we can allow an error to occur, and we are pretty focused on error prevention.*
>
> *Interviewer: 'But there is a high frequency of invasive procedures in the ICU I would think, and if you say, put in 100 central lines, inevitably, just by the numbers, there must be a reasonable probability that one of those might go wrong?'*
>
> *Participant: 'I think I can accept that to some degree, like there is risk involved in what we do. Sometimes you're going to encounter something that didn't go quite right.'*

Part of this involves understanding that there may be times when the intensivist should acknowledge the need for the perspective of others to maintain a full overview of a situation:

> *[Sometimes] the most important person to be skeptical of is yourself. Because you have a bigger blind-spot than you can possibly know, and so be skeptical of what you think and always be prepared to think that although that's the way you see it and you're probably right. But what if … What if that's not quite the way things are?*

and the ability to verbalize that to the team:

> *Speaking up, but also having the confidence to say, "I'm not comfortable at this point in time". So, recognising one's limitations and being comfortable to admit that you have limitations. You know, we've all got limitations. I run patients past my senior Consultants when I need to… "What do you think about this? This is what I'm thinking…", so I think that's important.*

So how do intensivists prepare themselves to handle a situation when things go wrong? Should they be cold, and stone-faced to cope, or can they be a resilient and caring human at the same time?

> *I think the day you stop feeling is the day you should completely give up clinical work. So, you don't want to decompensate, you don't want to get burnt out, you don't want to have nothing left to give to the next person.*

For longevity in the specialty, the intensivist needs to develop a plan of who to talk to and debrief with around the day-to-day as well as around specific clinical events. Every intensivist, no matter how senior, should have a mentor who they trust and who can give advice, not only medical advice but emotional too.

> *I think everyone should probably think about having (or think about who would be) a go-to person.*

> *... if I was advising myself, I would choose who I debriefed to. And sort of learn who those people are from experience … people with a bit of wisdom, who will give you a fair hearing; who aren't going to be too critical. Like some people who work in ICU are very clever, but sometimes I feel like they can't identify with the common man.*

The prepared intensivist should also look within themself to ensure that they stay grounded and cared for. Being fully committed to one's professional calling requires an equal commitment to knowing when to let it go and to invest in yourself and your friends, family, and community. This is the deep well of support that allows us to recharge and maintain our humanity. An intensivist bears witness to a lot in the ICU – serious illness, family strains, and lives ended prematurely. It takes a conscious effort to turn that experience into a source of simple gratitude rather than pessimism and despair.

> In terms of personal things, I would tell myself that you need to make time, you need to maintain your circuit breaker. Whether that be sport, your family, a hobby, non-medical friends to kind of break out of that circuit that can happen, particularly in ICU when you are stuck in here ... You're not walking around the wards, things like that. So, I think that's really important.

> To try and switch off in a better way and find strategies to deal with that and to switch off and not let professional life sort of creep into your personal life.

An element of this is managing fatigue:

> The hours of Intensivists here, and the hours of responsibility, are just insane. The amount of nights we have to leave home, we have to be worried that you're going to get called, you don't have time to be a free person. I think when you are younger that's cool and exciting for a while, but I think there is a big price. I think we all pay for it.

> Know when you are tired ... Have a sense of when you are burnt out. Be able to step back from cases.

For some people, the work can take its toll, and some intensivists felt it prudent to have an exit strategy:

> What you're doing, for the length of time ... It's a very hard time to sustain. And I knew that I had an expiration date at some point or another. I knew that there were other things that were going to pop up along the way that I was going to get interested in and would want to do and that was going to be hard, making those few commitments run together at a point, so I couldn't practice in the fashion that I wanted to practice. So, I went into it knowing that I had a timeline, an expiration date, for me anyway. So, I started making my exit plans before I ever actually got along the career path. So that I knew what I was going to do, down the road.

For some intensivists, having a second specialty (for example pulmonology or nephrology) may assist in preventing burnout, as they are able to work in each alternately. This may include both procedural activities as well as clinical activities:

> I think it's good to have another pathway, because you do get worn out doing all of the night call, and the weekends. So, I would encourage junior faculty to think about that - what it looks like. Because as strong as you think you are, you can't do that forever.

Forgiveness of an error is also something to contemplate, as it is needed to overcome the guilt of having made a mistake:

> To be less hard on yourself is probably a useful thing. To recognise that adverse events happen ... which may or may not be related to what you have done, even if you have done everything right, it's still going to happen. You are going to be in unfortunate situations where you come on and something else is happened or is presented to you after it has happened. And so, I think ... to be less judgemental of yourself.

At the same time, the intensivist also needs to develop self-confidence, self-belief, and a degree of assertiveness:

> *You can still work on that conceptual framework of self-reflection, kindness, humanity, compassion. But some people do it better than others. It comes to some people more naturally, to be compassionate.*

> *I would like to think I have become more assertive … not someone who you can ignore and disrespect. A bit more that 'This is my space, my unit, I'm looking after it, these are my patients, and you're communicating with me, and we are going to talk about this'.*

Conclusion

The intensivist needs to undertake a great deal of self-preparation and introspection in order to become a well-rounded, confident yet humble adaptable, resilient intensivist. This is founded on the ability to undertake emotional and professional reflective practice. This valuable habit contributes to the ability to remediate or modify one's own practice through peer review, consultation, and calibration. Developing a more intimate awareness of one's personal trajectory through career stages is aided by this process and allows short-term and longer-term preparation for professional challenges.

Reference

1. Wald EL. A fine line. JAMA. 2020;324(15):1501. https://doi.org/10.1001/jama.2020.19331.

Marc Romain completed his undergraduate medical studies and speciality in internal medicine in South Africa before moving to Israel, where he currently resides and works. He is a specialist in internal medicine, general intensive care, and nephrology. He is a senior physician in the medical ICU and the head of the Critical Care Nephrology and Nutrition Unit at the Hadassah Medical Centers, Jerusalem. His interests include multi-organ support therapies (CRRT, hemoperfusion, ECMO), aviation medicine, and educating the next generation of doctors, nurses, and intensivists.

Denise Goodman trained in pediatrics at Cincinnati Children's Hospital Medical Center and pediatric critical care at Children's Hospital of Pittsburgh. Prior to this she had had undertaken a BS(Physics) at Niagara University, her MD at the State University of NY at Buffalo (now Jacobs School of Medicine at University at Buffalo), and her MS (Epidemiology) at Harvard T.H. Chan School of Public Health. She spent 2012-2013 academic year as the Morris Fishbein Fellow in Medical Editing at JAMA. Her interests include delivery of care, outcomes, care of children with medical complexity, and medical editing. She considers it a privilege to accompany children and their families through some of the most difficult experiences in their lives, and to share both their joys and challenges.

Tracey Varker is a Senior Research Fellow in the Department of Psychiatry, University of Melbourne, and Phoenix Australia—Centre for Post-traumatic Mental Health. Dr Varker leads a team of researchers who focus on improving the lives of those affected by occupational trauma and stress. This includes emergency services and military personnel, healthcare professionals, and those working in heavy industry (e.g., mining and construction). Her research interests center on improving the lives of those impacted by occupational trauma and stress; using evidence synthesis to promote the recovery of those affected by trauma; and improving our understanding of, and the treatment of, problematic anger.

Chapter 24
This Is Where You Live

Mary Pinder and Marc Romain ⓘ

> *Primum non nocere (First do no harm)*
>
> *—Hippocratic oath*

Medical personnel are guided by the principle of 'first do no harm'. As a consequence, adverse events for patients or staff are a significant source of stress in intensive care practice. Clinicians experience fear of causing patient harm (trait anxiety) and guilt and shame in the aftermath of a critical incident (state anxiety) [1]. The nature of the workplace requirement for dealing with critically ill patients in a complex sociotechnical environment means adverse events are unavoidable, [2, 3]. This chapter explores advice around the attitudes and behaviours that intensivists attribute to helping them manage the confronting nature of the workplace and find meaning in their lived experiences.

Study participants described *acceptance of the inevitability* of medical error and patient deaths as a key factor in mitigating the emotional fallout associated with adverse events. This is not condoning complacency, recklessness, or a lack of concern for patient wellbeing. Nor does it abrogate all responsibility for our actions and blame shifting. Instead, it fosters a realistic attitude acknowledging the challenges of the workplace and is seen as important for intensivist mental health.

> *I think I'm more accepting of the fact that these things will happen. Not that… That sounds wrong because I would obviously work very hard to prevent anything…But that is part of the job and that you can't continue to take good care of patients if you let it break you. And that, if, in order to take care of the most children in the best way that you can, all we can do*

M. Pinder (✉)
Department of Intensive Care, Sir Charles Gairdner Hospital, Perth, WA, Australia
e-mail: mary.pinder@health.wa.gov.au

M. Romain
Department of Medical Intensive Care, Hadassah Medical Center, Faculty of Medicine, Hebrew University of Jerusalem, Jerusalem, Israel

D. Dennis et al. (eds.), *Stories from ICU Doctors*,
https://doi.org/10.1007/978-3-031-32401-7_24

is learn from these events. And I do think that processing them, and being upset by them and thinking about them is a necessary part of it. But that also, you just have to let it go. And to be vigilant.

I get to a point where I know that when you are dealing with such cases, errors should not happen, but they happen, because you are doing tons of critical things, making decisions, giving drugs, doing procedures, and errors can happen.

I tend to be quite objective about things, not so much subjective. So, I tend to rationalise why things go wrong. My philosophy is that medical science is not perfect and therefore complications will occur and not necessarily due to anyone's fault, that's my overall philosophy, and that's my attitude towards colleagues as well.

Part of the process of acceptance of adverse outcomes is the recognition of our own limitations and that there are events outside our control, and this may be facilitated by pre-existing personal beliefs and values.

Sometimes as an Intensivist, you can do everything right and the patient still dies. In much the same way, sometimes mistakes are made, and despite them, patients still live. The Intensivist doesn't hold all of the power in their hands – much of the time, survival comes from within the patient themselves.

You know one thing I would say ... I guess we're not superhuman. So, we can't fix everything – and of course this is where my [cultural] upbringing helps a little bit. I mean, we believe a lot in things going towards a predetermined end, and the choices that we make, and everything, are going to go the way it's gonna end. And sometimes that's helpful for me because it takes some of the burden off, in that I can't control ... I don't have full control over everything... Actually, I probably don't have much control over anything really, other than myself, and that is helpful for me.

In the interviews, participants also acknowledged *systemic factors* contributing to adverse events and that blame in these situations does not rest entirely with one individual.

I think people need to begin to realise that they are part of a big system. They are part of a big team. When things go bad, it's not all your fault. You can't take it all on yourself. If an issue goes downhill, it doesn't mean it's all your fault. You've got to look at it, you've got to analyse it, you got to start thinking it's not all me. I think, worldwide, people realise it's more about team and it's not the individual. So, it's like that whole Swiss cheese thing. You know, you have to go through a lot of mistakes for bad things to happen.

Critical incidents are seen as a key *learning* opportunity. This learning is important for eliminating errors in the future and as a way for all involved to find value and meaning in the experience and for personal growth.

I think we try to learn from each [event] because [you] don't only think about what you did wrong also think about you can fix it, how you can prevent it next time. Again, we discuss it, we remember it, we raise it once in a while, those situations. We tell people about the mistakes, I tell other people because they can also learn from my experiences. I think that the fact that we are trying to learn helps us professionally.

... not to be too harsh on yourself. And accept that this will occur, and when they occur, do your best to retrieve them. And sometimes things happen that aren't necessarily someone's fault. And yes, I think preparation, and then I guess learning from your own mistakes. Not repeating the same mistakes over and over again.

… you cannot grow without learning from your mistakes. I know now, what will happen if you do this, or somebody else does that. I know because I have seen it. It's not necessary by mistake. It's a decision. A decision can take you places. Other decisions will take you to another decision or another place. I know now what will probably happen if you take this decision. I can't teach this unless they experience it. Sometimes I stop them, but usually I let them continue. It's a skill, it is a profession, it's based upon the successes and failures. You have to learn from the failures in order to evolve. You have to. Otherwise, you are oblivious to the things that can happen.

Another coping strategy identified from the study participants' responses is maintaining a *balanced perspective* and recognising adverse events.

So adverse events will happen because of you; adverse events will happen around you; adverse events will happen to you. And that's normal. You're not less of a human being because of it. You are part of a system, and you are an important part of the system, and you need to recognize when you're functioning as well as you can, and when you're not.

Normalising the process includes acknowledgement that the experience is not unique and even happens to experienced colleagues.

I know that all of my seniors and all of my Intensivists, that they also have mistakes and they are having their bag also of their patients that they made harm or damage because they make decisions and I know that they have it also. I know I'm not the only one.

And so just to provide some reassurance that these events aren't singling you out, they are commonly experienced, and that the fact that they are happening around you, or to you is to be expected.

Another facet to keeping things in perspective is the recognition that error is unintentional and everyone strives to do their best and makes the decisions that seem right at the time. This is an important learning point that experienced specialists relay to junior staff.

… I say to them, 'How does it feel when you do something wrong?' And they go, 'It feels terrible.' And I say, 'But if you knew you were doing something wrong, would you have done it?' They go, 'No, of course not.' I say 'Right, so then the difference is, when you're doing something wrong, it feels like you're doing something right; it's only with hindsight that it becomes obvious.' … Nobody knowingly cannulates a carotid; nobody knowingly severs a vein; nobody knowingly sticks a needle into your heart when you think you're putting in a chest tube; you don't knowingly do it. And so that's really important to remember … If you think what you're doing is right, then do it. I will always support you if you can walk me through logically why you wanted to do something, so just do it. That's when your Fellowship is all about. This is your growth.

… always be meaningful and reassuring that no one comes to work to hurt anybody. And we sometimes play a really dangerous game in ICU, and despite everything we do, sometimes things happen.

I think we have to learn that it's okay (it's not okay) but it's okay to make the wrong decision or to practice your skills until you're very good at them, and to take into account that is not okay to make a mistake but it's part of your work. If you don't do procedures, you don't have complications, but if you want to do procedures, you will have complications. And I see for myself, and all of my colleagues, especially the youngsters, that the first, the second, the third mistake is a catastrophe. You want to die. You want to disappear. And then you need to realise that it's part of your progression. It's part of your evolution and it's not a sterile environment.

The study participants addressed the influence of *age and experience* in managing workplace stress. Seniority was seen for the most part as beneficial in helping intensivists be less self-critical and less emotional and gain a more balanced perspective following adverse events.

… something that I thought I could have done better, I think I would have mulled on that quite a lot. I mean, I still do but… I would have thought about it a lot more when I was younger.

I would say that personally, I think the fact that I am working with my age and experience, most probably both of them, I can deal with errors … in a less emotional way, I would say. And I get to a point where I know that when you are dealing with such cases, errors should not happen, but they happen, because you are doing tons of critical things, making decisions, giving drugs, doing procedures, and errors can happen. I think that with the experience, I am dealing with these errors, even if I did it, or even if another person is doing it, there is less of an emotional way and more of a professional way of interrogating what happened exactly.

I think that most of the time, people mellow and become very a bit more reflective about it, but I think when people like that are early in their career, they can be a little, or very critical, and [they] just can't understand that perfect medicine doesn't exist.

However, it was acknowledged that dealing with the process of adverse events is still as difficult for experienced intensivists, but they have learned the value of debriefing with colleagues.

I think I would tell them it doesn't necessarily get easier with time, and that's okay. That it doesn't get easier with time that processing things, processing events are important for yourself as much as it is for whatever like the actual medical event was. And that, I think I've learned more with time to find space and people to talk to about events, and I think I would probably encourage a lot younger version of myself to do that.

Experienced intensivists may have an additional burden of stress in that there may be a perception that errors are less excusable for them than for their junior colleagues. It was also recognised that the experience of senior colleagues has a foundation in the learning gained from making mistakes.

You can say that the older clinician should not make that mistake. And that the younger one is excusable because he has no experience. But I think that somebody who is making a mistake that can be avoided it doesn't matter if he is the younger one or the older one. I'm sure that… you are building your experiences on the mistakes that you have done.

Study participants also recognised the importance of *peer support and self-care* in maintaining mental health and helping to make meaning and facilitate closure after adverse events.

I think doctors are very self-judgmental. And to be less hard on yourself is probably a useful thing. To recognise that mistakes happen, or adverse events happen, maybe not mistakes. Which may or may not be related to what you have done, even if you have done everything right, it's still going to happen. You are going to be in unfortunate situations where, you come on and something else is happened or is presented to you after it has happened. And so, I think, I think, to be less judgmental of yourself.

… you have to be careful not to personalise everything that goes wrong. The cumulative baggage of that would just destroy you. And so, I've been able to, I think in a healthy way, absolve myself of things that I'm not, you know, personally responsible.

Lastly, study participants advocated maintaining a sense of *humility* and avoiding hubris. Intensivists should not take sole credit for successful patient outcomes or sole responsibility for adverse events:

If you become a Senior Intensivist and you are so arrogant to think that the second you show up, you'll figure it out… you're going to be a dangerous doctor. Kids can humble you in a second … I have gotten enough experience to be mature enough to know that even after my best efforts, I could have made bad choices along the way, and the child could die.

I often correct people when they say, 'Oh, what a great save' (laughs). And I think, if you say you saved, then do you also, when a child dies, say 'Oh, I failed!' I think it depends whether you really see yourself in that… whereas I do believe I have a skill set, and I do believe I can make a difference, I'm not so sure that I can interrupt destiny. I don't know that my ego is so strong to think that I interrupt destiny in such a powerful way … It is just a minute, and a blip. The child that you are able to successfully resuscitate; the hyperkalaemia that you recognise; the critical airway that you're able to … Great! That's what you're supposed to do!

I mean you can be the world best at something and things can still go wrong. Or you can do everything absolutely right in a situation and still have a problem; or you can be absolutely wrong all the time, but it doesn't matter what you do it doesn't make a difference, and you end up in the right place anyway.

Conclusion

To counteract the stresses imposed by the nature of the intensive care workplace and the inevitability of patient death and medical error, intensivists advocate maintaining a sense of perspective, accepting that, despite their best intentions, adverse events can and will happen. Using such events as a learning experience, remaining humble, and supporting each other without judgement or blame is the preferred approach.

References

1. Voultsos P, Koungali M, Psaroulis K, Boutou AK. Burnout syndrome and its association with anxiety and fear of medical errors among intensive care unit physicians: a cross-sectional study. Anaesth Intensive Care. 2020;48(2):136–42.
2. Donchin Y, Seagull FJ. The hostile environment of the intensive care unit. Curr Opin Crit Care. 2002;8:316–20.
3. Reason J. Human error: models and management. BMJ. 2000;320:768–70.

Mary Pinder is an Intensive Care Specialist and Director of Clinical Training based at Sir Charles Gairdner Hospital in Perth, Western Australia. She trained in intensive care in the UK and South Africa as well as Australia. She is on the Board of the College of Intensive Care Medicine of Australia and New Zealand (CICM) and roles with the CICM have included Chair of the Second Part Exam Committee, Chair of the Assessments Committee, and College President.

Marc Romain completed his undergraduate medical studies and speciality in internal medicine in South Africa before moving to Israel, where he currently resides and works. He is a specialist in internal medicine, general intensive care, and nephrology. He is a senior physician in the medical ICU and the head of the Critical Care Nephrology and Nutrition Unit at the Hadassah Medical Centers, Jerusalem. His interests include multi-organ support therapies (CRRT, hemoperfusion, ECMO), aviation medicine, and educating the next generation of doctors, nurses, and intensivists.

Chapter 25
Keeping Things Tidy

Peter Vernon van Heerden ⓘ, Sigal Sviri ⓘ, and Liron van Heerden

The most precious gift we can offer anyone is our attention.

—Thich Nhat Hanh

Intensivists need to cope with, and manage, a complex working environment to produce a product, healthy patients, at the end of the process, all without damaging our own health and/or impacting our relationships [1]. When things go wrong, the consequences need to be managed. However, everyone including our patients would be better served if we prevent adverse events from happening in the first place. This is the focus of the advice in this chapter.

One of the strategies for preventing adverse events is in effect controlling the complex environment as much as possible [2]. This means making sure that information is disseminated effectively to everyone involved in the care of the patient, even if it means repeating the information several times and, in various formats, such as verbal handover, written notes in the patient file or written specific instructions. This behaviour may come across as pedantic and prescriptive, but it will ensure the senior intensivist's instructions are noted and carried out, contributing largely to high-quality communication between specialist doctors. Important treatment details are also less likely to be "lost in translation".

P. V. van Heerden (✉)
General Intensive Care Unit, Department of Anesthesiology, Critical Care and Pain Medicine, Hadassah Medical Center, Jerusalem, Israel
e-mail: vernon@hadassah.org.il

S. Sviri
Department of Medical Intensive Care, Hadassah Medical Center and Faculty of Medicine, Hebrew University of Jerusalem, Jerusalem, Israel

L. van Heerden
University of Melbourne, Melbourne, VIC, Australia

There is a clear advantage to written instructions, in addition to verbal instructions, in medicolegal terms.

I decided that I'm going to 'over-communicate'… … I'm going to make sure that my communication is clear and consistent in just about everything I need to. And just keep going down that pathway, and just make everything as transparent and informed as we go along, to minimise the opportunities, that somebody could 'have a go' at me. So, I guess it's a self-defence mechanism in many ways, but also, I think it's in the patient's best interests. That everyone is having a shared model of what's happening…

Staff laugh at my daily care plans because they're very prescriptive. And it might say something like, 'Ultrasound right chest for drainage of an effusion'. Or 'once marked, don't move the patient'. And that's just from previous experience. I've come back in the morning and had people on high, 80% oxygen, and they were on pressure support, which in my personal view is not correct. So, I'll write on the daily care plan now, 'Maintain full ventilatory support' if I want that to occur. 'Until the FiO_2 is less than "x" or whatever', so I tend to be a little bit more prescriptive. But all that stuff is based around previous experience.'

When dealing with junior medical staff, the intensivist should not assume that they will know what to do. Indeed, they may not even have enough experience to know what to ask, let alone do, in a given situation. Hence, the information given should be pitched at the lowest common denominator. Trainees at different levels of training will ask questions and understand answers in keeping with their level of training as outlined by one participant:

The medicine I practice now is different from the medicine I practised twenty years ago, but I've surrounded myself with a cadre of incredibly bright, young specialist doctors who are always asking me questions. They want to know in their first year, 'Why am I doing it?' In their second year they become very fixated on 'How they do it' In their third year, it becomes about distinguishing what is important and what is not important: 'What should I be spending my time on? What direction should I be taking?' because they look at it with a much bigger picture.

Teaching a standardised way of handing over information or using checklists are effective ways of ensuring correct and comprehensive transfer of information, reducing communication errors, and improving patient safety and care:

I try to go through with my junior guys and teach them to be as thorough as they can to make sure that they don't miss something. And that means having proformas in their own head, for example starting with the patient from the top of the head and going down to the heels, just working through every single body system and saying with the nurse and with my team: 'This is what our issues are here; this is how we're dealing with it', so sharing the communication so that everyone is on the same line, but we're also going through things in a systematic way so don't miss something. So, I try and ingrain that in them.

We have learnt a lot about systems, whether it's checklists or having a routine that you stick to. If you think about a lot of the critical incidents that happen, it's because something has been assumed and steps have been cut often. So, I think that being careful in the way that you deal with those situations is useful.

Effective communication within and between the intensive care team and referring or consulting specialist doctors is part of the effective supervision of junior colleagues in the ICU by the attending intensivist. They are the leader of the team and take ultimate responsibility for what happens in the ICU and the outcome of the patient, as well as for adverse events in the ICU. Several participants described the need to be on top of every detail for every patient:

> A lot of the things you do to pre-empt any mistakes that might happen, because, if you just let everything run its course, I think a lot more mistakes would happen, and that's why you are there, in charge. And so, a lot of the communication, the way you set things up as to what's going to happen next… I talk through a lot about why we are doing this, what are we going to do, and I guess that is the whole point, is to pre-empt errors. So, everyone is aware of the upcoming play. So, I think around every procedure you do, you are mitigating potential errors.

> Again, to pay attention to detail. I stress that point. To keep caring for the patient at every point. Not to let it go when the patient becomes a little better because sometimes things happen…

> It's just, 'Ah, I've always being like this ever since I've been an intern'. I'd always, before I went home, even if we'd finished late, I'd always make sure that I checked all the blood results before I went home. I just always used to do that.

Senior clinicians can often foresee problems because of their clinical experience, theoretical knowledge, practical skills, and personal maturity. They've seen it all before. This is why effective supervision of junior colleagues in their decision-making and technical skills, combined with effective communication, is complementary and important.

> I'd like to think that every day, on every ward round that we do and with our checklists, we are in fact preventing, pre-empting, predicting the known knowns. But in terms of recognising the behaviours of others, and more directly intervening, it would be finding your way to constructively say, 'Are you sure you want to do that? Have you thought about why? Why don't we have a chat to someone else and see what they think?' And I try and openly say to trainees 'Are you sure?' as this is the most loaded and important question in intensive care. As soon as someone asks 'Are you sure?' you shouldn't be.

> An individual, say a trainee, who receives a piece of knowledge may not understand that the knowledge needs to be acted upon or needs to be propagated. The whole event can degenerate into a failure of supervision since the trainee didn't know they needed to be supervised on that decision, and you didn't realize that you needed to tell them.

Of course, obsessive attention to detail can be debilitating, but in the authors' experience, the more capable and comfortable the attending intensivist is in their environment, the less overwhelmed they will be by detail. This is all part of "growing up" as a senior doctor.

> I tend to be a little 'micro-manager'. I'm all up in everyone's business in the unit, and that may be a product of me still being relatively junior and so I still tend to have my hands in the water all the time, so I'm talking to families all day, every day.

> First week as Faculty I worked 140 hours; I couldn't leave the hospital because I was so wound up. Because there was no backup. Because I was finally ultimately responsible for the lives of the children I was taking care of.

Several participants emphasized the need to be sceptical about information provided by third parties—"trust, but verify"—for the safety and correct care of the patient and medicolegal reasons, as the person ultimately integrating the care plan and being responsible for the care of the patient.

So, one of the things that I teach registrars is to be skeptical of both others, and what they say to you, not in a disrespectful way but to question what they say.

And you always have to think about what is the worst-case scenario, and step back from there. And then use things to reassure yourself that it's not the worst-case scenario as opposed to the other way round: assuming that things are fine and then needing things to be escalated. So, I think starting out with the assumption that everything is going bad... I mean, look for the worst life-threatening thing and address that first... and then move backwards from there...

So, the job of the Intensivist talking to an adult emergency doctor is to confirm everything they say and take everything they say with a grain of salt; assume the worst, provide ample protection for the child; there are times when we can over-care for a child, but most of the time, giving more care is only in the child's best interests.

...and there was this very sort of legendary kind of grumpy adult ICU Doctor, and he would always say, 'Believe nothing; trust no one!' and I have always sort of taken that to be true, ...

Preventing adverse events is an excellent motivator to remain well-informed and up to date, both in knowledge and skills. This means routinely practising the procedures common in the ICU, such as central line and arterial line placement, intubation, tracheostomy, and thoraco- and abdomino-centesis. This is true for junior staff learning the procedures, senior medical staff teaching the procedures, and nursing staff assisting in the procedures, so that they become second nature. A good medical knowledge base is also clearly essential.

With complications of procedures that are performed, I tend to rationalise it by saying, 'Look, there are complications with any procedure, and if you do enough of them you will have complications from those procedures.' And that, as long as you can confidently say that you are current in terms of being able to perform that procedure safely, and that you've got enough experience... that complications will occur, and that is not necessarily anyone's fault it's just a probability.

Of course, in any team there will be individuals with different skill sets and abilities. The taciturn, less-than-perfect communicator may be the person most skilled in some or all practical procedures. Part of effective leadership in an ICU is to encourage people to their strengths and help them to self-awareness of their limitations. Regular team and individual assessments will promote a culture of self-awareness.

So, I would say self-awareness and situational awareness would be two of the top ones in that list because I think some of the other things flow on from those things. So, if you're not aware that there is a problem, you are not aware of whatever else is going on, then that leads to difficulties with communication, lack of teamwork, and those sorts of things.

And self-awareness is important because I think that many critical incidents result from task focus. Often Intensivists get sort of focused on putting a tube in, or getting the line in, or whatever, and they're not self-aware enough to say, 'Actually, something is going wrong here; I'm not handling this correctly; How should this go differently?'

Intensivists work in a team in the ICU and as discussed in Chap. 9 should recognise the strength of the team as a support structure, to ensure quality of care, quality improvement, and peer review [3]. Intensive care practice is one of the most "visible" and scrutinised medical specialties, with review by colleagues, visiting medical teams, and nursing and allied staff in real-time. Even when we don't all see eye to eye, it's important to promote the ICU team concept:

.. With really difficult cases, particularly patients who may not be going to get better or are facing a very long-term admission with poor quality of life, sometimes the nursing and medical staff separate quite a bit in terms of what's the goal of care. The nurses can do that because they don't actually have a responsibility of the final say, whereas the medical staff really do.

Triumphs are instantly visible, but so are incidents and accidents. Intensivists should nurture positive relationships amongst the ICU team for the benefit of patients and for the support they can offer each other. Collaboration is required for quality improvement initiatives to succeed and for successful healthcare delivery. If intergroup relationships are not built on the basis of respect, compassion, authenticity, and kindness, then disagreements may hamper communication about problems encountered and the success or failure of solutions.

If there was one thing you want to say, [you've] got to be kind to patients; to families; to colleagues; to nurses. You've got to think the best of them, you have got to be generous and kind... If you're trying to be tough, macho, or smart; and trying to be astute; and knowledgeable; and you're trying to do all of the trials; that isn't really going to sell it. I think being humane and kind, obviously you have to be competent that's a given, but it's more important than anything else in my mind...

And it's no good to be nice to somebody when you need them. They'll be able to tell. They'll say, 'What do you want?' You've got to be nice when you don't need them.

We are doing some of that, a support group. We used to do a few times a year, meetings of the intensive care outside of the hospital, going to a restaurant to celebrate something... And this suddenly shows you the other possibilities and you take it back with you to the ICU. You carry it back with you and you take it to a better relationship inside the ICU. So, I think one of the stress relievers is the support that you feel inside the ICU and if you have good relations with your nurses, with your colleagues, it's something that can help. You might not feel that threatened when you make a mistake. Even though, if you did a mistake, they will still be there for you. I know in the same way, I will be there for most if not all of my nurses, probably Fellows, and probably juniors that are in the unit. This relationship inside the microcosm of ICU is something that can relieve a part of the very high emotional stress - that you can develop from the mistakes. If the relationship is bad, when somebody makes a mistake, it will explode, because there will be only blame. So doing social activities out of the ICU and bonding of the team is important.

I want to have, first of all, a group meeting with the nurses and doctors together, to talk about cases that were end-of-life, young patients dying, family that were hysterical, cases that were very traumatic. To hear how they felt and what happened to them, how they coped. But also, what do they expect from me, and from the other doctors? How to bridge the gap between the doctors making the decisions and the nurses being there to take the consequences of the decisions that the doctors make. So, we come (doctors) and we say to give this, or give that, and go away. They [nurses] have to be there with the family and deal with whatever happens, whether it is good or bad. So I would like to bridge the gap. If they want to join the meetings, if they want us to explain to them, if they want us to ask them what they think. Whatever they want.

I think that the team-based training that we do is improving. In some situations, but we still do very little interdisciplinary team-based care. And so, I think that is something that would really help because I think that often things arise when there are clashes, and so I think that that would be helpful.

As well as building and nurturing our own teams in the ICU, it's very important to maintain good, nonaggressive, and nonconfrontational relationships with referring medical and surgical teams and indeed to develop and maintain appreciative regard, understanding, and empathy for their point of view and respect their skills [4]. This will help prevent adverse events in the ICU because of clear, open, and friendly communication, and better support for when adverse events do occur.

'And I think that's important to me, to deal with the fact that, most... a lot of the time, we do have to deal with either misjudgements or misadventures, and again I think that another thing that I often say to the Fellows and I actually believe myself, "Go into the operating theatre, watch what cardiothoracic surgery is like, sit there for three hours and see the skill that is involved. And if you do that, and the surgeons see you do that, you start a different relationship. I always joked with the Head of Cardiothoracic surgery, there was a complication or something, and I went to theatre with him, and he was doing some complicated aortic work, and I said that looks really hard. I promise, I will never make fun of cardiac surgeons again.

... They might have a patient who needs to come to intensive care, and they'll manage them on the ward, making the patient come to some risk, because you gave them a hard time. It doesn't help, and it doesn't solve any problems because people then become defensive, and no-one is focused on the problem anymore. 'You and me, mano a mano. Okay let's see who wins!' It's just pointless.

I think the thing that I've worked on the most is to try to learn how to see things from other people's perspective; because we are really in the ICU, the team leader; but that does not mean we are the owner of the team; and so, to see how other people - trying to stand in their place and see what they're seeing and be more of a cheerleader and not a dictator of the team. I've learned to not take offence when somebody disagrees or says something that you're wondering why, or where did that come from? And being confident in who you are, if someone disagrees with you, or doesn't really want to do the same plan, to be confident and flexible when things can be done in two different ways.

I actually tell the young guys all the time, 'You've got to call the surgeons when things are going well. Don't call the surgeons only when there is a problem. Just pick up the phone and take a photo of the patient say, on an intra-aortic balloon catheterisation, sitting out on a chair or walking with the physios, and say "check him out. He's walking around and looking great ..." That's all you have to do ... Otherwise they just associate your voice with trouble. It becomes like a Pavlovian reflex. it doesn't take much to call them up and say things are going well.

Unfortunately, sometimes despite our best efforts, we cannot achieve the quality of relationships we would like. We then have to navigate around these unsatisfactory working conditions.

Some surgeons, it just never happens, and you give up. In most cases, with time, there is a seminal event that happens where they realised that. 'Oh, somebody else has an opinion and can do it', and you start looking at each other eye to eye. But I think it's one of the stresses, your opinion not being respected.

Maintaining and valuing healthy family relationships and friendships outside of work will also increase job satisfaction, productivity, and efficiency, making us better colleagues and communicators and more attentive to our patients. This should hopefully also help us avoid incidents and accidents.

> *And don't ever forget or abuse your family, abuse as in, take them for granted - your family. Because I think without them, many Intensivists and particularly ... well this is about me... Would fall into a very deep dark hole very quickly, and not have the resources to get out.*

Conclusion

Due to the complexity of patients' conditions, the need for urgent interventions, and the considerable workload fluctuation in the ICU, the likelihood of medical errors, which can induce adverse events, increases considerably compared to those of other departments. Quality assurance becomes a complex task. This chapter discussed a number of preventative strategies, identified as highly valuable amongst intensivists, as key to developing a culture of patient safety within the ICU.

Prevention is the most appropriate intervention in the ICU. The backbone of preventing adverse events is controlling and curating the ICU environment to create a climate of leadership, teamwork, trust, openness, transparency, respect, and compassion for the ICU team to provide safe care. Through high-quality and effective communication, operating alongside effective supervision, self-awareness of errors, and support of individuals' strengths within the team can establish a positive environment. Further, establishing, fostering, and maintaining positive relationships within the ICU team, between medical teams, and with one's family and friends are of utmost importance. However, all of these objectives alone are insufficient to reduce the risk of adverse events. The litany of preventative measures described must be used in combination to create such a safety culture and to produce the most important product: healthy patients.

References

1. Alameddine M, Dainty KN, Deber R, Sibbald WJ. The intensive care unit work environment: current challenges and recommendations for the future. J Crit Care. 2009;24(2):243–8. https://doi.org/10.1016/j.jcrc.2008.03.038.
2. Sameera V, Bindra A, Rath GP. Human errors and their prevention in healthcare. J Anaesthesiol Clin Pharmacol. 2021;37(3):328–35. https://doi.org/10.4103/joacp.JOACP_364_19.
3. Ervin JN, Kahn JM, Cohen TR, Weingart LR. Teamwork in the intensive care unit. Am Psychol. 2018;73(4):468–77. https://doi.org/10.1037/amp0000247.
4. Misseri G, Cortegiani A, Gregoretti C. How to communicate between surgeon and intensivist? Curr Opin Anaesthesiol. 2020;33(2):170–6. https://doi.org/10.1097/ACO.0000000000000808.

Peter Vernon van Heerden   qualified as an anesthetist and intensive care specialist and has practiced in South Africa, the UK, Australia, and Israel. He is the Director of the General Intensive

Care Unit, Dept. of Anesthesiology, Critical Care and Pain Medicine, Faculty of Medicine, Hadassah Hospital and Hebrew University of Jerusalem, Israel.

Sigal Sviri is a specialist in Internal Medicine and Critical Care. She is the Director of the Medical ICU at the Hadassah Medical Center, Jerusalem, Israel, and was in charge of one of the COVID-19 ICU's at Hadassah Hospital during the COVID-19 pandemic. She has served as the Secretary of the Israeli Society of Critical Care and the Director of the Israeli Board examinations committee in Critical Care. Her interests include mechanical ventilation, prognostication in the ICU, ethics, and end-of-life decision making. She is part of the VIP Group (very elderly patients in the ICU) which studies prognostic factors, decision making, and outcomes in critically ill elderly patients.

Liron van Heerden has an undergraduate degree in neuroscience from the University of Western Australia, with honors from the Univ. of Melbourne. She did her experimental work at the Florey Institute of Neuroscience and Mental Health in Melbourne. She is currently undertaking a master's degree at the Univ. of Melbourne.

Chapter 26
Actions in the Moment

Nancy Tofil ⓘ and Matthew Anstey ⓘ

> *Want of foresight, unwillingness to act when action would be
> simple and effective, lack of clear thinking, confusion of counsel
> until the emergency comes, until self-preservation strikes its
> jarring gong - these are the features which constitute the
> endless repetition of history.*
>
> —*Winston Churchill*

Responding to real-time emergent situations can be one of the most stressful situations in critical care. Remaining calm, in charge, and open to suggestions from others is a skill that continues to improve throughout one's career. This chapter explores advice around four clinical considerations in these situations: shared decision-making; team preparation; familiarity of team members; and delegation.

N. Tofil (✉)
Division of Paediatric Critical Care and Paediatric Simulation Center, Children's of Alabama, University of Alabama at Birmingham, Birmingham, AL, USA
e-mail: ntofil@uabmc.edu

M. Anstey
Sir Charles Gairdner Hospital, Perth, WA, Australia

School of Public Health, Curtin University, Perth, WA, Australia

School of Medicine, University of Western Australia, Perth, WA, Australia

Shared Decision-Making

Sharing of decisions is a strategy to help respond to real-time events regarding better patient care. This can also be self-protective to enhance the intensivist's emotional well-being. Not feeling all of the cognitive and emotional burden of decisions oneself is helpful. Consultative and inclusive decision-making processes allow decision-sharing and shared responsibility, which offloads the weight of the moment.

> *Another thing that I have learnt from my practice that I have try to impart on others is, for example, in a resuscitation, to ask everybody in the room if they are comfortable stopping and that they can sleep at night as well as I can. So, that if someone says, 'I don't know why we did that resuscitation', I will say that, 'I also need to sleep at night', and it is important that we take our emotional well-being into account, and as a leader, we need to take into account everybody's well-being.*

> *Generally, it's a shared thing. Even in those events it's... a most important way, at least to decrease the stress, is to feel that everybody has the same opinion that this should have been done, that this treatment that we should give now... and to share the stress with others is very important. The treatment that was done by the cardiologist the treatment after that was a shared treatment between the cardiology team, the surgeon, the Intensivist, it's shared all the time.*

Sometimes it does take some time to reach shared decisions. Most situations allow for this time, and in the long run, it is very helpful for team dynamics.

> *So, bringing everyone around to the appropriate endpoint so that everyone is on board, usually you have got time to do that. Even if that means taking a bit longer than what would be ideal for what I would want. If it has to take an extra day, then that's not the end of the world.*

> *[If] I have three Consultants. I always ask them – not in every decision I make – but in a structural decision or in a strategic decision they are involved, and I always listen to what they have to say.*

Occasionally in pediatrics there are decision support tools or important studies that can help guide clinical decisions in a more objective and less biased way [1]. In adult intensive care, there are a variety of risk calculators available, and even though these tools were not necessarily designed for determining individual outcomes, they may provide reassurance as to clinical gestalt and, if available, should be considered.

> *In difficult decision-making, I try where possible to use some sort of objective tool, a risk assessment or something like that, so my decision-making is not, hopefully not, flawed by some bias.*

Above all else our participants identified the need for intensivists to be clear and respectful. Most times the team of people you are working with you will work with again. When people feel valued and respectful, they will share their opinions resulting in better patient care.

> *One, be respectful. Two, make your case pretty clear. Make sure that you're actually talking about the same thing. Have a common shared understanding of the facts, but perhaps not a shared understanding of what you should do.*

Preparation of the Team

The team in the intensive care unit is ever-changing. There is a large pool of nurses, and rotating junior medical staff, making it uncommon to have the same team attend each critical event. So, nothing takes the place of good preparation. Discussing contingency plans and predicting possible outcomes and ways to handle these helps the management of emergencies run smoother with fewer errors. Being deliberate and explicit is important [2].

> I would try to pre-empt all the different things that would happen ... 'Okay I'm going to intubate. I know that when I intubate potentially there's going to be a vagal response, potentially there's going to be a drop in blood pressure, potentially we're going to need fluids so I'll be the one intubating at this point, but if XY and Z happen I want you to do this...' so you kind of pre-plan going into it as to what potentially could happen...

> There is less chaos if people know where things are heading and what the next step in the management is, then they can facilitate not just better management but better communication and better outcomes for the patient. And not just patient outcomes - although they are obviously important. But outcomes also for the staff who feel like... well, the patient died but we did everything appropriate.

Know Your Team (Ad Hoc vs. Trained Longitudinal Teams)

Working as part of a team is one of the highlights of being an intensivist. When this team works flawlessly, it is an amazing and wonderful positive feeling that brings joy to all members. This helps intensivists' well-being and self-actualization. "Being in the trenches" with team members you trust builds a strong level of commitment. However, it is equally important we know our team as individuals, such as what they like and dislike, what their children's names are, and where they call home.

> Treat them as equal all the time, and then when the time comes for them to be potentially important for something you want to do, they will help you, because they feel you are a genuine nice person who is interested in them as people. If you don't do that, I don't think you're going to get the best out of your ICU.

> It's like any relationship, if you don't know each other you have to do the dance, you have to get to know each other. In general, you are able to get to the middle of the road with some level of mutual respect and confidence.

> So, doing social activities out of the ICU and bonding of the team is important. We do it a little, but maybe there's not enough effort to do that. We acknowledge the importance of doing it. Because of the support that you will get when you get to the ICU, when you deal with a stressful event. So, these are maybe the two things that can help relieve pressure.

Delegating

Knowing your team also comes from working with them and understanding the skills they contribute to different situations. The best teams function when all team members are actively involved in doing tasks they are competent to perform and asking for help when needed and when no team member has too much mental or physical work overload. Proper delegation of roles is crucial for optimal team performance. This has been shown in simulated pediatric cardiac arrest scenarios where the addition of a cardiopulmonary arrest coach helps decrease the workload of the team leader and improve team performance [3].

I would say just to be careful, and to role delegate, not to try to do everything yourself. Because I think standing at the end of the bed versus trying to assist with getting lines in or something when someone is struggling, that amount of time that you're losing is important.

You need to stand there, taking all the visual cues in and all the things are happening think about other things, and the team is good, the team will run a resuscitation without you doing anything, so trying to get them to have that ability to step away a little bit, but at the same time delegate tasks. And I think that it has taken me a while to get better at delegation, that's something that I try to teach my registrars.

High-performing teams from other industries (such as Formula 1 racing pit crews) train over and over to deliberate mastery together with explicit roles that need to be coordinated. This is not always possible in the ICU due to short-term and longer-term rostering, as multiple combinations of nurses or doctors can be thrust into any emergency situation. Having had previous experiences with them, previous simulation training, and a common understanding of roles, combined with appropriate delegation, can make those ICU crisis situations run smoothly.

I guess that's about being a good leader. Being able to stand back and lead, delegate a task and know that that task will be happening in the background, and then being able to move on.

Conclusion

There are many amazing moments of being an intensivist. Running a near-perfect code, saving a patient's life is truly transformative. Unfortunately, these are not common, and dealing with the more common ups and downs is crucial to long-term well-being.

References

1. Chapman SM, Maconochie IK. Early warning scores in paediatrics: an overview. Arch Dis Child. 2019;104(4):395–9.
2. Prince CR, Hines EJ, Chyou P, Heegeman DJ. Finding the key to a better code: code team restructure to improve performance and outcomes. Clin Med Res. 2014;12(1–2):47–57.
3. Tofil NM, Cheng A, Lin Y, Davidson J, Hunt EA, Chatfield J, MacKinnon R, Kessler D, for the International Network for Simulation-based Paediatric Innovation, Research and Education (INSPIRE) CPR Investigators. Effect of a CPR coach on workload during pediatric cardiopulmonary arrest: a multicentre, simulation-based study. Pediatr Crit Care Med. 2020;21(5):e274–81.

Nancy Tofil is a Professor of Pediatrics and the Division Director of Paediatric Critical Care. She is the Medical Director of the Paediatric Simulation Center at Children's of Alabama/University of Alabama at Birmingham (UAB). The Simulation Center has trained over 85,000 learners in almost 13 years. Our center has a focus on interdisciplinary learning and parent education. Professor Tofil is the Senior Associate Program Director for the Pediatric Residency Training Program. She obtained her medical degree from The Ohio State University College of Medicine and her Master of Education from UAB. She completed her pediatric residency and fellowship training at UAB.

Matthew Anstey is an intensivist and researcher at Sir Charles Gairdner Hospital, Curtin University, and University of Western Australia in Perth. He has a Master of Public Health from Harvard University, and was the 2010-11 Harkness Fellow in Health Policy, based at Kaiser Permanente in California. He was the past chair of Choosing Wisely Australia advisory group. His research interests focus on improving outcomes for ICU survivors (and built the survivors website mylifeaftericu.com) and improving the quality of care received by patients.

Chapter 27
Actions After the Moment

Michael Ruppe and Z. Leah Harris ⓘ

> *Death, of course, is not a failure. Death is normal. Death may*
> *be the enemy, but it is also the natural order of things.*
>
> —*Atul Gawande*

Mistakes happen. We call them "adverse events," "patient safety events," or "medical errors." Good people with excellent training make mistakes. And for the intensivist, mistakes are high stakes. They often equate to permanent disability or death. This chapter provides advice on managing these moments.

When Fellows are asked "What does it feel like to do the wrong thing?" inevitably they describe a list of emotions: guilt, remorse, anxiety, shame, sadness, fear. But when you are doing the wrong thing, it feels the same as doing the right thing – you don't know it's wrong, or that it isn't going to turn out the way it should have, until *after* it has occurred. Most adverse events and mistakes are unintended and difficult for the healthcare provider, as the person who caused the error, to process.

What is the "right" way to process a mistake that causes harm? How much emotional damage is appropriate for mistakes to cause? Is it okay to fear the legal or professional fallout of a mistake? The modern ICU environment is granted no special status. Outcomes are increasingly transparent. The funding viability of hospitals is increasingly linked to "quality of care" metrics. Public reporting platforms such as the Society of Thoracic Surgeons and the US News and World Report have

M. Ruppe (✉)
Division of Critical Care, Department of Pediatrics, University of Louisville, and Norton Children's Medical Group, Louisville, KY, USA
e-mail: michael.ruppe@louisville.edu

Z. L. Harris
Dell Children's Medical Center, Austin, TX, USA

Dell Medical School at The University of Texas at Austin, Austin, TX, USA

D. Dennis et al. (eds.), *Stories from ICU Doctors*,
https://doi.org/10.1007/978-3-031-32401-7_27

239

made it possible for consumers of health care to see how patient outcomes at various hospitals compare [1]. Rates of infections, surgical complications, and unplanned readmissions are internally tracked, and areas in need of improvement are "put under a magnifying glass" to find ways to change their practice.

Individual events leading to patient harm are reviewed with an evolving patient safety methodology. These processes are referred to with phrases like "root cause analyses (RCA)" and have structured reviews. The polished end-product of these evaluations is frequently showcased in a hospital-wide "morbidity and mortality" conference. Most hospitals have established risk management and legal mitigation teams to get ahead of events that could develop litigious fallout. Caught in the middle is the intensivist, often holding the smoking gun, disguised as a laryngoscope blade, central line kit, or an order entered into the electronic medical record.

And I think part of coping with intensive care is acknowledging that people don't mean to fail. Systems don't mean to fail. They do, and we build in catchers to catch it, and that's our role. And our role is not to be persecutory to those that haven't lived up to the best standard. It is to support the patient and then support our colleagues as well.

When a mistake happens, and after the immediate needs of the patient are addressed, the need for disclosing the medical error takes priority. This complex and essential conversation is increasingly emphasized for its importance in the education of future intensivists. The disclosure of most medical errors falls squarely on the shoulders of the intensivist. Prudence requires this intensivist to consider whether the error is substantive enough to involve a hospital-based risk mitigation legal team prior to disclosure. Omitting this essential step can have the unintended consequence of increasing the vulnerability of the intensivist and the hospital as a whole.

Once the risk mitigation strategy is decided, the intensivist should take several steps. First, a preparatory review of the salient patient records should be performed. This should start with a review of the medical records and include interviews with involved individuals. This allows the intensivist to have the most first-hand information prepared to address the family with facts rather than suppositions. Often this process requires time. Families should be kept apprised of the ongoing investigation and need close and detailed communication during this period. They don't need to know the individual results until all the data has been collected. Involving the family openly, honestly, and transparently is imperative to maintain trust.

Essential to this process is having all the members of the team speak with a unified voice and a single message. Families might try to get different members of the team to share opinions or data prematurely. All members of the team need to recognize how medical errors can fracture a relationship with a family and put members of the care team at risk for legal action.

As a conversation proceeds, several key components should be emphasized.

The best way we can honour that child and this incredible profession that we are part of, is to be as honest, as brutally honest, as possible.

The conversation needs to have transparent honesty along with compassion. Saying "I'm sorry" is very appropriate. Families should be given the opportunity to be upset. That is part of the process of responding to an injury to their loved one. Anger, rage, blame, disappointment, distrust, hostility, and condemnation are frequent patient and family responses that often fall squarely into the lap of the intensivist rostered for the day. This is an inevitable aspect of disclosing errors and contributes to the stress and emotional toll of the career.

As the conversation evolves, the intensivist should be aware of several essential components of this process. As expected, the tone of the conversation may move toward accusations such as, "How could you let this happen? What are you going to do about it?"

These painful accusations should be heard and considered as part of a natural response. Responding with "I don't know, and I'll find out" may be necessary. Describing the process for systematically reviewing patient safety events is appropriate and can leave a family with the sense that their tragedy is being given the appropriate attention that it deserves. Sharing that a systematic, constructive, and educational review is underway demonstrates to a grieving family the authentic priority that the event has triggered. There will be times when hospital and departmental leadership, in addition to risk management and legal representation, will need to be included.

The intensivist should refrain from adding assumptions or speculation when prodded to appease a family's request for answers.

… And I never want to throw my colleagues under the bus, you know? So, I would just present the facts that I know. I would not present any speculation or what I think happened or what I think could have been done differently

Being informed, compassionate, and complete in admitting faults without engaging in speculation or incrimination forms the basis of the conversation. An adverse event can have a profound impact on the well-being of the intensivist. Pledging an oath to "do no harm" is in direct contradiction to the inevitability of harm befalling their patients. These events can range from unpreventable, inevitable, and minimally impactful to an avoidable system failure that directly causes permanent disability or death to a patient who otherwise had the potential for a full recovery.

In no uncertain terms, the gravity of the events often weighs proportionally on the emotional distress of the intensivist. Paramount in recovering from an adverse event is engaging in a "growth mindset".

Trying to engender a 'growth' mindset, or 'learning' mindset to try and normalize that these things can happen but also that we are somewhat responsible to make sure they don't happen again.

This mentality is crucial to processing the adverse event and minimizing the likelihood of a similar error happening in the future. This can provide a framework for resilience. Redirecting the narrative from blame to learning, and then to tangible improvements, can serve to soften the emotional burden of the event [2, 3].

It is critical for a forum to exist for these adverse events to not only be discussed but for the provider involved to share what they have learned and how this will change their clinical practice. Often these conferences seem to be a review of errors committed by more junior intensivists with more senior intensivists opining. Having the most senior clinician present a case that reveals an error in judgment, regardless of whether there was an impact on the patient, helps to establish a safe culture for discussion and to frame the discussion as a learning event. Broadcasting events in a constructive, educational setting can expand the power of teachable moments and benefit many others.

A recent medical error at a prestigious academic medical center in the United States rocked the foundation for many frontline intensivists. A bedside nurse, RaDonda Vaught, was convicted on two charges of criminally negligent homicide and abuse for the in-hospital death of a patient under her care. Ms. Vaught's criminal conviction jolted nurses across the country.

Transparency has been the cornerstone of confronting medical errors. The American Nurses Association released a statement that read: "Health care delivery is highly complex. It is inevitable that mistakes will happen, and systems will fail. It is completely unrealistic to think otherwise. The criminalization of medical errors is unnerving, and this verdict sets into motion a dangerous precedent. There are more effective and just mechanisms to examine errors, establish system improvements and take corrective action. The non-intentional acts of individual nurses like RaDonda Vaught should not be criminalized to ensure patient safety" [4, 5].

When a medical error occurs, the family may lose trust in the intensivists taking care of them and their loved one. Families have been known to "fire" intensivists from trainees to seasoned faculty by seeking to exclude an intensive care clinician practitioner from the care of the patient. A highly functioning intensive care unit should work with an upset family and share that they cannot choose their ICU team. Allowing a family to refuse a nurse puts the nursing team in an awkward position if that nurse needs to be excluded from care every time that patient is admitted. Similarly, intensivist schedules cannot be juggled to match a patient and their family with their preferred specialist doctor team.

Leadership should support the critical care team and identify other systems to help the family feel supported and still have the same intensivists in place. Mediation with social workers, chaplaincy, pastoral care, nursing, and the intensivist team is often necessary.

Finally, intensivists tend to feel alone on their ICU "island," yet the world is becoming increasingly aware of these shared experiences. Seeking counsel from senior colleagues, commiseration from peers, and engaging in meaningful self-care activities all serve to help the intensivist address and process these events. Many hospital systems are aware of the impact of emotional burden and distress on clinicians and are providing increasing amounts of employee assistance and mental health services to address issues head-on.

There are several easy-to-implement processes to help mitigate the impact of an adverse event:

Hot Debrief

As discussed in Chap. 2, "hot" debriefs occur in the immediate timeframe of an event. There is a clear need for the healthcare team to be able to come together and discuss, in real time, the events that have just transpired and to review the impact of these events. If the adverse event resulted in a death, it is even more important to capture all the individuals involved in the care of the patient who has died or has sustained a severe treatment-related injury. It is important to hear the sequence of events from the medical leadership team on the unit at the time of the event. No individual should go home from a shift without some time to process the event that has occurred, especially if they might be asked to interview in the coming days asking for more information about the event. Many ICUs have a scripted debriefing process that can be used after any event and can be led by the team member most comfortable doing so [6].

Cold Debrief

The "cold" debrief (see Chap. 2) is a review of the adverse event with all the data collected and shared with all members of the team, often within the context of hospital patient safety and systems improvement processes. Although more frequent in the fields of resuscitation, these are extremely valuable to "close the loop" with individuals, to share the data with the original team at the "hot" debrief, and to describe the final shared understanding of the event and proposed current or future preventative system changes [7, 8].

Temporarily and Briefly Stepping Away

Unlike traditional jobs, the lengthy day of an intensivist does not typically have dedicated "coffee breaks" or "lunch hours." This often creates a relentless, fatiguing day without much-needed periods for refreshing or reflecting on the day's events as they occur. If staffing permits, allowing the nurse, respiratory therapist, and/or intensivist to step away from the ICU can help the individual involved process and come back more focused on the other tasks at hand. For many intensivists, there is no other staff to allow for this exchange and they become resigned to jumping back into the demands of the ICU. Eventually, the intensivist involved must take time to process the events to own what happened, learn from the mistake, and be prepared to come back the next day. Classically, small hospital chapels or faith/sacred spaces have been used by clinicians as a place of respite and private reflection. Many hospitals have built healing gardens or other green spaces attached to the hospital that can provide a similarly quiet, therapeutic environment. Sometimes just walking outside is sufficient.

While peer-to-peer counseling is often effective, utilizing trained psychologists, psychiatrists, or other mental health specialists is also of incredible value. The recent COVID-19 pandemic has helped to raise awareness and destigmatize mental health issues in healthcare providers [9]. In recent years, ICU providers have been faced with a myriad of challenges including critical nursing shortages, higher acuity of illness, and an increasingly transparent, outcome-driven environment. Career burnout among intensivists and its impact on patient outcomes is becoming increasingly recognized as the stressors of the ICU environment grow [10, 11].

Conclusion

As the name implies, the "intensivist" has chosen a vocation with extremes of acuity and stress. They are charged with making crucial medical decisions and performing procedures under any condition. They absorb the emotional strain of grieving families, the burden of medical complications, and the realities of critical illness. When patients suffer complications or harm, the intensivist is responsible for addressing the clinical fallout. They need to be experts at disclosing medical realities to loved ones and conducting reviews with medical staff. Integrity, professionalism, and compassion are the cornerstones of this process. But to sustain a career at this "intense" level, an evolved and prioritized understanding of the needs of the human inside the intensivist white coat is crucial. ICUs need embedded, proactive, and responsive psychological support systems. Future generations of intensivists will hopefully be equipped with these skills and capacities to take care of not only their patients but also themselves.

References

1. Miller BJ. What do we know about US news? Iowa Orthop J. 2022;42(1):15–7.
2. Chang S, Lee HY, Anderson C, Lewis K, Chakraverty D, Yates M. Intervening on impostor phenomenon: prospective evaluation of a workshop for health science students using a mixed-method design. BMC Med Educ. 2022;22(1):802.
3. Dwieck C. Mindset: the new psychology of success. New York, NY: Ballantine Books; 2007.
4. Statement in response to the conviction of nurse RaDonda Vaught. ANA Enterprise News release. 2022. https://bit.ly/3LcDdqC.
5. Kelman B. Former nurse found guilty in accidental injection death of 75-year-old patient. NPR March 25, 2022. https://n.pr/3JMYFY9.
6. Gilmartin S, Martin L, Kenny S, Callanan I, Salter N. Promoting hot debriefing in an emergency department. BMJ Open Qual. 2020;9(3):e000913.
7. Wolfe H, Zebuhr C, Topjian AA, Nishisaki A, Niles DE, Meaney PA, Boyle L, Giordano RT, Davis S, Priestley M, Apkon M, Berg RA, Nadkarni VM, Sutton RM. Interdisciplinary ICU cardiac arrest debriefing improves survival outcomes. Crit Care Med. 2014;42(7):1688–95.

8. Mullan PC, Wuestner E, Kerr TD, Christopher DP, Patel B. Implementation of an in situ qualitative debriefing tool for resuscitations. Resuscitation. 2013;84(7):946–51.
9. Greenberg N, Docherty M, Gnanapragasam S, Wessely S. Managing mental health challenges faced by healthcare workers during covid-19 pandemic. BMJ. 2020;368:m1211.
10. Bourgault AM. The nursing shortage and work expectations are in critical condition: is anyone listening? Crit Care Nurse. 2022;42(2):8–11.
11. Mangory KY, Ali LY, Rø KI, Tyssen R. Effect of burnout among physicians on observed adverse patient outcomes: a literature review. BMC Health Serv Res. 2021;21:369.

Michael Ruppe is board certified in pediatrics, internal medicine, and pediatric critical care and is an attending physician in pediatric cardiac critical care at Norton Children's Hospital, Louisville, Kentucky, USA. He completed medical school at the University of Toledo College of Medicine followed by a combined internal medicine and pediatrics residency at the University Hospital of Cleveland/Rainbow Babies and Children's Hospital. He then completed a pediatric critical care Fellowship at the Children's Hospital of Philadelphia. During this time his interests translated into research and publications in end-of-life decision making and medical ethics. In 2009 he moved to Louisville, Kentucky, and is active in quality improvement, point-of-care ultrasonography, international health, and pediatric cardiac critical care.

Z. Leah Harris currently serves as Professor and Chair of the Department of Pediatrics for the Dell Medical School at The University of Texas at Austin, Director of the Dell Pediatric Research Institute, and Physician-in-Chief at Dell Children's Medical Center. She is a proud practicing pediatric critical care medicine physician, lifelong learner, and multidisciplinary supporter.

Part VII:
Doctors Don't Exist in a Bubble

Foreword: Through Our Eyes

Liz Crowe ⓘ

My own eyes are not enough for me. I will see through those of others.
—C.S. Lewis

I write this foreword from a number of perspectives. I am an experienced paediatric intensive care (PICU) social worker who spent two decades of her life sharing the highest highs and the saddest of tragedies alongside skilled and compassionate paediatric intensivists. I have a PhD and numerous research papers investigating and exploring the risks and protective factors for burnout and well-being for healthcare professionals working in critical care. I am also the wife of a much-adored paediatric intensivist. So, I write as a clinician, a researcher, and a partner, acutely aware that it is difficult for us to separate these spheres of our lives as the following chapters demonstrate.

Sharing long hours and days side by side with intensivists contemplating and experiencing the life and death of others has created a deep intimacy and respect for the women and men who have chosen to commit their lives to an intensive care speciality.

The narratives that follow share several themes. Firstly, intensive care, whilst led by the intensivist, is a team sport. Each member of the intensive care multidisciplinary team has a role to play in the care of the patient and their family. When the intensivist can acknowledge and utilise the broad range of skills offered by the ICU team hopefully the burden of responsibility can be experienced as shared. It is my experience that as teams strengthen and psychological safety grows so too will humour, fun, and a sense of belonging, which naturally lightens the mood and the load of the ICU experience. There is a tacit wisdom that grows across an ICU career. Junior intensivists need to be patient with this development and lean into their colleagues for support and guidance. The only people who will ever truly understand the ICU environment are your colleagues. Intensivists should create space and a

L. Crowe
Royal Brisbane and Women's Hospital, Brisbane, Australia

culture to talk with their colleagues across the multidisciplinary team, seek feed-back on conversations and communication, and foster a debriefing culture (formal and informal) and space for personal reflection. This will grow you as an intensivist and as a human. When each member of the team walks on to a shift, the first question asked is "which intensivist is on?" Everybody knows that the intensivist sets the tone of the day. Be the intensivist that encourages collaboration, education, psychological safety, and fun. From a well-being perspective the literature is very clear. Belonging to a team where you feel safe, respected, and included is one of the strongest pillars for well-being and long-term resilience in critical care.

The second theme demonstrates the heavy sense of responsibility endured by the intensivist. While the intensivist carries ultimate responsibility for patient care it is important to remain cognisant that every member of your team is invested and is striving to deliver their best. Collaboration shares the responsibility and decision-making, increases creativity, and improves patient outcomes. Use your team widely, respect their skills, and encourage everyone to focus on the process not the outcome. Often in an ICU people arrive too injured or ill to survive or live without severe morbidity. However, if we focus on excelling in the process, use contemporary and evidence-based medicine, view each patient as a whole person, including family and friends in communication, engaging with compassion and an intention to listen and support patient goals and dignity, then whatever the outcome we can be proud.

Thirdly, being an intensivist is a deeply meaningful and privileged career that does impact every aspect of your life. There will be enormous sacrifices to achieve the training and accreditation, followed by decades of sacrifice due to shift work, long days and nights, and all-encompassing emotional and physical fatigue. Equally however, as an intensive care specialist you have the opportunity to save and change lives, to create a space for sacred and meaningful deaths. Patients and their families will remember you and revere you for your skills and intellect, your warmth and humour. Remember that your family and friends are on this journey with you and will also make sacrifices for your career. Allow them to share in your stories so they can, on some small level, appreciate why you are absent, distracted, tired, and grumpy. Let them read the cards and notes of thanks from families and colleagues. Let them know the part they played in enabling you to have this career, to have these precious and extraordinary moments with patients and your team. If you are too tired to talk to your kids, sleep beside them for a while at night. If you have no words left for your partner hold their hand while they watch TV and you doze through the show. Absence does not have to equate to distance or silence. Thank them repeatedly for their role in your career. Then during holidays or precious days off engage fully with those who love you. Surrender yourself to games and silliness. Build memories, be your best self, take photos, laugh, and invest heavily in filling your own cup so that your career can be a long, rich, and meaningful one. Then when you retire from this line of work you will continue to have a life full of people and hobbies that sustain you.

Liz Crowe Dr Liz Crowe is a staff well-being specialist who has worked as an advanced clinical social worker for over 20 years in the paediatric intensive care specialising in crisis, trauma, and end-of-life care with children and families. In the last decade Liz has expanded her expertise to include research and clinical work on the well-being of healthcare professionals, which was the focus of her PhD. In 2021 Liz published an extensive resource for the ANZ College of Anaesthetics on 'how to respond to a critical incident and conduct debriefing and support for staff'. Liz is a passionate and humorous educator and podcaster who regularly speaks internationally. Liz is the successful author of *The Little Book of Loss and Grief You Can Read While You Cry* and the co-host of the podcast 'Five Things Nursing'.

Chapter 28
Nurses Know

Shelly Ashkenazy and Annette O'Higgins

A healer is someone whose hand the patient wants to hold.

—Aude Mermilliod

Florence Nightingale, "the Mother of Nursing," was a nurse, a role model, and an educator for patient health and comfort [1]. This is the example nurses follow while taking care of patients, especially in critical conditions where they undergo procedures and intensive treatment to survive critical-illness sequelae. The ICU is a stressful environment for patients, families, and clinicians. However, nurses and intensivists choose to work in such an environment, with some of them making it their whole career. There is no doubt that the nursing profession is physically and emotionally demanding. This is even more prominent in the ICU where there is a high level of distress in the atmosphere and working as a team is essential.

To cope with the intense environment and demands characterizing the ICU, the nursing staff are required to develop "ICU resilience." This resilience is established from an individual's initial psychological predisposition, as well as the experience gathered over the years. Resilience is positively associated with the development of coping skills, a social support framework, and the overall well-being of the nurse [2].

Negative effects are mainly due to stress, posttraumatic stress disorder (PTSD), and burnout. Moral distress or moral injury, which also harms resilience, may result from the singular or continuous exposure to critical clinical decisions, such as end-of-life discussions and prolongation of artificial life support. When confronting

S. Ashkenazy (✉)
Hadassah University Medical Center, Jerusalem, Israel

A. O'Higgins
Social care division, Dalkey Community Unit, Dalkey, Co, Dublin, Ireland

D. Dennis et al. (eds.), *Stories from ICU Doctors*,
https://doi.org/10.1007/978-3-031-32401-7_28

251

these stressful situations, nurses may feel unable to care for patients according to their beliefs and may feel powerless, since they can voice their opinion, yet are not making the final patient care decisions related to morally complicated debates. A nurse said:

> *I am in distress, we are an instrument, a tool, we are subject to decisions that we do not agree with, and this is frustrating. I can handle it if I am not drawn into it and just do my job.*

In contrast, an intensivist said:

> *You know I am going to live my whole life with the decisions being made for this patient, and I will do everything to make sure that I took everything into account while making end-of-life decisions.*

Why is the doctor-nurse relationship important in the ICU? It's because we need each other to do our jobs well and to ensure the best outcome for patients. We need to listen to each other, using good, knowledgeable, clear, fun, sad, interesting, timely, and, most importantly, professional communication.

Both nurses and intensivists have the same goal: high-quality care and comfort for their patients. Teamwork and good relationships are essential to promote and achieve this goal as part of a team. Sometimes a team member might be a bit "odd" or their thinking may not be mainstream. Don't be dismissive of their opinion and keep an open mind. Listen to them; their words may be gold!

When conflicts occur, emotional burdens and moral distress appear. ICU nurses do have their way of ventilating their emotional distress and confronting these situations. Below is one nurse's advice to help cope with nurse clinicians' distress in the ICU:

> *Trying to look for the positive, trying to look for the good things, when you believe that what clinicians want to do at the end is positive for the patients, it reduces the emotional burden. If you see the logic and the reason, it helps. When you know to ask for help and you have a place to vent your distress it helps. But mostly what helps you cope is when you know why you are here.*

The most important thing is not to leave matters unresolved. Otherwise, the difficulty of coping and solving the dilemma will become stronger. In order to solve dilemmas and prevent useless arguments, good communication between doctors and nurses is essential to create a better atmosphere in the ICU. Since each clinician group has its philosophy, disputes sometimes arise during stressful environments or events, which is normal. The best advice for junior and senior doctors to cope with such difficulties is to preserve positive collaboration between nurses and doctors, as one nurse reflected:

> *Years of working in the ICU is like growing up together in the same neighborhood, you stay together at night shift, you work during holidays and weekends while you gave up your family meetings. Sometimes it is quiet, sometimes it is hectic. It will not work without a good relationship, without respect from each other. The situation that we are involved in is sometimes like soldiers in a war. They count on each other. They cooperate as a team. Each has his duty but also cares for each other's. The relationship between us is so important in our stressful workplace since the decisions [which have] been taken are critical, between life and death.*

Therefore, it is recommended that doctors ask nurses for their opinion. They know their patients and their families well, even if they do have different opinions. Share your thoughts on the treatment plan, be open-minded, and listen:

We are working hard to take care of those critical and complicated patients, and when the doctor does not share the plan of care with us it feels unrespectable.

The other thing is to listen to your intuition. Pay attention to your sixth sense in the ICU, your gut. If you have a feeling about a patient, and it's a bit too silly to say what it is, pay attention to that emotion; don't ignore it. If anything, take it as a sign to be extra observant of the patient during that shift.

The ICU can be an intimidating area for both doctors and nurses – the noise, monitors, alarms, dialysis machines, infusion devices, and ventilators can all be daunting. It may seem paradoxical to say but try to keep it simple. When faced with all that equipment, keep in mind that the equipment is only as good as the person using it. The two most important pieces of equipment in any resuscitation are the Ambu resuscitator bag attached to oxygen and the suction machine. You can save or maintain a person's life with just those two pieces of equipment, so do not be over-whelmed by all the other machines and equipment you encounter. However, do not be ashamed to call for help.

At the start of your time in the ICU, it can seem stressful, hence the importance of a strong induction, preceptorship program, in-house education sessions, and buddy systems which all help create a positive learning environment, which reduces stress. Knowing "what" and "why" you are doing something is important. And then, reflect on your practice. Use the tools provided by your employers, such as debriefing, employee assistance programs, and counseling if they are needed.

Humor, having a laugh, family, having outside interests, sleep, being in support-ive relationships, eating well, and physical activity all help you balance your life when you work in the ICU.

One nurse said:

We develop dark humor which is something that makes us laugh and helps to cope with the stress.

Each one of us chooses his way of coping; each one of us has a different person-ality. One nurse reflected on different personality types:

The verbal person will probably share thoughts, frustration, and wonders with other clini-cians while working or at any social opportunity. The conversation enables clinicians to hear other opinions that will verify and support the person's feelings and might ease the emotional burden. The introverted personality will find an activity that comforts the distress.

Like doctors, nurses that work so hard with such intensity in the ICU setting need to find things outside of the hospital that helps them with their well-being. There also needs to be a separation of work from everything else. One said:

I also prepare myself mentally before I enter and leave the hospital, like a dream time. It eases the mental and physical shift between the intensive environment and the home. Also speaking with other colleagues and trying to negotiate the situation, and not confront the situation.

And another:

You must separate work and outside ICU walls. When you go out of the ICU door, there is a whole world. Not everything ends in a disaster. It will help you recover from any stressful shift.

When you understand the importance and the meaning of your profession, it improves your resilience and helps you cope with the distress. A nurse reflected on the privilege of the job:

Birth and dying are amazing. It is something special when you attend at a time someone is separated from our world. Therefore, I feel I have the privilege to be there and accompany the patients, whether they die or not. This gives meaning to our profession. It strengthens our resilience, and when we do not succeed in saving a life, you can still see the meaning when I am there, and holding the patient's hand. This is the summit of my work, and it gives me the ability to cope and respect every decision clinicians make. The understanding that this work is not for everybody mentally and physically helps to overcome a difficult situation. So, my advice is to remember you are a human being and to be there with your humanity is much more than the regular nursing tasks. When the doctor is clear with the meaning and reason for his work, he will be able to cope better with difficult and distressing situations.

There was also recognition of the need to consider the patient holistically as a person, not a diagnosis or a jumble of numbers:

Look at the patient not just on the numbers. It will help to increase empathy.

Remember it is a person in the ICU bed, so do not be afraid to look, touch, and talk to them and look at their skin, nails, eyes, and hair. These things tell you how a person is doing: are they getting worse? Are they responding well to the treatment plan? Always go back to the basics: skin temperature; heart and respiration rates; oxygen saturation; pupillary reactions; urinary output; enteral feed absorption. Are they constipated? Always look at these parameters first. Assess the patient, not just the equipment and numbers. The small thing that you miss can be a big problem later for the patient.

And acknowledgement that efforts to provide care to both patients and their families may be just as important as patient outcomes:

The recognition that we tried everything. We gave the patient a high quality of care that the patient could not get in a regular ward, even if [they] decease.

Help the family to pass the stressful time in respect, be there for them then you get satisfaction, and it will help you to overcome the event.

Respect and support for each other will facilitate an open relationship. Do not hesitate to ask the nurse questions when you do not know. It does not detract from your own expectations. Since nurses are near patients' beds 24 h a day, be aware that your clinical decision affects the nurse's plan of care daily. Therefore, share them with the nurse in advance before giving orders.

Remember that each profession has different knowledge, skills, and point of view. However, everybody has the same aim while taking care of critical care patients. To achieve all clinicians' goals, it is essential to have a good relationship and a positive atmosphere in the ICU. A nurse reflected on her experience:

After twelve hours of hectic shift with prolonged resuscitation, you go out and think why does it work so well together? This is because, at that time, open-mindedness was to everybody, nurses, and doctors. Listening to each other brings all efforts together and leaving the ego behind, aiming to the main goal, saving the patient life.

So, dear doctor, from ICU nurse to ICU doctor, face-to-face and with candor, some advice:

We are both dedicated professionals doing difficult and demanding jobs. We also love what we do. Remember, we are members of a team – we understand that you have many things on your mind, and you are taking care of multiple patients during the day. We remind you that we are spending all day looking after one or two patients and we know them very well. We also interact with their families for much longer periods. So please, respect our concern when we are worried about our patients and ask for your review and advice.

Follow the policies, standard operating procedures, and guidelines of your ICU. Remember it is very difficult to protect a staff member who does not follow policies. Always ask when you don't know something, it is the intelligent thing to do.

Be honest. Errors can happen anywhere in a hospital, and by anyone; however, errors in the ICU can sadly have dire and even fatal consequences. Be transparent about any mistake, and report it immediately. We are in compassionate professions, so be compassionate when mistakes are made.

The team will go through many ups and downs as we care for our patients, remarkable successes, and dismal failures. We should celebrate together and commiserate together – but we should always support each other. Most days, thankfully, are routine (despite being hard work). Even then, kindness and good humor make the day pass much more pleasantly, and time and experience influence coping skills:

When I was young, there were events that were hard to see, but today I have developed a resistance to it. This is also a change in my attitude towards death. A father of a friend died, and I look at this differently now in light of my professional development. My perception was changed compared to people outside the profession. I see a privilege in the fact that I can support families and patients in extreme situations. This may be an unforgettable time for them, and I am there. This is something that gives me the strength to continue. I understand that when I am speaking to patients and families, I can change the experience and the situation of pain and the experience of death. Talking to families, I mainly try to combine the message that their beloved had deteriorated with leaving a place for comfort.

You may have studied longer than us, but many of us have been working in the ICU for years and have seen and heard everything. As well as being health professionals in our own right, we have experience. Do not ignore our concerns and warnings about deteriorating patients – we are telling you we are worried because we care.

We should support each other, our patients, and their families and learn from our mistakes. We value being part of the debrief after an adverse event and having our voices heard. We are a part of the team. We really appreciate you, doctor, and from the history, we described at the beginning of this chapter, we hope you appreciate us too, as we have a strong professional tradition.

Conclusion

The ICU is a shared experience that creates and maintains wonderful friendships with both colleagues and patients that the passage of time and the moving of place will not impact. People from outside of the ICU world and walls will never understand how we manage to survive this stressful work and lead our lives. They will also never understand the satisfaction of saving a life or providing support at the end of life. We are proud to be a part of this; be proud of it too.

References

1. Karimi H, Negin Av. Florence nightingale: the mother of nursing. Nurs. Midwifery Stud. 2015;4(2):e29475. 1–3.
2. Yu F, Mackay RD, Smith MK. Personal and work-related factors associated with nurse resilience: A systematic review. Int J Nurs Stud. 2019;93:129–40.

Shelly Ashkenazy has worked as a registered nurse for the last 24 years. She is licensed and worked in Israel and Illinois, USA. Most of her career has been spent working in the ICU at Hadassah University Medical Center, where she has served as deputy head nurse and trauma coordinator. Since 2021, she has served as a head nurse in the general ICU. Shelly earned her PhD in Nursing at the Hebrew University of Jerusalem studying pain and discomfort in mechanically ventilated ICU patients. She has published articles in various medical and nursing journals. She is a member of the organizing committee of the Israeli Association of Cardiac and Critical care Nursing.

Annette O'Higgins is currently the Director of Nursing in a residential care unit. Her critical care experience has included neurological, general, and cardiac ICUs in Ireland, Australia, and Bahrain. Her mantra is to know that your health is your wealth, and treat people as you would like to be treated.

Chapter 29
Allied Health Can Help

Diane Dennis ⓘ **and Tracy Hebden-Todd**

> *Don't sacrifice yourself too much, because if you sacrifice too much there's nothing else you can give*
>
> —*Karl Lagerfeld*

The interpretation of what it means to be an Allied Health Professional (AHP) is complex and arguably different depending on where you are in the world [1]. Nonetheless, alongside medicine and nursing, AHPs have long been recognized as a key workforce embedded within the intensive care specialty [2], with a significant presence every day of the week. Further, as AHPs are proportionally fewer in number compared to their nursing and medical colleagues, they may have comparatively more continuous individual contact with long-stay patients. For this chapter, a number of dieticians, pharmacists, physiotherapists, and speech therapists were asked what advice they would offer to doctors embarking on a career in the intensive care specialty.

One of the most important pieces of advice from AHP was for doctors to be aware of the significant impact that an intensive care career choice has on their life, both inside and outside of the workplace. Doctors coming into the specialty therefore need to anticipate, prepare, and plan for the stressors of the environment in order to achieve a satisfactory work-life balance.

> *It [work in ICU] has a significant impact on their life, so is that what they want to do? With long hours, on-calls and those sorts of things...*

D. Dennis (✉)
Department of Intensive Care and Physiotherapy, Sir Charles Gairdner Hospital,
Perth, WA, Australia
e-mail: Diane.Dennis@health.wa.gov.au

T. Hebden-Todd
Physiotherapy Department, Sir Charles Gairdner Hospital, Perth, WA, Australia

257

It was also identified that the pressure on junior doctors to advance their career paths can be overwhelming. It was thought that although on one level, an accelerated career trajectory might reflect personal success, it may also present the possibility of missing important lived clinical experiences – and learning the coping strategies that come from such events – that ultimately create a high-functioning intensivist. One participant's advice was:

Don't get caught up in the exams. Don't get caught up in what the expectations of the College of Intensive Care wants. Don't get caught up by the expectations of all the senior Consultants around you that you need to be here, or you need to be there. Don't place that pressure on yourself. Get through them in your own time, you'll get there; just take your time. Don't have the pressure—don't run. Don't let the pressure run you.

In terms of dealing with AHPs, the first piece of advice to doctors was that they develop an understanding of the skill level of the AHPs they work with. Allied health staff employed in the ICU are often highly experienced professionals in their own right. They need to attain advanced skill levels within their own field as a prerequisite to working autonomously in the ICU environment. It was felt that this level of expertise can be underestimated by junior doctors, and this may present a lost opportunity to harness best practices for evidence-based high-quality healthcare in the setting. The advice to doctors was to consider the expertise of AHPs, seek their opinion, and engage them in shared decision-making.

There's usually a number of allied health that have been in the area for a number of years and would have seen a lot of things. Acknowledge their expertise, yeah and maybe just be aware that they probably know a bit—might know more than you think we do. Don't underestimate the value of experience.

I think with increased understanding comes an increasing acknowledgement of what your Allied Health team members can actually offer a patient.

The AHPs acknowledged the increasing cognizance of multidisciplinary roles in undergraduate medical training; however, this understanding was seen as perhaps narrow.

Sometimes maybe they don't know exactly what we do as well. They can only learn a certain amount at medical school.

Gaining a broad understanding of the scope of individual AHP team members and then the cumulative impact of the group was recommended as serving to widen the intensivist's situational awareness related to patient care.

Get to know others' roles. I think sometimes there's a very shallow understanding of what each discipline does.

The ICU is a niche and ever-evolving specialty for all health professionals. Within this context, AHPs are passionate about staying abreast of contemporary practice; a pharmacist might know a better medication option than the treating doctor; a physiotherapist might present an alternate mode of weaning mechanical ventilation; a dietician might be more knowledgeable about the latest approaches to nutritional insufficiency in the ICU clinical setting. In other words, the local AHPs may be more "current" with the evidence-based practice pertaining to their specialty. The advice was that this could be harnessed by doctors if they utilized holistic and inclusive working relationships. In this environment, the AHPs also feel valued and enjoy being a part of the team.

I think just knowing that we're up-to-date with the latest in our area and what we actually do.

We try and do lots of teaching and training with training registrars, so they see that as they're coming through, and that's made a difference.

I think that it's a very multi-disciplinary environment that you really do need to value your team. If you treat everyone with respect and make them feel like they're really part of the team and have something to give that they're going to give that back to them. You'll work really hard for them and have good communication with that team member.

I find the intensivists extremely collaborative and welcoming of the multi-disciplinary team, which is really nice. I think it's so important too. Everyone wants to feel like their work is valued, and, even if you have that intrinsic value and know that it's valuable and see the patient making gains, to have that acknowledged and respected by other team members, particularly a Consultant, is really important. When Consultants are more willing to speak to all the team members extensively about the patient's journey and where they're at medically, it can only help you clinically to develop goals and things.

The AHP team recognized that being collaborative and communicating simply were desirable qualities of an intensivist:

[You need someone] who can collaborate with you and listen. Yeah, who's prepared to answer questions and give you time.

The junior doctors explain things in ways that facilitate understanding for other junior staff. I think the more experienced you become, the more you lose insight into how complex things sometimes are, and you might explain things at a different level. I think sometimes go into joint sessions with Allied Health if you have a chance. I think they're pulled in a hundred different directions and busy, but I think sometimes even doing things like that can really facilitate their understanding.

They felt that multidisciplinary meetings present an opportunity to both share and gather important information which may otherwise be missed. They also facilitate relationship and team building:

I think multidisciplinary team members' meetings are really important because it just encourages that communication when, sometimes during the day, it's really hard to all meet at once. I think we unpack a lot when we meet just weekly, so that's quite important too.

I like that inclusivity and consideration of what everyone has to offer. We all have our niches, and we've all got something to bring to the table … moving away from a very medically focused, sit-down round, looking through all bloods and X-rays and scans, to actually having it as a multidisciplinary team meeting where they're literally going around discipline by discipline in relation to the patient.

In terms of clinical practice, leading by example in not being afraid to ask for help; having the willingness to learn; and the fallibility of being able to admit when you don't know something were all identified as valuable traits of the intensivist:

The Consultants were incredibly collaborative and inclusive where they had certain layers of safety within their own clinical expertise. These were Consultants who had been working for over 20 years and were experts in their field. What was humbling for me to watch was that they called for help from their colleagues, from the—the junior anaesthetist, other specialties as they had a deteriorating patient, even though they had the skills and knowledge to be able to manage it, they got help immediately. I would say, for me it was like, what a great example. We don't need to rely on our own skills, let's use what we have around us.

A willingness to learn; a willingness to admit when they don't know something. I think the most dangerous point of a junior doctor's career is when they don't have the knowledge, say, that a Consultant has, but they're not willing to acknowledge that, and they're trying to live up to their role. I think that that willingness to be vulnerable and to accept what we don't know [is important].

The AHPs felt that although the intensivist might presume overall responsibility for the patient journey, they were strong of the opinion that this accountability is shared by all professions. There is therefore an obligation by all to relay pertinent information related to any decision such that it is informed and, further, that the burden of any poor outcome is shared.

I think there's definitely a strong onus on them, but I think at the end of the day, we're all here and responsible for the patient; physio, speech therapists, the patient care assistants, the clerical staff. The whole journey of a patient from admission to discharge or even further, into the community, it's multifaceted. It can't be one.

I think our team is responsible for the wellbeing of patients. I think the doctors are responsible for their patient's medical care. I think the whole team looking after a patient is responsible for the patient's wellbeing. Patient wellbeing is a shared responsibility.

I guess that's where the buck stops at the end, so they have that ability to override anything else, but I do feel like that every team member has a responsibility.

The intensivists voiced their sense of responsibility for the well-being of the whole team – including AHP personnel – and this was seen as valued by everyone. It was also recognized that, despite acknowledging their position within the "ICU family," AHPs have the opportunity to seek support elsewhere within their professional network in the event of significant clinical and nonclinical challenges.

I see myself as responsible for my wellbeing, but should I need support in this working environment then it's my managers… Other heads of departments…

Conclusion

Allied health professionals work across all aspects of the intensive care environment and consider themselves an integral part of the team that delivers healthcare to high acuity patients. In doing so, they value the knowledge, the expertise, and the incredible commitment of the doctors and nurses who specialize in the area. Working together they experience both the highs and lows of the specialty and create lifelong relationships that extend far beyond the bedside.

References

1. Chadwick M, Larmer P, Smythe L. The history of allied health: an international perspective. J Allied Health. 2020;49(4):285–9.
2. Ridley EJ, et al. Surge capacity for critical care specialised allied health professionals in Australia during COVID-19. Aust Crit Care. 2021;34(2):191–3.

Diane Dennis has been employed as a researcher in the ICU setting since 2008, with an interest in simulation and human factors in the safe delivery of healthcare services. She has been exploring the well-being of medical staff in the specialty since 2018. With a background in clinical training as a physiotherapist, she has taught as Co-Lead of Simulation and Senior Lecturer at Curtin University and is currently acting as Deputy Head of the Physiotherapy Department at Sir Charles Gairdner Hospital in Perth, Western Australia.

Tracy Hebden-Todd is currently the Head of the Physiotherapy Department at Sir Charles Gairdner (SCGH), Perth, Western Australia. She began her 30-year career working in Pediatric and Adult Intensive Care units both at SCGH and at the Princess Margaret Children's hospital in Perth in 1987. Prior to that she worked in the UK, Saudi Arabia, and New Zealand. She has been privy to the most humbling moments, experienced remarkable human survival, the fragility of life, and grief; she has observed and experienced the deleterious effect of compassion fatigue and burnout and the impact these have on the individual and relationships. She is very proud to have worked with such extraordinary people and is thankful for this opportunity to contribute to this very important story.

Chapter 30
Family Matters

Paula Kosowitz, Megan Knott, Fiona van Heerden, Robert Gradidge, Adam van Heerden, Isabelle Gius, and Liron van Heerden

> *As we express our gratitude, we must never forget that the highest appreciation is not to utter words, but to live by them.*
>
> —*John F. Kennedy*

Introduction

Paula Kosowitz

Being an intensivist is not a family-friendly occupation. The sacrifice of things that really matter – like those precious family occasions, the graduations, the birthdays. Those around them must often wonder why anyone would choose such a

P. Kosowitz
Department of Intensive Care, Sir Charles Gairdner Hospital, Perth, WA, Australia

M. Knott
Rosanna, VIC, Australia

F. van Heerden (✉)
Melabev Home Care for the Aged, Jerusalem, Israel

R. Gradidge
Floreat, WA, Australia

A. van Heerden
Inner Spark Psychology, Melbourne, WA, Australia

I. Gius
London School of Economics and Political Science, London, UK

L. van Heerden
University of Melbourne, Melbourne, WA, Australia

career—with all those years of study; the exams; the pressure of obtaining a consultancy position; and the day-to-day stressors of the job itself. Although there may be rewards in facilitating a patient's recovery, the emotions that intensivist experience are at times heart-breaking to witness. I've seen doctors fight back tears with families when they had tried every procedure possible to help, without success. I've seen them searching their souls considering if anything could have been done better or whether they had missed something. There is certainly a lot that is never openly talked about, and this must take its toll on these truly amazing individuals—I'm sure some carry enormous unspoken burdens. However, the intensive care group is a family of its own, and the rewards of belonging to such a team are huge. In this chapter we hear from the family of intensivists as they celebrate their relationships, the highs and the lows, and the pride they take in knowing that their family member belongs to this special club.

Mother of Her Intensivist Son: "Proud, Yet Concerned"

Megan Knott

The majority of high achievers who undertake medicine do so with the best intentions of wanting to help others, but whether they really realise the long-term impact on their own health and well-being is questionable. From a parent's perspective, I have seen the hard work and dedication of one such student who has carried the burdensome impact on personal health and well-being for 25 years. The impact is not only personal for the medico, but it also affects their parents and their developing family in its formative years. I wonder how much longer it can be done. These medicos learn to absorb the pressure environment of an ICU and hospital but more so if they have a more sensitive and empathic temperament.

Making quick, difficult, and frequently life-threatening decisions requires a level of tenacity and self-sacrifice not found in other professions. At the end of a long shift, not unusually well over 12 hours or even 30 hours, the mental fatigue, let alone the physical fatigue, can be extreme. Then having to unwind before they return to family, if possible, can be difficult. This means endeavouring to turn off after having gone through the emotional drain of difficult decisions, talking to distressed patients and relatives, and dealing with shortages in the hospital system due to under-resourcing.

The pressure on the clinician's families and parents as the fatigued medico returns home often results in fatigue-related grumpiness, irritability, or withdrawal from family dynamics, merely to survive. The family situation often involves young boisterous families, so, at times, the mental and physical reserves are exhausted before they even get home. It is not uncommon for depression to set in, while trying to navigate the two disparate environments. As a parent of this person, and wanting the best for one's child, I endeavoured to fill in the breach of babysitting, supporting, debriefing and listening, and balancing sitting back while family time is given priority.

Keeping healthy with exercise and sports is very difficult, so physical health is compromised. They can say goodbye to a team sport, which is unfortunate if that is your passion—shift work quashes consistent participation in that. Physical health suffers.

I have often commented at the end of a very long shift or after night shifts, which have not unusually followed the day shift, that I would not like to be the personal recipient of any of my child's end-of-shift clinical decisions! The unnecessary and unreasonable expectations here are both risky and dangerous. I have been at the dinner table when a phone call has come in, while on consultation for the night shift, requiring an immediate response. I saw my child physically slump in the chair with mental and physical distress at the situation. The anguish and anxiety could only be resolved with a return to the hospital to assist with the situation.

Living with human error: I don't think anyone really realises the impact on the medico when they *think* that they may have made an error of judgement, whether it be human error or more especially from a fatigue-induced mistake—let alone an actual error. It can be catastrophic to the medico—for the concerned doctor—implications for the patient and family and possibly hospital reporting, medicolegal, and coronial implications. The impact ripples out to the immediate family and parents, who worry for the mental health of this person in their role as their child, partner, parent, and friend.

I am proud of the dedicated concern that my child gives to patients and their families, none of whom I will ever know, but I constantly worry about the impact on the health and well-being of this type of continuing work on my child.

Wife of Her Intensivist Husband: "Privileged Challenge"

Fiona van Heerden

It has been a privilege to be married to an intensivist. I witness so many wonderful gestures of gratitude from "strangers" that he has treated or from the relatives of patients he has treated, and I am constantly proud of the wonderful work my husband does. There are however certain disadvantages.

My husband and I met in the anatomy dissection hall during our second year of studies. I was an occupational therapy student and he was a medical student. He was a shy young man, always cracking jokes to conceal his shyness. We married in 1984. I worked as an occupational therapist at a general hospital in Johannesburg, and he was finishing his degree at the teaching Hospital. After completing his studies, he was enlisted into compulsory army service, which entailed 2 years of service at a military camp away from home. This marked the start of our married life—one coloured by separation and a husband away from home due to his devotion to work and study. I was undertaking a master's degree in neuroscience while working, and he and I were both busy. When I was 6 months pregnant with our first child, we went to Exeter, to a job my husband took as a registrar to continue his specialist studies.

He arrived in the UK before me, and I followed afterwards on my own. I flew to London, caught a train to Reading and the coach to Exeter, pregnant, alone, and carrying my luggage to a foreign destination where we would remain for at least a 2-year period.

He studied for his anaesthetic exam and wrote his primary exams in Ireland. Initially we stayed in hospital accommodation, but this was only a short-term solution. We needed to find our own accommodation. Our only option was to buy a small house; as first-time buyers, this was all we could afford at the time. Even renting something was too expensive for the meagre salary.

Our first child was born, and on the same day, we were discharged from the maternity hospital; we moved into our sparsely furnished home, sharing walls with the neighbours. I remember the first day so clearly. Daniel slept in his cot, I unpacked all our clothes, a light sleet was falling (end of November 1989), and my husband was on call at Exeter Hospital. I also remember him studying for his exam. He was upstairs in the house, while I kept our son occupied downstairs, trying to be as quiet as possible.

Shortly thereafter, I was pregnant with our second son. The night my waters broke my husband had undergone a taxing night on call and only just managed to utter: "I'm so tired, any possibility of prolonging the pregnancy? I really need some more sleep". As a doctor, he seemed to struggle even more seeing my discomfort in both pregnancies and ordered an epidural, despite my being adamant I wanted a natural birth. Luckily, I was able to deliver both boys with minimal intervention. For our daughter's birth 6 years later in Australia, it was second nature to him. My waters were breaking, and he offered me a cup of tea.

My husband's father advised him never to bring his work home with him. True to this advice, when he was home, he never did much work—unless of course he was on call. He managed in a very efficient way to complete his work while at the hospital. He was however often very tired at home. I was tasked with taking the kids to school and extra-mural activities and maintaining the household. I recall a visiting couple asking him where our nearest supermarket was and he replied, "I have absolutely no idea".

On another occasion, my eldest son was absent-mindedly hitting electrical wires with a metal stick. Sparks were flying, and I was unsure what to do. I phoned my husband at work, but before I could say anything he said, "I can't talk right now, I'm in the middle of a resuscitation". On a positive note, I became an independent woman who knew there were times I simply could not call on my "intensive care specialist husband".

There have also been many perks to being the wife of an intensive care specialist. We have travelled to a number of exotic places for international conferences. Even now on his sabbatical year, his locum work has taken us to some rural Australian towns that we have never seen before. Our family has always been well looked after medically, getting special treatment at various specialists' offices.

However, in our household you have to be very ill before you receive medical treatment (the cobbler's children go barefoot!). We rarely have Panadol or other very over-the-counter medicines on hand. In the early 2000s, I was quite ill and coughing excessively at night. Since he was working hard as usual, and needed a good night's sleep, I was sent to sleep in the lounge. This went on for a few nights. He was so unperturbed by my coughing; I had to eventually plead with him to pay me some attention. He then organised for me to have an X-ray. The radiologist was shocked I was still upright and informed me that I had severe pneumonia.

Being the wife of an intensive care specialist has been both a privilege and a challenge. I am incredibly proud of the work my husband has accomplished over the years. He has worked humbly and efficiently and has recently been at the forefront of the COVID treatment response in Israel. On the other hand, he is often emotionally and physically "spent" by the time he comes home, and I accommodate him by allowing him to rest, as well as doing many activities without him. This has given me the chance to socialise with my friends and engage in my own creative pursuits. My independence has been hard-earned, but I wouldn't have it any other way.

Husband of His Intensivist Wife: "Nurturing with Pride"

Robert Gradidge

My wife was already working as an intensive care specialist when we met, so I've never known her do anything different, and my biggest challenge has been to understand how stressful and demanding the job can be. I know that communicating with patients' families is one of the most stressful parts and it helps that I'm trained as a family counsellor, so when she needs to offload and talk about her day I can listen and make suggestions if she asks for advice on what to say. I know she finds it helpful to talk about stuff and debrief when there's something troubling her, although she doesn't feel the need to share every detail of every day.

My wife tells me she passes on what I say to her colleagues: for example, she came home one day worrying that she was getting older and losing her edge and that her younger colleagues were leaving her behind in terms of knowledge and skills. When, after some time, she'd finished venting, I just looked at her and said it would be a sad day for her specialty if the people coming after her weren't smarter and better, and those few words helped shift her mindset. I know she tells that story a lot—I think everyone has probably heard it by now!

We're lucky in that we are really close as a couple and are a great team—there's no competitiveness or jealousy or resentment between us. I'm happy to do all the household duties so she can just chill and relax when she's home. She'll agree that I'm the far better cook in any case! We don't have children, just a very demanding rescue dog, and that makes it easier, but I guess we would have worked it out if we'd had kids.

The most stressful thing for me is worrying about her health when she's at work for long hours—not eating properly and not getting enough sleep. My coping mechanism is to make sure she has decent food at home and snacks to take with her—that's my nurturing instinct coming out.

It still surprises me how insecure and unsure of herself she can be, after everything she's achieved and still doing. She always accuses me of having rose-tinted spectacles, but I think she's truly an amazing person and I couldn't be more proud.

Son of His Intensivist Father: "Generous with Sacrifice"

Adam van Heerden

Growing up, I had a strange familiarity with hospitals that was distinctive in my circle of friends. My Dad always made a concerted effort to give us a glimpse into his work by introducing us to his colleagues and patients. I wistfully recall being led around the intensive care ward as both a child and a curious teen. I was intrigued by the various life support and resuscitative machines and inquired about the condition of each patient. This curiosity culminated in a week of high-school work experience that my Dad generously organised for me. While fellow classmates were answering phones and stapling documents, I aided in tracheostomies and witnessed an open-heart surgery. I believe my Dad wanted us to understand the critical nature and poignancy of his work.

In retrospect, it was only fair we were given some insight into the work that intruded on our family life. Before I could articulate it verbally, I had the sense that my Dad's work was unquestionably important and worthy of sacrifices from the family, predominantly in terms of quality time spent together. When prompted to draw a picture of my Dad in Year 1, I depicted him working at a desk with an inordinate number of desk legs. Even then I understood that his work was both important and taxing. As a child, I was uncertain whether he would return for dinner or remain at the hospital tending to patients. And as a teenager, I wished he would modify the division of his social energy. It seemed his colleagues and patients received a gregarious doctor, while we had inherited the reserved and overworked father.

I now understand that the emotional toll and sheer gravity of his work often meant my Dad did not have the energy or patience to engage in generous conversation upon returning from the hospital. This seems to have set the tone for the rest of the family. Weeknight dinners were typically conducted in front of the television as this required minimal social effort. While this provided an opportunity for my father to share his penchant for stand-up comedy and the Simpsons. My sister and I have often discussed our shared longing that our family would engage in richer conversation together.

As a family of Jewish descent, Friday night Sabbath meals stood in stark contrast to the perfunctory family meals throughout the week. I relished these meals as they were festive and sacrosanct in nature. My father took the time to bless each of his children individually, and we would all sing a song of gratitude to our mother for maintaining the household with munificence. I listened attentively to my father's anecdotes and later traded these with friends as if they were precious jewels. As our family became more religious, this time together was further safeguarded from the demands of my father's work. Unless he was on call, my father was prevented from checking his phone or work emails from Friday night until Saturday night. This opened up time for playing cards and board games together and shared reading time where we could simply bask in each other's presence. There is an old saying that "more than the Jews kept the Sabbath, the Sabbath has kept the Jews". This is certainly true of my family. The Sabbath brought us together and acted as a buffer against the immense stress my Dad experienced each day in the intensive care ward.

It is a mixed experience growing up as the son of an intensivist. My Dad has provided a model for enacting meaningful work in the world, yet this has often come at the cost of spending quality time as a family. I've noticed how much calmer and emotionally receptive my Dad is during his Sabbatical this year. He is far more attentive with friends and family than after prolonged periods of regular work. As my own career progresses, I notice my own tendency to become preoccupied with work to the detriment of relationships. I try to balance this by socialising with friends and engaging in hobbies on a regular basis.

It is telling that all three children sat the Graduate Medical School Admissions Test (GAMSAT), and maybe just as telling that none followed through in becoming medical practitioners. We have witnessed the meaning our father derives from such critical work, as well as the sacrifices necessary to sustain a career as an intensivist. Notwithstanding, our father's work ethic has been indelibly imprinted upon us, and we have each sought to cultivate successful and ethical careers.

As a psychologist, I strive to embody my father's unassuming and collaborative approach to care. Despite his numerous accolades, he takes the time to explain procedures clearly and simply to patients and their family members. He goes out of his way to put a smile on the face of his patients and has a constant eye on cultivating the development of early career doctors. This generosity of spirit brightens the hallways of any intensive care ward my father steps foot in, and it is this generosity I seek to emulate.

Daughter of Her Intensivist Mother: "Is There Blood; Is There Bone?"

Isabelle Gius

In hindsight, growing up with a mother who was also an intensivist meant that my childhood was different from the other kids around me—not that I knew any differently. Medical terminology at the dinner table, 12-hour workdays, and coming home in scrubs have always seemed normal to me. Like any other job, though perhaps more intensely, my Mom's work impacted my life and shaped my understanding of the world.

My relationship with health was definitely strange and contradictory. I remember the two questions that I would hear over the phone if I ever called my Mom about some illness or injury: "Is there blood? Is there bone?" If the answer was no, as it usually was, then it could wait until she came home. Activities at summer camp that my friends loved, like go-karting, would never be the same after hearing about the horrible accident that landed a girl my age in the PICU.

I was used to my mother working long hours: getting up early and staying up late, nights on-call, and vacations that were never really vacations. My Dad and I settled into a familiar routine, ordering pizza whenever she was working nights. I knew it had been a rough day at work when there was a break in her usually calm demeanour. Sometimes she needed to talk about it, sometimes she couldn't, but it was clear that something horrible, more horrible than usual, had happened.

Although as a child I wanted nothing more than to be picked up from school—a rare occurrence with two doctors as parents—I don't have any lingering resentment. I understood, though perhaps not always as clearly as I do now, the importance of the work my Mom was doing. How many children had been given more time with their own families because of her? How could I complain? The best memories I have of my Mom growing up were the times that we found balance within her busy schedule: going out for early morning breakfasts and her taking the day off to spend time together. Those moments were so rare and special because of my Mom's job, not in spite of it.

My mother being an intensivist helped make me into a feminist. My Dad is also a physician, and yet I was keenly aware from a young age that it was my Mom's career that stood out, eliciting rude comments from other mothers or questions from friends at playdates. I am certain my Dad was never questioned about why he worked so much or who took care of the kids. My Mom taught me that the balancing act of being a working mother was possible, although difficult—more difficult than it should be.

I am incredibly proud of my mother's achievements, especially because it's a job that I could never handle. I am in awe of her dedication, work ethic, and strength. Yet I also realise that she is human, that being an intensivist means growing accustomed to a lack of sleep and being familiar with death. A career in medicine was never in the cards for me, but it was powerful to grow up with a mother who was doing exactly what she was meant to be doing. My Mom's job inspired me to fearlessly imagine what my own future could look like.

Daughter of Her Intensivist Father: "Honour and Reward"

Liron van Heerden

I have been incredibly fortunate to have, not only an intensivist as a Dad, but also to have one who is held in such high esteem and who is well-regarded in every hospital he has graced with his presence. Growing up I was very proud to say, "My Dad, the intensive care specialist", and as I matured, this feeling of pride not only prevailed but has grown tenfold with an increased understanding of what this profession truly entails. The time, effort, and consideration it takes to perform these duties and still have the capacity to show up for your family has been an inspiration for the person I strive to be.

I fondly look back at the times when my Dad would take me to the hospital with him and show me around the wards. I would love to see the faces of his fellow employees, patients, and families of patients light up with glee to meet the daughter of the renowned professor. They would exude gratitude and tell me how lucky I was to have such an incredible Dad. He would teach me about his patients and the challenges of their conditions, and I would hold on to every word, astounded by his knowledge, expertise, and the way he would conduct himself with such humility, compassion, and efficiency.

There have been a great number of benefits to being a family member of an intensivist. I have had the privilege of being included in some gifts of gratitude from patients, including a lavish degustation meal at the famous King David Hotel in Jerusalem, a holiday stay at a villa in Bali, situated right in the rice paddies, and many intensivist conferences around the world where, without fail, my Dad would introduce me with pride and gush over my accomplishments to his friends and colleagues. Concurrently, his humility would extend the length of his greatest achievements. In 2019, we travelled to Cairns as a family for a conference and to accompany him at an award ceremony. We were told it was a small award, not hugely important, and the ceremony would mostly pertain to the graduating class of intensivists. This "not hugely important" award was in fact the College of Intensive Care of Australia and New Zealand Medal, which acknowledged his contribution to Intensive Care in Australia and New Zealand—one of the highest honours for an intensivist in Australia and New Zealand. I watched on in awe as recent graduates swamped him, celebrating him and his achievements, and as he accepted this incredible honour with grace and self-effacement.

My Dad's achievements have imparted in me a pressure to succeed, high expectations that have been both prescribed and self-imposed. At times, this pressure to excel in academic studies and pursue well-regarded professions has been a challenge. However, the value of education and the pursuit of excellence have been deeply instilled in me, allowing me to develop an incredibly strong sense of determination, aspiration, and motivation to strive for nothing short of my best efforts.

While it has been an immense privilege in the grand scheme of things, at times, it has been a bittersweet reward. The unimaginable mental and physical toll it takes to deal with patients that require critical care, the long hours, the intensive requirements, and the unfortunately unavoidable loss of patients has sometimes meant my Dad has justifiably needed time for himself and time to replenish his energy sources.

Furthermore, while the family has benefited from innumerable medical connections, ease of finding specialists, and free medical advice, the latter has proven to be more accessible for family friends than for personal use at times. Ironically, there was a scarcity of medicines and medical supplies at our house. If our condition was not dire or "intensive", it could take some time to convince my Dad that we required tending to our wounds.

All in all, however, it has been highly auspicious, rewarding, comforting, and an enormous privilege to have the honour of having an intensivist as a Dad. The way in which he has performed his responsibilities and fulfilled above and beyond the requirements of the job has taught me immeasurable qualities I am truly so thankful for. I am incredibly fortunate to learn a deep sense of obligation to the well-being of others, to learn patience, resilience, compassion, and drive.

Paula Kosowitz has been a receptionist for the Intensive Care Department at the Sir Charles Gairdner Hospital, Perth, since 2007. She came to healthcare from the Oil and Gas industry after working on the North West Shelf Project in Western Australia. She is an active member of Toastmasters and enjoys teaching leadership and communication.

Megan Knott is a retired teacher who has had a career in both Primary and Secondary teaching, reaching the position of Assistant Principal in the public education system in Victoria, Australia.

Fiona van Heerden qualified as an occupational therapist, with a master's degree in neurological occupational therapy. She also qualified as a counsellor and as a reflexologist. She volunteers at a cancer centre in Jerusalem and undertakes home OT assessments for the frail and elderly.

Robert Gradidge completed a BSc in agricultural economics at the University of Pietermaritzburg in South Africa, migrating to Australia for love in 1999. He then had a career change and was awarded BCoun through the University of Notre Dame, specialising in drug and alcohol and family counselling.

Adam van Heerden works as a psychologist at Inner Spark Psychology in Melbourne. He is interested in nature and is a practitioner of capoeira.

Isabelle Gius is currently an MSc student at the London School of Economics and Political Science, studying Gender, Development, and Globalisation. Previously, she was an intern at *The American Prospect*, a national politics and policy magazine, and she has also interned with the Institute for Advanced Studies in the Humanities and several nonprofit organisations.

Liron van Heerden has an undergraduate degree in neuroscience from the University of Western Australia, with honours from the Univ. of Melbourne. She did her experimental work at the Florey Institute of Neuroscience and Mental Health in Melbourne. She is currently undertaking a master's degree at the Univ. of Melbourne.

Part VIII:
The Journey Moving Forward

Foreword: Where Did We Come from, and Where Are We Going?

Diane Dennis ⓘ

Learn continually. There's always 'one more thing' to learn.
—Steve Jobs

This project had its origin in an idealistic, side conversation between Dr Cameron Knott and me at a simulation conference about the possible inoculation of future intensivists from the stressors of the workplace. We pondered how to do this? Could we somehow assess workplace stressors, then develop and package up some sort of pre-emptive, hands-on educational experiences, perhaps utilizing simulation as the modality of choice? We find ourselves a long way from that goal, and far more pragmatic about the complex and unpredictable nature of the ICU environment.

Our team have explored the diversity of "normal" responses experienced, coping mechanisms employed, and the common internalized expectation of omniscience, and ultimate responsibility for patient care that intensivists seem to commonly bear. Our goal has therefore shifted, and now lies more in advocating for the positive well-being of intensivists, by normalizing and generalizing common responses so that those individuals know they are not alone if they are experiencing these in seeming isolation.

Through the conduct of this research and having completed human research ethical reviews at seven institutions where we were explicitly required to engage with the psychiatry specialty, we were aware of the potential impact we might have on individuals participating in the research. As participants often demonstrated unexpected and considerable emotion in their recount of their experiences, we began to ask the question at the end of each interview, "Are you okay?" and "How does it feel to be asked about these things?" The consistent response from intensivists was that it felt good to be asked about their feelings and coping strategies, and that there was

D. Dennis
Department of Intensive Care and Physiotherapy, Sir Charles Gairdner Hospital,
Perth, WA, Australia
e-mail: Diane.Dennis@health.wa.gov.au

a shared mutual recognition of the importance of the work, and the need for support to be provided to everyone—perhaps not just to those who reach out for it.

The chapters that follow in this final part of the book explore some of these perspectives and highlight the need for an open, well-judged system of support that is normalized across the specialty. With this in mind, we also explore the desirable attributes of potential intensive care training candidates to facilitate high functioning trainees in the future.

Diane Dennis Dr Diane Dennis has been employed as a researcher in the ICU setting since 2008, with an interest in simulation and human factors in the safe delivery of healthcare services. She has been exploring the well-being of medical staff in the specialty since 2018. With a background in clinical training as a physiotherapist, she has taught as Co-Lead of Simulation and Senior Lecturer at Curtin University and is currently acting as Deputy Head of the Physiotherapy Department at Sir Charles Gairdner Hospital in Perth, Western Australia.

Chapter 31
Is It Okay to Ask?

Natalie Henderson and Courtney Bowd

> *One day in retrospect, the years of struggle will strike you as the most beautiful.*
>
> —*Sigmund Freud*

Well-documented links exist between ICU admission and post-traumatic stress symptoms, complicated grief, and other symptoms of psychological distress for both patients and their relatives [1–3]. Although increasingly recognised, the impact on and the experiences of healthcare professionals working within the ICU environment have been less considered. By extension, the doctors working in the specialty are rarely questioned about their mental health and well-being:

> *Interviewer: 'When were you last asked about it? When were you ever asked about it?'*
>   *Participant: 'Never!'*

Intensive care medicine is one that is wrought with opposing feelings: Being viewed as 'okay' with the weight of the job, versus actually 'being okay'. Because of this, intensivists, both in the paediatric and adult disciplines, often do not discuss their feelings, nor are they frequently asked about how they are feeling. This was acknowledged in the interviews, with participants suggesting that this could be due to perceptions of 'how they are supposed to be'.

> *I think it's really interesting, and I think it's probably a topic in medicine that hasn't been explored because we're supposed to be... The way that I described to you is I think the 'way we are supposed to be'. Now, I think for me, it is relatively easy to fit that mould...*

N. Henderson
Division of Critical Care, Department of Pediatrics, University of Louisville, and Norton Children's Medical Group, Louisville, KY, USA

C. Bowd (✉)
Phoenix Australia – Centre for Post-traumatic Mental Health, Melbourne, VIC, Australia
e-mail: courtney.bowd@unimelb.edu.au

Intensivists learn to balance the care of the sickest of humans. Coping mechanisms vary between individual intensivists with some openly discussing their struggles and stressors, while others are less likely to share. The inconsistency in handling the stressors can often increase burnout and intensivists exiting the critical care profession.

> *Because there's a lot of people that leave their jobs because they're internally just boiling over ... because they just have no way to look after themselves.*

Others endorse the ability to separate the hard situations and stressors in ICU from their personal lives.

> *Yeah, like I said, I compartmentalise really, really effectively, so it doesn't hurt me to go back and look at them. There are still some where I'll say that I wish I had changed something a little bit, but it went where it went, and most of the time was okay; sometimes it may not have been. But there was not much I could have done in the acute phase that would have been any different with what I had at the time.*

Throughout the process of data collection for this book, paediatric and adult intensivists who undertook the interviews also demonstrated a range of responses to the experience of being interviewed. As such, understanding the effect of the actual interview, not the job of being in the ICU, yielded interesting and varied responses worth exploring.

Cathartic Effects of the Interview

Holding the balance of life and death, health, and sickness each day is not without emotional weight on the managing intensivists. The goal of intensivist interviews was to qualitatively explore the experiences of intensivists, discussing content that was quite personal in nature, such as burnout, trauma, psychological distress, and coping. However, while the response to the actual interview varied, two effects were notable. First, many participants felt the interview assumed a cathartic or therapeutic venue for their stressors:

> *It has actually been really therapeutic.*
>
> *I think it's good to chat through it. Again, it's not like you're a psychologist or psychiatrist, you sort of take what's given and sort of ask follow-up questions, but you're not trying to get into my psyche too much...*
>
> *I actually think it's really fascinating to think about, because I don't spend a lot of time actually thinking about how I cope with things, and so I think that it's kind of nice... This has been very therapeutic for me. It's been kind of nice.*
>
> *I talk about these things a lot. I think our group is probably more vocal than a lot, so I don't think there's a lot of people that I work with that don't have an outlet.*
>
> *Personally, I think it's good to make yourself talk about these sorts of things; that you can heal from those sorts of things.*

Others acknowledged, outside of the interview setting, that talking about or discussing work-related traumas and patient encounters can be beneficial. This is from both a reflective experience and helping to prepare others for the experiences they are likely to have as part of this career.

> *I think it's important from like 'maintenance' point of view.*

> *I think it's been helpful. I think there is some value to thinking about past experiences and what your perspective is on them. So, I think to that extent it's been helpful.*

> *Yes. Well maybe it does help a little. I think it is really useful to talk things through and even if you feel like, 'Oh I can now use this really horrible experience to make someone feel better in this moment,' then I think that that is worth it.*

On the whole, the cathartic and therapeutic experiences of the participants provide a basis for the benefits (or lack of perceived harms) of this type of research and investigation moving forward, to better understand the experiences of intensivists within the unique environment that is the intensive care unit.

Unremarkable Emotional Effects of the Interview

While many intensivists felt the interview elicited some cathartic feelings, others did not find the interview had any impact and none indicated that they found the process to be intrusive or problematic. Like many studies of this nature, concern existed in the study design that the interview itself could further add to burnout or distress by discussing workplace trauma. However, while appropriate mitigations and supports were put in place, this concern did not seem to bear out in the data.

> *Yeah, again, I mean I was actually talking with a colleague about some of these similar issues... Like you said, how the bag of heavy cases weighs on you, and how you process that, recently, so we didn't unearth anything that I'm too bothered about.*

> *No! Gosh no! I'm fine! [Laughs] But you know, this is so fun, I can't imagine being in tears. For me this is sort of... I feel... I feel selfish... it's sort of a 'high' that you get to sort of think, and reflect and talk about the pieces that come together...*

> *Interviewer: 'I want to know whether or not you are okay, and whether or not you are okay with the process of the interview itself?'*
> *Participant: 'I'm definitely okay in both. As I said, I was worried you were going to start by saying, 'Think back on a bad outcome, you know, we'll use that as our taking off point' and I would be like, 'Bahhh? Bahh? ...' So, I actually... Like I said I would never be able to remember everything... but as I said, I thought... 'Well, there was that kid... and then there was that other kid.... and then...'*

Others expressed that while they may not always acknowledge their underlying feelings surrounding the events experienced in the ICU, they were not negatively impacted by the interview.

> *We laugh about that in our Morbidity and Mortality conference, we have that monthly, and so you finally have moved on from the bad situation and you have to re-discuss it again and it's like, 'Okay, here's the Band-Aid, let's rip it off; we finally let it heal and now we gonna open it up!' No, I think the fact that we talk a lot at work; we talk about things and it helps; No, I'm okay with it...*

I think I'm distanced enough now in time from them that I don't have the strong emotions that I used to. And I unpacked them quite often over time, and so now [there are] no new emotions... and it hasn't... So neither good nor bad. It's just rehashing of some things that have happened, so I don't find this upsetting or cathartic either... just 'to be expected.' I was a little worried that I'd actually be more upset about things, but this has been fine.

So, I worked at trying to remember examples so that I would have something ready [for the interview] and in doing so I really did that... and worked through them... and that was a couple of weeks ago.

Conclusion

The interview and data collection processes allowed intensivists to share their experiences in ways in which they are not typically invited outside of conversations with colleagues. While responses to the interviews varied, the majority either felt that the overall process was a cathartic experience or that they were not at all affected by the encounter.

This range of responses highlights the importance of conducting qualitative interviews with this population in the future (in accordance with relevant human research ethics statements), to better understand the experiences of intensivists and to help identify their needs.

Yeah, because I would rather get this out in dribs and drabs, than have a big cathartic blow-up. I think it's important to be connected to... again, I don't take my errors and put them in a box and hide that box away; I would leave the box in plain sight; because I have to be able to revisit it, to be honest. It's important. Honesty and integrity are really important to me. My buddy did some personality tests on me, and it all came down to that integrity is the only thing that matters to me. If somebody doesn't have integrity.... If something has integrity, even if I disagree with it, but it has integrity, I inherently respect it. So for me, there is an integrity in saying, 'Yes, these were errors I was involved in. These were errors that I observed.' I can objectively talk about them because there's stuff to be learned there, and there is an integrity with that I can live with. I'm very happy to live with, I yearn for. That that's how I want to live my life. So, it is useful for me to talk about these things. I also think that, as I alluded to, like, that managing our grief over bad events that we were involved in or had no responsibility for. Just managing that grief, it comes in waves, but it is best managed, I think, continuously, rather than just dealing with it at the time. I'm aware of my emotional burden related to that boy. I don't feel guilty about that anymore. But I can access it. I can tell you his name; I'll never forget it...

I wouldn't say necessarily that I feel that it's been helpful. I do think that there is an acknowledgement within our group that 'wellness' is very important. We have a wellness committee, and we talk about wellness, and do those things – like some are superficial things like you know, parties or get-togethers, or showing slides, but there is that openness and acknowledgement that wellness is important. So, I don't feel like I live in a space where people don't appreciate that. Or to some of your other questions, where I couldn't go to at least some of my other colleagues, and say, 'This is a hard job...' I wouldn't do that to all of my colleagues, but some of them I would. So, I feel neutral about it.

References

1. Davydow DS, Gifford JM, Desai SV, Bienvenu OJ, Needham DM. Depression in general intensive care unit survivors: a systematic review. Intensive Care Med. 2009;35(5):796–809. https://
   doi.org/10.1007/s00134-009-1396-5.
2. Parker AM, Sricharoenchai T, Raparla S, Schneck KW, Bienvenu OJ, Needham
   DM. Posttraumatic stress disorder in critical illness survivors: a metaanalysis. Crit Care Med.
   2015;43(5):1121–9.
3. van Beusekom I, Bakhshi-Raiez F, de Keizer NF, Dongelmans DA, van der Schaaf M. Reported
   burden on informal caregivers of ICU survivors: a literature review. Crit Care. 2015;20(1):1–8.

Natalie Henderson is an attending critical care physician at Norton Children's Hospital. She
spends her time in the Just for Kids Pediatric Critical Care Unit as well as well as the Jennifer
Lawrence Foundation Cardiac Intensive Care Unit. Clinically, she participates in multiple committees related to cardiac critical care. She serves at the Associate Fellowship Program Director for the
paediatric critical care fellowship program. She has an interest in education and, along with two
colleagues, has developed an end-of-life curricular to improve the education around end-of-life for
trainees. She serves as the Medical Director for the palliative care service line at Norton Children's
Hospital. She also spends time teaching at the medical school where she also serves as an advisory
dean for more than 30 students each year.

Courtney Bowd completed her undergraduate degree at the University of Queensland and has
recently completed the Master of Public and Social Policy at Macquarie University, Sydney,
Australia. She is currently a Policy Specialist at Phoenix Australia—Centre for Post-traumatic
Mental Health in Melbourne, Australia, where she works across a range of knowledge translation,
training, and policy review projects, with a particular focus on supporting disaster impacted communities and the recovery workforce. Prior to joining Phoenix Australia, Courtney worked as a
change management consultant for a professional services firm.

Chapter 32
Future Travellers

Mary Pinder and Eileen Tay

> *Our offensive philosophy is to simply find a way to get the ball into the hands of our team's best player.*
>
> —Kelvin Sampson

Trainee selection for specialty training programs is a challenging and increasingly complex process. This chapter focuses on trainee selection for intensive care training programs and explores the study participants' reflections on the requisite range of professional skills and personality traits for successful intensive care practice. We explore how much of these are considered to be inherent in the individual or able to be learned.

The aim of trainee selection for intensive care training programs is to ensure the recruitment of junior doctors with the potential to complete the training programme and who have, or will develop, the relevant professional skills for the competency of specialist intensivist practice. Inherent and learned personal attributes are needed to manage the stresses of the job.

> *…if you can clearly see that someone doesn't have the right personality to work in the stressful environment, and particularly in ICU where, if you get stressed about looking after one patient, often what happens is in a busy unit, you've got multiple things going on at the same time, and some people just can't do that. It's clear. Unfortunately, it's not something you can learn. If you're going to get anxiety or stressed about small things, sometimes it's very hard to unpack, or to lose.*

M. Pinder (✉)
Department of Intensive Care, Sir Charles Gairdner Hospital, Perth, WA, Australia
e-mail: mary.pinder@health.wa.gov.au

E. Tay
Faculty of Forensic Psychiatry, RANZCP, Melbourne, VIC, Australia

Faculty of Psychotherapy, RANZCP, Melbourne, VIC, Australia

Cultural diversity within the training programme members and amongst the program's trainees is important for the process of identity formation and maturation for medical trainees. Identity formation is a progressive developmental process throughout a doctor's career. Role models from similar cultural and racial backgrounds have been shown to be beneficial and helpful for doctors' overall health and well-being. Myers [1] echoes the observation that professionally 'you can't be what you can't see'.

The study participants reflected on crucial intensivist professional individual knowledge, skills and attitudes, and their importance for functioning as part of a multi-disciplinary team. Communication skills, appropriate empathy, and managing stressful work environments require an openness to learning and the capacity to self-reflect on their resilience to stress and cope with the death of patients. Good communication is a complex skill which encompasses verbal and non-verbal components, as well as empathy for other team members and the wider hospital environment. It is essential for effective teamwork and forms the basis of trust between team members.

> *…in intensive care, you have to like to be part of a team; you can't want to be a person who does it on their own…I need to be able to communicate with my team, and help the team on the ventilator understand what we're doing, and what we need to look for. And I need the nursing staff to understand what we're doing. I need to raise the awareness of the team, so that the team can collectively anticipate problems, and then treat them together. Also, lots of times in the intensive care unit, for example, a bad thing happens, a kid desaturates, and something happens, the bells go off, blah blah blah, we all run there…. By the time I get there, it's all over. I didn't see it. I need to be able to communicate with the team that trusts me to listen, and has the right vocabulary to explain to me what happened, so I can figure out how to make it not happen again…*

Other important professional skills discussed included achieving a balance between confidence and humility, an ability to be decisive and not be too proud, to acknowledge one's mistakes, and to be willing to review and revise our management plans in the face of errors or omissions.

> *I think a balance of confidence and humility, because you need to be able to be confident in your plan, and implement it, and help the team understand what it is you want to do. But your humility will allow you to revisit that and revise it if you identify that you are missing something, or that there is new information that changes the model. So, I think those are important traits to have in concert with another*

High 'emotional quotient' (EQ) was described as an essential attribute that should be a factor in trainee selection. It was seen as an important skill for managing critically ill patients as scientific knowledge and technical ability.

> *So, I think one skill is the EQ skills, but we don't, we don't recruit for. We have poor tests for choosing it, but we don't recruit for it. So, I think someone that is… I think that's a really necessary skill. If you don't have those skills, then you may be brilliantly knowledgeable, you may be brilliant at managing patients and rescuing the lady downstairs in ED with the two kids, however every other conversation that you have with either the treating team, or a family, may be conflict-driven and you may not care or have the skills to even recognise that.*

There was a need to understand the stresses of colleagues, contextualise poor behaviour, and avoid interpersonal conflict to prevent adverse patient care.

> … I think you really need to be quite grounded in yourself to be a good Intensivist. Only because you're either dealing with grumpy transplant surgeons, which is not personal, it's just the way it is, or we get surgeons who are very upset, and you can virtually see them go through the… it's the 'A,B,C' of grieving. You know they're at the denial stage. They'll be at angry in two hours. You know, you can see it, so you need to have a really good understanding of other people.

Potential trainees in any specialty need to reflect on their personal characteristics in deciding on a training pathway and choice of future career. The observation was made that there is a bias to obsessive compulsive personality/disorder (OCP/OCD)-type traits as the dominant personality type amongst intensivists. An aphorism for illustrating the differences in the acute care specialties is that if you like working in chaos, choose emergency medicine; if you like a controlled environment choose anaesthesia; and if you like a bit of both, choose intensive care medicine.

> I laugh with some of the trainees when they ask for advice about what sort of specialty they should choose and are thinking about something… I will take a little tangent here, if I may… Thinking about Emergency Medicine versus Critical Care for example. And I look at them and I say, 'Look at yourself in the mirror, and tell me do you feel like you have more OCD type traits, or more ADHD [Attention Deficit Hyperactive Disorder] type traits? Because if you have more ADHD type stuff, I would suggest that you consider Emergency Medicine; if you have more OCD type traits, Critical Care is probably where you're going.' Because I think we're all totally OCD in the ICU. There might be a tiny bit of ADHD as well, off the record.

There is clearly a responsibility on the part of the educational institution oversee-ing the training programme to meet its obligations. It must ensure the training pro-gramme is fit for purpose and select trainees who are capable of its successful completion. Traditional methods of trainee selection using a curriculum vitae, refer-ences, and interviews are universally recognised as poor predictors of subsequent performance.

Training programs are now incorporating strategies such as crisis management simulation scenarios, situational judgement tests, and personality testing into the selection process [2, 3]. Study participants opined that the importance of a reliable metric to assess personal attributes remains elusive. A crucial point was the influ-ence of the training program: is the end-product of an excellent intensivist because of the quality of the training programme or the innate qualities of the trainee?

> Does Harvard have the best astrophysics program because they train people well? Or is it because they take the world's best pre-astrophysicists? So, I think there's a huge upfront selection bias. We absolutely have to take people in the front door that are 'in touch' with their empathy and have reasonable emotional IQs. If we fail to do that we will struggle as a field. So, there has to be some method, metric or understanding of the importance of these traits when we screen people, and I think we have to recurrently expose people to both the opportunity to witness and to lead with supervision in these encounters. Neither of these things will guarantee the outcome, but I think that's the only thing we have to use.

Conclusion

It is essential that any trainee selection process promotes equity, inclusion, and diversity to improve the culture of the workplace and to best serve our communities by ensuring the cultural background of trainees is representative of those of critically ill patient populations. To this end, trainee selection pathways must include strategies to mitigate unconscious bias and institutional racism [4].

Participants in this book have articulated the prescient Sir William Osler's summary of the essence of being a doctor in the concept of 'equinamitas': 'Acquire the art of detachment, the virtue of method, and the quality of thoroughness, but above all the grace of humility'.

References

1. Myers MF, Gabbard GO. The physician as patient; a clinical handbook for mental health professionals. Washington, DC: American Psychiatric Publishing; 2008.
2. Cociante AG, Nguyen MN, Marane CF, et al. Simulation testing for selection of critical care medicine trainees: a pilot feasibility study. Ann Am Thorac Soc. 2016;13(4):529–35. https://doi.org/10.1513/AnnalsATS.201601-012OC.
3. https://www.cicm.org.au/CICM_Media/CICMSite/Files/Training/T-1-Trainee-Selection-Policy.pdf (downloaded 5 March 2022).
4. Simone K, Ahmed RA, Konkin J, et al. What are the features of targeted or system-wide initiatives that affect diversity in health professions trainees? A BEME systematic review: BEME Guide No. 50. Med Teach. 2018;40(8):762–80. https://doi.org/10.1080/0142159X.2018.1473562.

Mary Pinder is an Intensive Care Specialist and Director of Clinical Training based at Sir Charles Gairdner Hospital in Perth, Western Australia. She trained in intensive care in the UK and South Africa as well as Australia. She is on the Board of the College of Intensive Care Medicine of Australia and New Zealand (CICM) and roles with the CICM have included Chair of the Second Part Exam Committee, Chair of the Assessments Committee, and College President.

Eileen Tay is a Consultant Psychiatrist in Perth, Australia. She is interested in developing further supervision skills for medical practitioners and is currently undertaking additional training in this field of work, as supervision is an increasingly recognised discipline in the helping professions. She has been involved in doctors' health for over 20 years as part of an advisory and treating clinician network. She is also developing comparative Psychotherapy education modules for psychiatry trainees.

Chapter 33
Future Destinations

Peter Vernon van Heerden ⓘ

> *In the long run, we shape our lives, and we shape ourselves.*
> *The process never ends until we die. And the choices we make*
> *are ultimately our own responsibility.*
>
> —Eleanor Roosevelt

And so, we come to the end of this narrative. The project resulting in this book was the brainchild of Dr. Diane Dennis. She conceived the work and has been the driving force and energy behind the completion of the project, the publication of several papers on the topic, and the writing of this book. For me, one of the main outcomes of the entire endeavour has been to show us two things; one, there are shared/common experiences for all intensivists and we are not alone in dealing with the challenges of a difficult career path; and two, we don't talk about these matters nearly enough.

The way the career path is organized for intensivists varies from country to country. In Australasia, intensivists are privileged to work in a system that has recognized critical care as a separate specialty since 1976, with a well-defined career path, sufficient human resources, and support structures. This allows for adequate opportunities to take leave and welfare support for both trainees and specialists who are under stress. This is not the case in other countries where critical care medicine is still somewhat of an orphan specialty, staffed by enthusiasts from other base specialties, such as anaesthesia or surgery. This is notwithstanding the greater respect for and understanding of the role of intensivists since the COVID-19 pandemic.

Intensivists work in a demanding environment and there is a human toll. Clearly there is room to improve the lot of the intensivist. Improvements should include

P. V. van Heerden (✉)
General Intensive Care Unit, Department of Anesthesiology, Critical Care and Pain Medicine,
Hadassah Medical Center, Jerusalem, Israel
e-mail: vernon@hadassah.org.il

© The Author(s), under exclusive license to Springer Nature
Switzerland AG 2023
D. Dennis et al. (eds.), *Stories from ICU Doctors*,
https://doi.org/10.1007/978-3-031-32401-7_33

improved public relations—patients and their families have very little knowledge of the work being done in the ICU until they personally experience it. We should be out there telling people what we do.

Even amongst colleagues, the understanding of what the ICU is for is not clear. For many of them, it is a place to send patients to, in order to reduce their own anxiety and stress, when things get difficult. So dear colleague, imagine what it's like when all those stressful patients are collected together in one place and the intensivist has to look after them, day in and day out, and where up to one in five will not survive.

Other improvements in the lot of the intensivist include providing sufficient resources—beds, ventilators, and syringe pumps. By all means, ask us to do a challenging job—please give us the tools to do it. This aspect is becoming more and more relevant as we see two important qualities developing in the population we serve. The elderly population is growing, presenting to the ICU with increasing frailty and more co-morbidities, making for longer and more complicated ICU admissions. Secondly, advances in medicine, such as more complex surgical procedures or cancer therapies, mean more demand for ICU beds and services.

Complex healthcare technology is also advancing (e.g. ECMO) and is increasingly being used. ICU services are increasingly being provided outside the walls of the ICU through the use of rapid response teams, medical emergency teams, central line teams, tracheostomy teams, post-ICU follow-up teams and clinics, amongst others. In some North American institutions, 20% or more of hospital beds in acute care hospitals are ICU beds. Therefore, we need the resources, infrastructure, equipment, and human resources, to deal with the increasing demand for ICU beds and services. Even more importantly we need the time and opportunity to build effective teams to manage the complex sociotechnical work of the ICU. We need to 'play as we train'.

One of the things we learned during the recent pandemic is that suddenly putting together doctors, nurses, and allied health staff who don't know each other to run an ICU and look after critically ill COVID-19 patients does not work very well. It takes time for the team to build and coalesce before effective work can be expected.

To answer, 'Where to from here?', I have the following two-part offering:

Firstly, critical care is here to stay, is growing, and will continue to do so into the future. As intensivists, we need to advertise our skills and services and claim the recognition these skills deserve. Secondly, those of us within the specialty, and those without, have to recognize the challenges we face as intensivists. We must demand the support we need to perform, to the best of our ability, to the benefit of our patients.

This means we must start a conversation about the stresses intensivists face in their career, especially around the occurrence of adverse events. We need robust strategies to deal with them. There is no one set of answers suitable for everyone

Starting the conversation is important—we hope this book is the beginning of this conversation and that the dialogue will lead to better health for intensivists and their patients. Intensive care is a young specialty and there is room for improvement and development as it matures. We should concentrate on the human aspects (our intensivists and our patients) as much as we do on technological advances in our very demanding workplaces as we move forward. We hope the words in this book serve as an inspiration to the next generation of intensive care professionals.

Peter Vernon van Heerden qualified as an anaesthetist and intensive care specialist and has practiced in South Africa, the UK, Australia, and Israel. He is the Director of the General Intensive Care Unit, Dept. of Anesthesiology, Critical Care and Pain Medicine, Faculty of Medicine, Hadassah Hospital and Hebrew University of Jerusalem, Israel.

Glossary[1]

Attending In the context of this book, Attending is sometimes used as a synonym for intensivist

Abdominocentesis Where a needle is inserted into the abdominal (belly) cavity to drain excess fluid

ADHD Acronym for 'Attention deficit hyperactivity disorder'

Adverse event An unintended undesirable outcome of a medical intervention or decision

After-hours Any time after routine daytime work hours

Ambu-resus bag A self-inflating resuscitation device used to support the ventilation of a patient

Anaesthesia The process of producing non-awareness to noxious stimuli, such as surgical incision

Anaesthesiologist The medical practitioner who administers medications to induce and maintain anaesthesia

Anaesthetist See Anaesthesiologist

ANZROD Acronym for the 'Australian and New Zealand Risk of Death' score. A score that predicts mortality (death) in acutely unwell patients.

APACHE Acronym for 'Acute Physiology and Chronic Health Evaluation'. A score that estimates ICU mortality (death) based on a number of laboratory values and patient signs, taking into account both acute and chronic disease processes

Arterial blood pressure monitoring Measuring and displaying the results of the blood pressure in the arterial system of the **patient, may be done invasively or non-invasively**

Arterial line placement Insertion of a soft nylon catheter into the radial (usually) artery of a patient for the purpose of **arterial blood pressure monitoring**

---

[1]This glossary aims to provide consistency for terminology used in different geographical zones for the structure and practice of intensive care teams. The editors have purposefully standardized the terminology in the text to allow consistency around comparable roles or functions. It is not intended as advocacy to replace usual descriptive words in different geographical zones.

D. Dennis et al. (eds.), *Stories from ICU Doctors*, https://doi.org/10.1007/978-3-031-32401-7

Blood smear Placing a thin drop of blood on a glass microscope slide in order to examine the cellular make-up of the blood

Brain dead A legal definition of when there is no evidence of brain function and the patient is declared deceased

Cardiac arrest Cessation of cardiac/heart function either due to absence of electrical activity (asystole) or chaotic electrical activity (e.g. ventricular fibrillation)

Cardiac catheter laboratory A hospital room or suite where catheters are advanced into the heart of patients under the control of X-ray devices called image intensifiers by trained cardiologists. Often abbreviated to the 'Cath Lab'

Cardiac pacing Insertion of wires into the heart chambers (implantable) or electrical conduction pads (external) to the chest wall of the patient and then connected to a device which provides electrical 'shocks' to the heart to maintain as normal a heart rhythm as possible.

Cardiopulmonary arrest **See Cardiac arrest above**, plus cessation of any respiratory effort by the patient

Cardioversion Application of an electrical charge to the heart to abolish an abnormal heart rhythm and replace it with a normal rhythm

Care conference A meeting of all team members from a number of disciplines if necessary to decide on an appropriate plan of medical management for a patient

Catheter A long hollow tube usually made of plastic/nylon which can be inserted into a body cavity

Central line A hollow plastic/nylon catheter placed into a large vein or the right atrium of the heart within the chest cavity via the internal jugular or subclavian veins for the purpose of measuring venous blood pressures or administering medications

Central line kit The equipment needed to safely place a central line

Charge nurse The head nurse in charge of the section or unit

Chest compressions Compression of the sternum in the front towards the spine at the back in order to compress the heart in between and so provide some blood flow in the patient who has suffered a **cardiac/cardiopulmonary arrest**

Chief resident Usually the most senior trainee doctor in the department who takes additional responsibility for teaching and administrative tasks (such as rostering of duties)

CICU Acronym for 'Cardiac Intensive Care Unit'

Clerical staff Non-medical staff who undertake administrative duties

Clinician Doctors and other medical and allied health personnel who are primarily occupied with patient care

Code Another way of saying the patient has suffered a cardiac/cardiopulmonary arrest (he/she has 'coded')

Cold debriefing Discussion of a clinical event at a time distant from the actual event, 'once the dust has settled'

College The body responsible for the training of intensive care specialists

College of Intensive Care of Australia and New Zealand See **College**

Co-morbidities Illnesses/conditions the patient may have which may or may not contribute to the current critical illness

Conscious state The level of awareness of self and surroundings (may range from awake/conscious to drowsy to asleep to unconscious)

Continuous veno-venous haemodiafiltration A mode of renal replacement therapy commonly used in the intensive care unit for patients with kidney failure

CPR Acronym for 'Cardiopulmonary Resuscitation'

Crisis management simulation scenarios Practice sessions in how to deal with unexpected medical emergencies

Critical care medicine The branch of medicine dealing primarily with organ support for patients with life-threatening conditions

Critical incident An event which threatens the life or limb of a patient

Dean The academic head of a college

Debrief; Debriefing Discussion after the event in order to clarify the issues surrounding the event, such as causality and possible prevention in the future

Desaturate A decrease in the concentration of oxygenated haemoglobin in the blood

Disclosure Revealing the details of an incident to all parties involved

Diuretic A medication used to increase fluid and salt output via the kidneys

ECMO Extracorporeal membrane oxygenation, the removal of the blood from a patient, oxygenating it across a semi-permeable membrane and then returning the blood to the patient's circulation—a treatment which replaces the function of the lungs and/or heart artificially

Elective surgery Surgery which is planned and is usually non-urgent (e.g. hernia repair)

Electronic medical record Patient details and a record of the treatment received which is recorded by means of a computer and not on paper charts

Emergency dialysis Urgent treatment for kidney failure using a machine to artificially purify the blood of toxins which are usually removed by the kidneys

Emergency medicine The branch of medicine which deals with all acute presentations to the hospital

Emotional quotient (EQ) The level of a person's emotional intelligence

Faculty A sub-division of a college or university dealing with a defined subject, e.g. Faculty of Intensive Care Medicine

Fellow This has slightly different meanings in Australia/Britain where it refers to a trainee doctor who has completed training and examinations to be a specialist and in the USA and Israel where it means a doctor still in specialist training who is undertaking a period of study in a specific speciality

FiO$_2$ The 'Fraction (or amount) of Inspired oxygen' being delivered to a patient

Frailty A decline in physical and cognitive reserves that leads to increased vulnerability

Functional reserve The amount of capacity for dealing with added demands on a body or body system

Goal(s) of care The agreed and desirable outcomes of a specific treatment plan

Haemodialysis A process of removing toxins from the body usually removed by the kidneys

Hospice An institution for providing palliative care for patients with terminal/end of life conditions

Hospital-based risk mitigation The hospital/institutional system for reducing adverse events

Hot debriefing Discussion of the causes, consequences and possible prevention of an adverse event during or immediately after the event

Human factors All the aspects of care that relate to human nature and human activity

Hyperkalaemia Abnormally high concentration of potassium in the blood

ICU Acronym for 'Intensive Care Unit'

Inotropes Medications administered usually intravenously to improve heart function

Intelligence quotient (IQ) A standardized measure of intelligence

Intensive care medicine See **critical care medicine**

Intensivist A medical doctor qualified in the independent practice of caring for critically unwell patients. Other terms used in the world are: 'intensive care physician', 'intensive care attending', 'intensive care consultant'.

Intra-aortic balloon catheterization Placement of a catheter with a balloon in the descending aorta for the purpose of improving heart function using mechanical means

Intubated/intubation Placing a hollow tube into the trachea/windpipe of a patient to facilitate connection to a mechanical ventilator

Invasive Meaning entering a body space such as the chest or abdomen or a blood vessel

IV Abbreviation for administrating intravenous fluids, or a 'drip' in lay terms

Laryngoscope A hand-held medical device used for viewing the larynx/entrance to the windpipe

Lasix The trade name for furosemide/frusamide, a diuretic medication

Latent safety events Events with the potential to compromise the safety of a patient or a health care worker

Laryngoscope blade The (usually) metal blade attached to a laryngoscope which allows visualization of the larynx (opening to the windpipe) for placement of a hollow tube to facilitate mechanical ventilation

M&M Acronym for 'Morbidity and Mortality' meetings that discuss patient outcomes

Mechanical ventilation The act of replacing or supporting the lung function of a patient using a machine (ventilator)

Medical officer A qualified doctor, but not necessarily a specialist doctor

Metoprolol A beta blocker medication used to slow heart rate

Morbidity and Mortality Meetings Meetings held specifically to discuss adverse outcomes, either additional illness/burden or death

Nephrology The medical speciality dealing with kidney disease

Next of kin The person legally most closely related to the patient

NICU Acronym for 'Neonatal (or newborn) Intensive Care Unit'

Non-invasive A device or procedure which does not breach the skin of a patient

Obsessive compulsive disorder (OCD) A personality disorder in which the person has a tendency to excessive orderliness, perfectionism and great attention to detail

Occupational therapy The allied health profession dealing with physical and mental disabilities through use of structured activities

On-call Being available in person or on the telephone to deal with urgent matters arising in the intensive care unit

Open disclosure See **Disclosure**

OR Acronym for 'Operating room'

Oxygen monitoring Measuring and displaying the results of the oxygen concentration or partial pressure in the blood either non-invasively (e.g. with a finger probe) or invasively (e.g. by taking repeated blood samples)

Oxygenation The state of the oxygen concentration or partial pressure in the blood of the patient

Palliative care Providing care and symptom control for patients with terminal (end of life) conditions such as advanced malignancy

Patient care assistants Workers with no medical training who provide support for clinical staff such as nurses by undertaking tasks such as feeding patients, washing patients, moving patients

Percutaneous Via/through the skin of a patient

Peritoneal The space within the abdominal cavity

Personal care attendants See **patient care assistants**

Personality testing Specific psychological tests to determine personality types

Physical therapist/physiotherapist The allied health profession dealing with physical disabilities or lung conditions through use of structured physical activities and exercise

Physician A qualified medical doctor (in Britain/Australia it might also signify a specialist in internal medicine)

Physio See **Physical therapist/physiotherapist**

PICU Acronym for 'Paediatric Intensive Care Unit'

Preceptorship A period of structured transition to guide and support newly qualified practitioners from student to autonomous professional

Provider Usually a registered medical professional entitled to provide medical services

Pulmonology The medical specialty dealing with lung diseases

Recovery The area of the hospital where patients recover for a short period after a surgical procedure (Recovery Room) or the act of getting better from a certain condition or illness ('he is in recovery from pneumonia').

Recovery trajectory The expected rate of recovery of the patient from a condition/illness

Registrar In Britain/Australia this means a junior/trainee doctor who is undertaking training in a medical specialty

Renal function The level of function of the kidneys

Renal replacement therapy Artificial means of doing the work of the kidneys in removing toxins from the blood, e.g. by haemodialysis

Resident In Israel/USA this has the same definition as **registrar** above, while in Britain/Australia it means a junior doctor before he/she enters specialist training (a rank below registrar).

Respiratory failure Failure of the lungs either to adequately transfer oxygen to the body or remove carbon dioxide form the body

Respiratory therapist An allied health professional who deals with treatments for the lung, such as oxygen therapy and mechanical ventilation

Resuscitation The act of providing urgent support for heart or lung function in the event of cardiac/cardiopulmonary arrest or urgent treatment of a life-threatening condition such a very low blood pressure due to sepsis

Root cause analysis Careful analysis of an event or series of events in order to determine the underlying cause/s. Often abbreviated to RCA

Routine surgery Surgery which follows the expected path, whether it is elective or urgent surgery

School of Intensive Care An institution set up for the purpose of teaching intensive care/critical care medicine

Situational awareness Knowing where you are and what is going on around you/ not having too narrow a focus

Situational judgement tests These are psychological tests which present the testtaker with realistic, hypothetical scenarios and ask them to identify the most appropriate response or to rank the responses in the order they feel is most effective

Speech therapists Allied health professional who deals with speech, communication and upper airway reflexes (swallowing)

Sternum The breastbone

Suction Applying negative pressure (e.g. via a tube), in order to remove secretions from the patient's airways

Syringe pumps Mechanical devices which empty syringes containing medication at a preset and continuous rate

Telemetry Being able to view patient physiological parameters (e.g. blood pressure) at a distance from the patient. This may be in another room or across the world

Terminal End of life

Thoracocentesis Drainage of fluid from the chest cavity (the space around the lungs)

Trache Short for tracheostomy

Tracheostomy The insertion of a hollow tube into the windpipe/trachea via an incision in the front of the neck

Trisomy 21 A genetic disorder also known as Downs syndrome, often involving defects in the heart

TTP Abbreviation for 'thrombotic thrombocytic purpura', a serious condition of the platelets in the blood

Vagal response A parasympathetic response due to stimulation of the vagal nerve characterized by nausea, sweating, low blood pressure and a slow heart rate

Ward round A formalized bedside review of each patient in the ward by the treating team

Weaning The act of liberating the patient from life support measures such as mechanical ventilation by slow and stepwise reduction of the support until the patient no longer needs it

Index

© The Editor(s) (if applicable) and The Author(s), under exclusive license to
Springer Nature Switzerland AG 2023
D. Dennis et al. (eds.), *Stories from ICU Doctors*,
https://doi.org/10.1007/978-3-031-32401-7